IMMUNOLOGICAL ASPECTS OF ALLERGY AND ALLERGIC DISEASES

VOLUME 8
Allergic Responses to Infectious Agents

IMMUNOLOGICAL ASPECTS
OF ALLERGY
AND ALLERGIC DISEASES

Edited by E. Rajka and S. Korossy

IMMUNOLOGICAL ASPECTS OF ALLERGY AND ALLERGIC DISEASES

Edited by

E. RAJKA

and

S. KOROSSY

Department of Dermatology
István Municipal Hospita l
Budapest, Hungary

VOLUME 8

Allergic Responses to Infectious Agents

SPRINGER-SCIENCE+BUSINESS MEDIA, B.V.

© Springer Science+Business Media Dordrecht 1976
Originally published by Akadémiai Kiadó, Budapest in 1976
Softcover reprint of the hardcover 1st edition 1976

ISBN 978-1-4684-0918-5   ISBN 978-1-4684-0916-1 (eBook)
DOI 10.1007/978-1-4684-0916-1

Library of Congress Catalog Card Number 75-34966

LIST OF CONTRIBUTORS
TO VOLUME 8

GYÖRGY BÁNKI, M.D.

Research Officer, National Institute for Hygiene, Gyáli út 2–6., 1097 Budapest, Hungary

ENDRE FEJÉR, M.D., C.Sc. (med.)

Late Dermatologist-in-Chief, István Municipal Hospital, Budapest, Hungary

ISTVÁN FÖLDES, M.D., D.Sc. (med.)

Professor and Director, Microbiological Group of the Hungarian Academy of Sciences, Pihenő út 1., 1529 Budapest, Hungary

MÁRIA JANKÓ, M.D.

Head, Department of Parasitology, National Institute for Hygiene, Gyáli út 2 6., 1097 Budapest, Hungary

KÁLMÁN KIRÁLY, M.D., C.Sc. (med.)

Professor and Head, Department of Dermatology, Semmelweis University Medical School, Mária u. 41., 1085 Budapest, Hungary

SÁNDOR KOROSSY, M.D., C.Sc. (med.)

Honorary Assistant Professor, Head, Department of Dermatology, István Municipal Hospital, Nagyvárad tér 1., 1097 Budapest, Hungary

GYÖRGY MAKARA, M.D.

Retired Head, Department of Vector Control and Disinfection, National Institute for Hygiene, Gyáli út 2–6., 1097 Budapest, Hungary

GÁBOR NYERGES, M.D., C.Sc. (med.)

Honorary Assistant Professor, Head of Department, Central Municipal Hospital for Infectious Diseases, Gyáli út 5–7., 1097 Budapest, Hungary

GEORGETTE NYERGES, M.D., C.Sc. (med.)

Deputy Chief of Department, National Institute for Hygiene, Gyáli út 2–6., 1097 Budapest, Hungary

ISTVÁN RÁCZ, M.D., C.Sc. (med.)

Assistant Professor, Department of Dermatology, Semmelweis University Medical School, Mária u. 41., 1085 Budapest, Hungary

KÁROLY SIPOS, M.D., C.Sc. (med.)

Retired Assistant Professor, Department of Dermatology, Szeged University Medical School, Lenin körút 18—20., 6720 Szeged, Hungary

IBOLYA TÖRÖK, M.D., C.Sc. (med.)

Registrar, Department of Dermatology, Semmelweis University Medical School, Mária u. 41., 1085 Budapest, Hungary

CONTENTS OF VOLUME 8

CHAPTER 71

ALLERGIC REACTIONS IN ACUTE BACTERIAL AND VIRAL INFECTIOUS DISEASES AND ACTIVE IMMUNIZATION PROCEDURES

by

G. NYERGES AND GEORGETTE NYERGES

INTRODUCTION

Infectious agents and their products are usually antigenic for higher organisms, inducing an immune response in the immunologically competent cells. Consequently, the reactivity of the infected organism to the infectious agent is altered, i.e., using the term first introduced by von Pirquet, the organism becomes allergic. The altered host reactivity is usually manifested in protective and functional immunity to the same agent, i.e. in non-susceptibility to the invasive or pathogenic effects of a foreign organism or to the toxic effect of an antigenic substance [103]. In this way the organism is protected against the pathogenic agent by

1

virtue of this altered reactivity. The concept of allergy in this context, however, should not be restricted to heightened reactivity, to antigen and resistance to subsequent infections. There are a number of clinical manifestations known which all have been supposed to have an allergic background. The altered reactivity of the infected organism is demonstrable experimentally by its response to the artificial introduction of the microorganism or its antigenic product. This is utilized in intracutaneous tests performed for the detection of infectedness or immunity and occasionally also for diagnostic purposes. Vaccines with active effect, containing microbial antigens may evoke allergic reactions in part of the subjects.

ALLERGIC ASPECTS OF THE PATHOGENESIS
OF INFECTIOUS DISEASES

Infectious disease is a result of the interaction of an infectious agent (microorganism or virus; in the following, microorganism) with the macroorganism. The pathology of the disease is determined primarily by specific properties of the microorganism, such as its organotropism, direct cell- and tissue-damaging effect, furthermore, its ability to interfere with the different protective mechanisms of the host organism. The degree and quality of this interference is characteristic of the microorganism. Thus, most of these diseases are specific for the microorganism, i.e. agents of the same species usually give rise to similar pathological processes and clinical manifestations. The severity of the disease, on the other hand, will be influenced by the virulence of the microorganism, as well as by the immune reactions of the macroorganism, determined by genetic and/or environmental factors.

In the pathogenesis of a number of infectious diseases factors such as the site of the pathological process within the organism, functional disorder of the involved organ(s), and the non-specific protective mechanisms of the host may play a role. In other diseases, particularly in those having a long incubation period, the specific immune reaction of the host should be added to the above factors. This is usually indicated by the appearance of specific antibodies and/or tissue allergy concurrently with the clinical symptoms. Symptoms resembling those seen in non-infectious allergic diseases may also indicate an allergic pathomechanism, and this may be further supported by histological findings of allergic type. In some organic lesions developing as late complications of certain infectious diseases pathogenic microorganisms may be absent; nevertheless, the time of appearance of the complication and/or the character of the histological changes may suggest an allergic pathomechanism.

As regards the pathogenetic role of allergic reactions, a sharp distinction must be made between primary diseases and their complications, namely, if allergic mechanisms are involved in the pathogenesis of the basic disease, this must be a regular response given by every individual to the specific agent. Allergic complications, on the other hand, only arise in a portion of the patients, indicating that individual disposition plays an important role in their development. Another fundamental difference is that in the basic disease the allergy is directed against the pathogen, while in the complications apparently the autoallergy evoked by the pathogen is of pathogenetic importance.

BACTERIAL DISEASES

The role of allergy in primary diseases

Bacterial diseases may be classified into two groups depending on the participation of allergic mechanisms in the pathogenesis of the *basic* disease.

1. In the first group the incubation period is short and the pathological process may be readily explained by the direct tissue-damaging effect of the pathogenic agents and their toxins and by the non-specific protecting mechanisms of the body. Purulent or fibrinous inflammation is usually found first at the site of entry of the pathogen. Bacterial toxins give rise to degenerative changes in remote organs and are responsible for most of the systemic symptoms. Some pathogenic agents may break through the barrier formed due to the non-specific inflammatory reaction around the site of entry, and may give rise to purulent inflammation in other organs which they reach via the blood of lymphatic circulation. The clinical picture is dominated by local symptoms, which are accompanied by systemic manifestations of variable severity.

In these diseases allergy against the pathogen and/or its products usually develops and is readily demonstrable. It is, however, unlikely that an allergic process would play any role in the pathogenesis of the basic disease. In fact, when the allergy appears, the most important pathological events of the primary disease have usually taken place and the allergic mechanisms are mostly involved in the development of some late complications only.

Most of the acute bacterial diseases belong to this group, e.g. staphylococcal, streptococcal diseases, diphtheria, dysentery, non-typhoid salmonelloses, etc. It has been suggested, but not unequivocally proved, that allergy might play a pathogenetic role in several symptoms of these diseases. For instance, scarlet fever is supposed to develop only in subjects who have been sensitized to the erythrogenic toxin, due to a previous infection [86a, b, 227]. This might account for the relatively low contagiosity of scarlet fever and for its rare occurrence in infants. It has also been shown that new-born babies not possessing antitoxic immunity of maternal origin do not respond to the intradermal injection of Dick's toxin [33]. Nevertheless, most authors attribute the rash in scarlet fever to the direct toxic effect of the erythrogenic toxin of *Streptococcus pyogenes* on the capillaries.

It was supposed earlier that allergic reactions were operating also in malignant diphtheria [209]. However, the fulminant course can also be explained by the rapid absorption of large quantities of the toxin, promoted by other invasive products of *Corynebacterium diphtheriae* [173, 178].

2. Several infectious diseases with long incubation period, e.g. typhoid fever, brucellosis, tularaemia, etc., belong to the second group. Clinical features include protracted course often tending to chronicity, frequent relapses, and severe general symptoms in face of the relatively insignificant manifestation in the individual organs. The histological picture is characterized by granulomata with mononuclear cellular reaction and by the presence of epitheloid and, occasionally, giant cells. Although humoral antibodies regularly appear in the patients' blood, they apparently have no significance in the process of healing. Immunity develops

slowly and is frequently transitory. Considering their pathogenesis, the diseases of this group show many common features with the chronic bacterial diseases (tuberculosis, leprosy, syphilis).

The infectious diseases of this group were termed cyclic diseases by Höring [109a, b], who distinguished them from the 'local' diseases belonging to the first group on the basis of the site of multiplication of their pathogenic agents: in group 1 this occurs extracellularly, while in group 2 in the cells of the RES. The intracellular location of the pathogen has been proved histologically in typhoid fever [183], brucellosis [93a, 217], and tularaemia [66]. Model experiments on the chorioallantoic membrane of the chick embryo have unequivocally demonstrated that streptococci, staphylococci, and C. diphtheriae multiply extracellularly, while S. typhi, Brucella and M. tuberculosis multiply intracellularly [84].

The pathogenesis of the cyclic diseases is determined decisively by the allergic state and consequent inflammatory reactions [109a, b]. The frequent relapses may be explained by the intracellular multiplication of the pathogenic agents. Namely, the pathogens may hide from the immune response, and at a time when immunity has weakened, they may reappear in the blood, causing relapse.

The allergy in brucellosis has been thoroughly studied. The symptoms of this anthropozoonosis, showing protracted course and undulating temperature, may be attributed, first of all, to an allergy developing during the 1 to 3 weeks of incubation to decomposed bacterial products [218].

Patients with brucellosis respond with severe local and general reactions when injected with killed Brucella or its extract. The reactivity to Brucella antigen of tissue cultures and leukocytes derived from infected subjects is significantly increased as compared to tissue cultures from healthy individuals [97, 129a, 153a]. Hypersensitivity persists even after clinical healing, therefore, reinfection is followed by symptoms appearing after a very short incubation period and lasting sometimes only a few hours [218]. Although the histological changes, particularly at the initial stage of the disease, are due to the direct toxic effect of the bacterium on the vascular wall and parenchymal organs, in the subsequent phase of the disease reactive reticuloendotheliosis develops with granuloma formation, resembling tuberculosis and indicative of an allergic pathogenesis [10, 218]. The same may be stated about the synovitis, serous meningitis, polyserositis and transient exanthema developing in brucellosis with acute onset and rapid disappearance [10, 176]. In protracted brucellosis, the ameliorating effect of vaccine desensitization also points to the involvement of allergic factors. As in other allergic diseases, corticosteroids are also helpful in controlling severe acute symptoms of brucellosis [218].

Allergy might play a pathogenetic role in typhoid fever [109c]. Although numerous symptoms of this disease appear to be in accordance with an allergic origin, the role of allergy is not so clear as in brucellosis. While in brucellosis allergy can be readily demonstrated by intracutaneous tests, such attempts have so far failed in typhoid fever. The severe reactions occasionally observed in patients immunized during the incubation period of typhoid fever are suggestive of an allergic mechanism operating also in this disease.

The clinical manifestations of tularaemia may resemble typhoid fever or brucellosis. The histological changes and the positive intracutaneous tests indicate that allergy is involved in the pathogenesis of this disease.

4

Bacterial diseases may be accompanied by symptoms strongly indicating an allergic origin. These are first of all various cutaneous manifestations, rapidly disappearing inflammatory reactions in the joints and on serous membranes all of which are similar to the symptoms of diseases with known allergic patho-mechanism, e.g. serum sickness. Also the shock observed in some fulminant infections may raise the suspicion of an anaphylactoid pathogenesis.

There are three relatively well-defined diseases which may develop after acute bacterial infections and have by all probability an allergic pathomechanism. These are acute glomerulonephritis, rheumatic fever and Reiter's syndrome. As the first named disease has been discussed in Chapter 53 (Volume 5), only the other two conditions will be dealt with in the following.

Acute rheumatic fever. The disease is an active inflammatory process which affects, most commonly and in variable combinations, the heart valves, myo-cardium, and pericardium. Carditis is usually associated with other symptoms like fever and arthritis, but may also develop insidiously in association with vague general symptoms or may appear in a fulminant form, particularly in children [126]. The concordance rate for rheumatic fever (in monozygotic twins it approaches 20 per cent, whereas that for dizygotic twins is approx. 2.5 per cent) suggests that genetic factors may be of some importance, although they are obviously not the sole determinant [96].

Although the exact pathogenesis of rheumatic fever is still unknown, its relationship with *Streptococcus pyogenes* of Lancefield group A (hereafter referred to as Str.) now seems to be sufficiently proved on the basis of the following observations:

1. In the majority of cases, Str. infection occurs 2 to 3 weeks before the onset of rheumatic fever.

2. Epidemics caused by Str. are accompanied by an increased incidence of rheumatic fever in the same population [249] and rheumatic fever follows about 1 to 3 per cent of Str. infections [42, 136, 196, 213, 252].

3. Streptococcal infection has been proved by bacteriological and serological tests in patients with rheumatic fever [28a, b]. Depending on the technique, Str. can be demonstrated in pharyngeal smears in about 50 to 60 per cent of the cases [27b]. Elevated anti-streptolysin-O and anti-streptokinase titres of serum were detected in 80 to 90 per cent of rheumatic fever cases, indicating streptococcal infection [27a, 221].

4. Treatment of the Str. induced disease with penicillin significantly reduces the subsequent incidence of rheumatic fever, and prophylactic use of penicillin has proved to be of considerable value in preventing recurrences [16, 24, 25, 42, 158, 195].

The relationship between Str. infection and rheumatic fever has been repeatedly demonstrated; nevertheless, the means whereby streptococcal infection produces tissue damage is not clear; streptococci have only occasionally been recovered from cardiac tissues of patients who died of rheumatic fever and have never been found in synovial fluids of the involved joints [103]. Furthermore, attempts to prove the role of the direct tissue damaging effect of Str. or streptococcal products have failed. Streptococci produce a wide variety of toxins some of which have cardiotoxic properties *in vitro* and *in vivo* [200]. The antibody levels to several streptococcal toxins and enzymes are at or near to their peaks when the manifestations of rheumatic fever appear. This finding contradicts the direct causal role of toxins in the lesions of rheumatic fever [96]. The concept that rheumatic fever is a disease of allergic pathogenesis is supported by the following clinical, immunological and experimental observations:

1. A hypersensitivity reaction to group A streptococci.
2. The interval between the primary Str. disease and the onset of rheumatic fever corresponds to the time necessary for the maximum rate of antibody production to be attained.
3. The clinical symptoms of fibrous tissue inflammation involving chiefly the heart and the joints are in many respects similar to those of serum sickness. The disease may be recurrent like allergic diseases in general.
4. Pathological changes found in rheumatic fever (fibrinoid degeneration, necrosis of fibrous tissue, Aschoff bodies, nodules consisting of necrotic fibrous tissue surrounded by macrophages, lymphocytes and plasma cells) [103] closely resemble the histological findings in various allergic diseases in man and experimental animals [166].
5. The higher the titre of anti-streptolysin-O following Str. infection the more frequent the incidence of rheumatic fever will be [221, 226]. This observation suggests an enhanced immune activity in patients with rheumatic fever. Very few patients will fail to show an increase in streptococcal antibody when two or more such tests (anti-streptolysin-O, anti-hyaluronidase, anti-streptokinase, anti-DNase, anti-NADase) are performed.
6. Patients with rheumatic fever do not exhibit an active protective and functional immunity to Str. Reinfection leads to recurrence of the disease [217].
7. In experimental animals, pathological changes resembling those in human rheumatic fever need several injections of Str. to develop [167].
8. It has been shown using the immunofluorescent technique that antisera produced in rabbits against group A streptococci were capable of binding to cardiac muscle [120b].
9. As non-specific evidence of immunological reaction, the C level in the serum of patients with rheumatic fever is usually found normal or elevated [34], or shows a considerable fluctuation around the normal value. This has been considered to be the result of increased consumption or production of C [151]. The observation that $\beta_1 C$ and $\beta_1 E$ globulins are attached to the sarcolemma of the myocardium [80] supports this interpretation. Another acute-phase reactant, the C-reactive protein, is often elevated.
10. ACTH and corticosteroid therapy is as beneficial in rheumatic fever as in allergic diseases. However, this benefit seems to be attributable to the anti-inflammatory effect of these drugs.

If the theory of allergic pathomechanism is accepted, we have to answer two questions: (*i*) what kind of antigen is responsible for the allergy? and (*ii*) which type of allergy is involved?

The antigen is still unknown. The patients' sera contain different antibodies

6

reacting with various Str. antidens, and patients with high levels of so-called 'anti-streptococcal antibodies non-cross-reactive with human tissues' [96] are likely to develop acute rheumatic fever. It is conceivable that the tissues are damaged by (i) a Str. antigen or (ii) an immune complex consisting of a Str. antigen and the corresponding antibody, e.g. a streptolysin–antistreptolysin complex [89], which acts as a new antigen, or (iii) a conjugated antigen formed from streptococcal and tissue components. It is also possible that rheumatic fever is a result of reinfection by homotypic Str. This assumption seems to be supported by the observation that the frequency of rheumatic fever was found to be equal to the expected frequency of homotypic reinfection. Considering that according to Griffith's typing each Str. type bears a distinct M protein, it has been suggested that M protein is accumulated in the tissues, then, having coupled with the anti-M-protein antibody, gives rise to the tissue damage [238b]. The pathogenetic role of the streptococcal M protein is supported also by the finding that immunization of the patients with M protein was followed by a fresh outbreak of rheumatic fever [156]. However, the presence of M protein in the tissues of patients could not be proved so far and the antibody to purified M protein does not react with human myocardium [96]. Furthermore, penicillin given as late as on the 9th day of Str. infection was found to be effective in preventing rheumatic fever [25]; this time would certainly be sufficient for the deposition of M protein in the tissues and for the formation of specific antibodies. More recent studies have, however, indicated that the antigen in question is widely distributed in group A Str. strains including those containing little or no M protein. Furthermore, pathogenetic role has been attributed to a streptococcal lipoprotein likely to bind to collagen [246]. It has been suggested that the streptococcal antigen in question may be present both in the cell and in the membrane; that it acts as a hapten; and that different carrier proteins (e.g. M protein) are of importance, depending on the source of the antigen.

Intracutaneous tests have also failed to provide information about the nature of the antigen. So far no standardized technique has been elaborated for the performance of such tests in rheumatic fever [27b]. Positive intracutaneous reaction with streptococci and their extracts can be obtained in a great number of healthy subjects, for the majority of the healthy population have been infected by Str. at some time during their lives. The percentage of positivity is not significantly different from that for patients with rheumatic fever. Although the positive intracutaneous reaction was found to be slightly enhanced in the acute phase of rheumatic fever [225], this observation is of little value in understanding the pathomechanism of the disease. The ability of developing positive cutaneous reaction (delayed hypersensitivity) can only be transferred passively with immunocytes [141]. The intracutaneous test performed with the nucleoprotein fraction extracted from Str. has been invariably positive in patients with rheumatic fever and negative in healthy subjects [246, 247].

Lymphocyte transformation with streptolysin S preparations was found to be positively correlated with that obtained with phytohaemagglutinin, but not with the serum inhibitor of streptolysin S [36], indicating that the transforming activity of streptolysin S preparations is not due to streptolysin S, but to other streptococcal products present in these preparations.

The autoimmune pathogenesis of rheumatic heart disease is dealt with in detail in Chapter 38 (Vol. 3). Nevertheless, it seems to be justified to discuss several aspects of this complex problem here, too.

There are several theories concerning the development of so-called 'anti-heart autoantibodies non-cross-reactive with Streptococci' [26c, 125, 203, 238b]. In response to the damage caused by some specific streptococcal cardiotoxins [129] attached to cardiac muscle fibres various substances (slightly modified native heart muscle, cytoplasmic cardiac components) are produced which differ in their antigenic structure from the 'normal' tissue constituents. These substances may induce autoimmune antibodies. Reinfections and non-rheumatic cardiac injuries might lead to an enhancement of heart-reactive autoantibody production, accounting for relapses as well as the postcardiotomy and postmyocardial-infarction syndrome.

Another theory suggests that rheumatic fever is due to cross-reacting antigens in Str. and in the heart muscle. Antibodies cross-reacting with a spectrum of soluble antigens of different species were demonstrated in human sera with high anti-streptolysin titres. Most of the positive precipitations were obtained with human heart antigens. Reactions with extracts of human skeletal muscle and kidney were demonstrated less often. Antigens of animal origin showed low incidence of positive reactions. In addition, a correlation was found between the increase in positive precipitin reactions and the degree of anti-streptolysin-O titres [250].

The so-called 'anti-streptococcal-cell-wall antibodies cross-reactive with human glycoprotein' [96] react immunologically with human heart valve and synovia, i.e. with connective tissue, and do not react with muscle [81]. Such antibodies have been demonstrated in a small number of children suffering from rheumatic fever [96].

The 'anti-streptococcal-cell-membrane antibodies cross-reactive with human cardiac muscle, skeletal muscle and arteriolar smooth muscle' [92] cause muscle damage (e.g. myocarditis, arteritis) [117, 123, 124, 255a, b, 256]. It is of significance that rheumatic and non-rheumatic heart tissues bind this antibody with equal intensity; it is not species-specific, but is moderately tissue-specific [96].

In fact, sera of patients with rheumatic fever have been shown to contain antibodies that react with constituents of the human myocardium; this has been demonstrated with C fixation [17], passive agglutination of collodion particles [26a], tanned red cell agglutination [238a], anti-human-globulin consumption test [219], platelet consumption [49], immunofluorescence, and precipitation [120a]. Such antibodies are present in 60 to 70 per cent of the patients during the first attack of the disease, the percentage increasing with the number of relapses [49]. There is no relationship, on the other hand, between the severity of rheumatic fever and the presence of autoantibodies. In myocardial biopsy specimens from patients with rheumatic fever γ-globulin attached to myocardial fibrils, vessel walls and, to a lesser extent, the interstitial tissue has been demonstrated [122, 126]. Deposition of immunoglobulins (IgG, IgA and IgM) was mainly found in the sarcolemmal and sub-sarcolemmal areas, and this is the most specific for the disease. However, similar deposition was found in vascular smooth muscle and interstitial connective tissue, too. Unlike the myocardium, the valves only bind IgG. Normal myocytes are strongly resistant to penetration by immunoglobulins, only antibodies reacting with surface (sarcolemmal or intercalated disc) antigens might be expected to be capable of any primary cytotoxic activity [120c]. Some authors have succeeded in showing in Aschoff's bodies C fixing substances which were thought to be antigen–antibody complexes. Cavelty [26b] induced autoreactive anti-heart antibodies and a tissue reaction resembling human rheumatic inflammation in a considerable number of animals, by injecting them with a mixture of Str., cardiac muscle, synovial and connective tissue extracts. Myocardial lesions were also produced in animals by prolonged immunization with heterologous or homologous cardiac muscle extracts in adjuvant [121]. According to other investigators [39], the inflammatory lesions which develop in the heart tend to be rather sparse and unimpressive. Furthermore, there is very little correlation between the titre of circulating anti-heart antibodies and the severity of the experimental cardiac lesion.

The non-toxicity for mammalian heart cells of the heart-reactive antibodies present in sera of patients with rheumatic fever [228] suggests that these antibodies have no primary pathogenic role; they are formed as part of an immunological response to heart tissue which has been damaged by some unrelated cardiotoxic agent [229]. The humoral anti-heart antibody only became cytopathogenic in those experimental animals in which the myofibre-cell barrier had been broken down by treatment with isoproterenol [74].

Since the nature of the allergen in rheumatic fever is still unknown, it would be premature to define the type of the allergic reaction involved. On account of the absence of eosinophilia, the relatively high erythrocyte sedimentation rate, the beneficial effect of salicylates and aminopyrine, and the inefficiency of epinephrine and antihistamine drugs [37] a type I anaphylactic allergic reaction (according to the classification of Gell and Coombs) can be excluded. A type II cytotoxic mechanism [80] seems to be more likely.

In summary, there is no doubt that (i) group A *Streptococcus pyogenes* is involved in the aetiology of rheumatic fever, and (ii) the pathogenesis of the disease is allergic or autoimmune. The allergen (autoallergen?) involved in the immune reaction and the type of the reaction have not so far been exactly defined. It is important to distinguish carefully between cause and effect [229].

Reiter's syndrome mainly occurs in young males and is a relatively well-defined clinical entity supposed to be an allergic complication of infection. Since the first description of the disease by Reiter [199a] numerous papers have dealt with this syndrome [106, 198, 199b, 240]. A search for an infectious agent was initiated by numerous authors. Reiter supposed that the disease was a spirochaetosis, and subsequent investigators suggested that it was a secondary consequence of staphylococcal, enterococcal, pseudodiphtherial, gonococcal, or shigella infections. In recent years the interest has been focussed on the mycoplasma and Bedsonia-group agents. Several workers succeeded in demonstrating inclusion bodies in epithelial cells of the conjunctiva and of the urethra. It seems that Reiter's syndrome is a secondary allergic condition following a variety of infections, primarily bacterial dysentery; it has been noted to occur relatively infrequently [240].

Diarrhoea, the earliest symptom of the disease, is generally followed by the well-known triad of symptoms: urethritis, conjunctivitis and arthritis, accompanied sometimes by cutaneous manifestations, uveitis and prostatitis, in about 2 to 4 weeks. The disease is associated with fever, loss of weight, normochromic anaemia, and increased erythrocyte sedimentation rate. It heals spontaneously within 1 to 7 weeks.

Allergic pathogenesis of the disease is supported by the following observations:

1. The interval between the primary disease and the onset of the syndrome is 2 to 4 weeks.

2. No specific pathogen is demonstrable.

3. The arthral manifestations are similar to those seen in other diseases of allergic origin.

4. Lymph node extracts or synovial fluid from Reiter patients induce a tuberculin-type cutaneous reaction in patients with Reiter's syndrome.

5. Sera of over 50 per cent of patients suffering from Reiter's disease agglutinate erythrocytes sensitized with prostatic extracts [85]. The significance of these antibodies is unclear.

VIRAL DISEASES

Viruses are intracellular parasites: their replication can damage or destroy the infected host cell. Recently, data have accumulated showing that pathological changes in viral diseases can only partly be explained by this direct viral impact on the host's cells and the role of virus induced immunopathological processes has been analysed [251]. Different mechanisms may be involved in immunopathological tissue damage in the course of virus infections. Certain viruses replicate in the cells of the immune system, inhibiting or, occasionally enhancing humoral or cellular immune response. Viruses and specific antibodies may form antigen–antibody complexes, which together with C may cause tissue damage and thus give rise to immune-complex disease. The cytotoxic effect of antiviral antibodies and C is due to their interaction with new surface antigen of the cell induced by the virus infection. Reaction of sensitized immune cells with viral antigens may also lead to tissue damage. Viral infections may have a pathogenetic role in autoimmune diseases, too.

The possible role of immunological processes in the pathogenesis of human viral diseases has been most thoroughly studied in three groups of diseases, i.e. in viral diseases with rash, in neurotropic virus infections and more recently in infectious hepatitis. The former two will be discussed here, the latter has been dealt with in Chapter 52 (Volume 5).

Viral diseases associated with rash

The list of viral diseases with rash is continuously increasing [144a, b, 244]. Some common features in their natural history deserve attention. The symptomless incubation period varies between 9 and 21 days. The onset is sudden and the general symptoms are followed by eruption. The elements of the rash follow a well-defined pattern of development from first appearance to healing. At the time of, or immediately after, the onset of the eruption specific antibodies may be detected in the blood. In the majority of these diseases delayed hypersensitivity develops against the viral antigens. Although the diseases included in this group can usually be distinguished on the basis of the severity of the general symptoms, characteristics of the eruption and the accompanying symptoms, the common features of the clinical course point to an identical or similar pathomechanism.

The concept that the exanthems have an allergic pathomechanism is due to von Pirquet [192b, c, d]. He vaccinated subjects without previous variola vaccination on different areas of the skin every day. The lesions caused by vaccination developed independently from one another, however, 8 to 11 days after the first inoculation, a uniform inflammatory reaction appeared around each lesion. Von Pirquet attributed this reaction to the coupling with the virus of antibodies produced in response to the first vaccination, which were present in all the vaccination lesions. In his opinion, not only the vaccination disease but also measles and other diseases with rash have an allergic pathomechanism: the pathogen multiplies in the mucous epithelium of the upper respiratory tract and initiates antibody production therefrom. The antibodies begin to 'digest' the virus at the end of the incubation period; toxic degradation products termed 'apotoxins' are liberated, which are believed to be responsible for the fever and the inflammatory reaction; the eruption is caused by agglutination of the pathogen in the capillary loops of the skin.

Although, owing to numerous unclarified questions, the exact pathogenesis of viral diseases with rash is still unknown, it is most likely that allergy plays an important, if not exclusive, part in it.

Vaccinia has been extensively studied from the aspect of allergic pathomechanism, and the significance of such a mechanism has been verified in both clinical studies and animal experiments. In patients with alymphocytic congenital agammaglobulinaemia, vaccination leads to progressive vaccinia [112] whereas it takes the usual course in children suffering from agammaglobulinaemia, but possessing normal lymphocyte function. The latter group, like normal children, acquire immunity to revaccination [82]. Progressive vaccinia cannot be inhibited by antiserum but heals in response to local injection of lymphocytes derived from a freshly vaccinated subject [128].

In immunotolerant rabbits vaccination failed to produce the typical lesion, and many of the animals died of generalized vaccinia infection [63]. Guinea pigs in which the production of humoral anti-vaccinia antibodies had been prevented by X-ray irradiation exhibited the same vaccinia lesions as the untreated controls [69]. If, however, anti-mononuclear serum had been injected around the site of vaccination, the reaction and typical lesion failed to develop, although the virus multiplied in the skin, and the blood of the animals contained haemagglutination inhibiting antibodies. Delayed-type sensitization to killed vaccinia virus was also presented by anti-mononuclear serum [191].

The phenomena observed in patients with agammaglobulinaemia and in animals rendered immunodeficient have unequivocally shown that the normal development of the vaccinia lesion is governed by cellular reactions and not by circulating antibodies. Furthermore, since allergy against the inactivated virus becomes demonstrable only after the vaccination lesion has fully developed, it is most likely that both are due to the delayed hypersensitivity of the organism.

According to Mims [163], the normal development of the vesicle is based on delayed hypersensitivity, whereas the regional inflammatory reaction suddenly appearing 8–11 days after vaccination is caused by humoral antibodies. He demonstrated the significance of the latter in experiments on rabbit myxomatosis. The virus was injected intradermally and anti-myxoma serum was administered intravenously on the 3rd postinfection day, when the lesion was still in the papular phase; one hour after the injection of the antiserum, an erythema appeared around the lesion, similar to that observed on the 8th day without antibody injection.

It has also been suggested, on the basis of experiments on guinea pigs, that neither humoral antibodies, nor delayed hypersensitivity, but local accumulation of interferon, plays the main role in the healing of vaccinia lesions [70].

The allergic pathomechanism of *measles* has been generally accepted, for numerous characteristics of the disease could be readily explained by such a mechanism, e.g. the incubation time, the appearance of exanthems, etc. However, measles virus has been shown to cause damage in cultured cells closely similar to that found *in vivo* [56, 223]. This observation has made some investigators [157] to abandon von Pirquet's theory.

As to the role of allergy in the pathomechanism of measles, there are substantially less data available than there are for vaccinia. During the development of the exanthem, the corium becomes oedematous with mononuclear infiltration [231]. By the 72nd h after the eruption the epidermal lesions disappear while the perivascular cellular infiltration persists. This reaction may be a manifestation of delayed hypersensitivity.

The allergy inducing effect of the virus is also indicated by the observation that several years after vaccination with killed virus natural infection may give rise to a severe reaction with atypical exanthems [73, 94, 168]. Subjects who had been vaccinated with killed virus responded with severe local reaction to injection of the attenuated virus [22, 72, 159]. In such individuals, intracutaneous test with the killed virus demonstrated delayed hypersensitivity [142, 143, 171] although some authors considered it to be an Arthus-type reaction [22]. It appears that the delayed-type hypersensitivity is due to the lipid fraction of the measles virus [101].

There seems to be little evidence favouring the concept that in measles the exanthems correspond to an Arthus-type reaction occurring between the humoral antibodies and the virus in the tissues. The observation that large doses of γ-globulin given on the 7th or 8th day of the incubation period may accelerate the eruption in measles (eruption on the 12th day) seems to support such a hypothesis. It may be assumed that under such circumstances the reaction between the passively introduced antibody and the virus which is already present is responsible for the rash. In this case the mechanism is supposedly the same as that operating under natural conditions when the exanthems appearing later are ascribable to the active antibodies [20]. The development of the measles exanthem can be prevented locally by the injection of convalescent serum [40] which, again, contradicts the above theory.

The role played by the reactivity of the organism in the development of the rash is indicated by the observation that in children suffering from certain chronic diseases measles appears in the form of giant-cell pneumonia without any rash [55]. Supposedly, in these cases the absence of the characteristic symptoms is the result of a reduced responsiveness of the organism.

During the disease the allergic reactivity to other impacts substantially decreases while the susceptibility to other infectious diseases is often strongly enhanced. It was already known by Preisich [194] and von Pirquet [192a] that tuberculin positivity may be lost during measles. The loss of tuberculin hypersensitivity has been verified also with the lymphocyte transformation test [217].

In the first four days from the onset of measles rash the rate of blastic transformation induced by phytohaemagglutinin in the patient's lymphocytes *in vitro* is also reduced [216]. It is known that nephroses with an allergic pathomechanism may transiently improve in response to measles or after measles vaccination [113, 254]. For this phenomenon there is no satisfactory explanation available at present. The increased susceptibility to infections may be attributed to the rapid decline of the serum IgG and IgA levels after the appearance of the rash. They reach the lowest values on the 3rd day after the appearance of the eruption, then IgG returns to the normal level by the 6th or 7th day, while IgA by the 8th to 10th day [150]. Parallel with the appearance of the rash serum properdin also falls to an unmeasurably low level, while during convalescence it returns to normal [179]. Since the decline in the immunoglobulin and properdin levels coincides with the reduction or disappearance of tuberculin hypersensitivity, it is conceivable that measles affect the entire immune apparatus at about the same time. The increased susceptibility to infections during measles, however, seems to be mainly due to the suppression of cellular immunity, since no changes in specific antibody titres explaining this susceptibility could be found [174c].

Recent investigations have also shown that delayed-type reactions to various antigens are suppressed by live attenuated measles vaccine similarly as by the disease itself [61].

The pathogenesis of viral diseases associated with rash may be outlined as follows, based on model animal experiments [59, 211] and on a line of different observations. During the incubation period, the virus multiplies at the site of entry and the regional lymph nodes; then they spread via the blood stream to different organs (primary viraemia). The virus undergoes further multiplication in these organs, and by the end of the incubation time a secondary viraemia develops. The primary viraemia and virus multiplication in the lymphatic organs set the stage for humoral and cell-mediated immune reactions. The manifestations of the disease result from the interaction of the following four factors: cytopathogenic effect of the virus; non-specific inflammatory reaction; Arthus-type reaction arising as a consequence of the interaction of humoral antibodies and viruses; and delayed-type reaction as a result of the interaction between sensitized lymphocytes and virus carrier cells [21a]. The relative significance of these components seems to be different in various diseases, contributing to the variability of the clinical picture. The type of rash also depends on the localization of the virus in the skin; viruses multiplying in the endothelium of the capillaries give rise to maculo-papular lesions, while those multiplying in epithelial cells cause vesiculo-pustular eruptions. The general symptoms may be attributed to the viraemia or to the toxic effects of cell debris. Recovery is not related to the appearance of the specific immune response; interferon production seems to be a more important factor of healing. The allergic reactions occurring during the disease may in some instances mitigate other specific responses.

There are two basic pathological processes involved in these conditions: neuronal destruction and regional inflammation. While the first is mostly the consequence of the direct cytopathogenic effect of the virus, the inflammatory reaction may be regarded as allergic in nature.

Immunological processes in the pathogenesis of neurotropic virus infection have been most extensively studied in the *lymphocytic choriomeningitis virus (LCMV)* infection, which is a characteristically virus-induced immunopathological disease [177b, 237]. LCMV replicates in tissue culture or in animal cells without being cytopathic. Adult, susceptible mice infected with LCMV remain symptom-free for 5–7 days, though virus replication can be demonstrated in their viscera and meninges. After that the inflammatory cells infiltrate the sites of viral replication causing clinical symptoms and death. Surviving mice are immune against LCMV reinfection. The occurrence of these pathological changes coincides with the onset of the immune response of the infected animal; a causal relationship between the two events may be postulated. The symptoms and fatal outcome of LCMV infection of mice could be considerably reduced and prevented by X-ray irradiation prior to infection [31], or by giving methotrexate [146] or by a diet deficient in folic acid [88]. Similarly acute disease could be prevented by neonatal thymectomy or administration of anti-lymphocyte serum [164].

The LCMV disease of mice infected transplacentally or at birth differs from the adult type infection. In these animals a virus 'carrier state' develops. This is not a real state of immune tolerance, however immune response is depressed: antibody production is delayed and poor [237], and the cell-mediated immune response is also weaker than in adult mice [177b]. These animals are free of symptoms. Later, however, as a result of the appearance of anti-virus antibody, a chronic illness may develop with chronic glomerulonephritis, focal necrosis in the liver and disseminated lymphoid infiltrates. In mouse strains whose immune response is very poor these pathological changes do not develop [177a].

It seems that both humoral and cell-mediated immunity play a role in the development of pathological changes in adult-type infection. Transfer of LCMV antibodies to carrier mice results in acute necrotizing inflammatory lesions followed by chronic mononuclear infiltration in regions of viral persistence. Cellular transfer from hyperimmune donors to carrier mice initiates and/or intensifies tissue injuries [177d]. Splenic cells from immune mice have a cytotoxic effect on LCMV-infected tissue cultures [152]. This may be attributed to a cytotoxic factor released during the interaction of the virus with the immune cells [177c].

Chronic carrier state can be produced also in adult mice by cyclophosphamide treatment. Splenic cell transfer from immune animals to these carriers leads to death, the pathological changes being quite similar to those seen in natural infection. Transfer of immune serum to these carriers produces less severe pathological changes [30].

The pathogenetic role of specific immune response of the host has been demonstrated in other neurotropic virus diseases, too. In animals infected with Venezuelan encephalitis virus [13] or Japanese B encephalitis virus [251] pathological changes in the nervous system were initiated or intensified by immune serum given at an appropriate time after the infection. In neurotropic virus infections,

14

in general, the intensity of the inflammatory reaction can be substantially reduced by administering corticosteroids prior to the appearance of the specific antibodies [79, 242].

The immune response, however, probably plays a lesser part in the pathogenesis of neurotropic virus diseases other than LCMV infection. This animal disease is, however, a suitable model for studying virus induced immunopathological changes. There are neurotropic virus infections in which the virus induced cell destruction is the major clinical feature (e.g. poliomyelitis); however, immune response is involved even in these cases.

Webb and Gordon Smith [242] have proposed the following hypothesis about the pathogenesis of viral diseases of the nervous system. The virus first multiplies in extraneural tissues, probably in lymph nodes; from there it enters the blood stream, where its multiplication continues in leukocytes, wherefrom other susceptible cells of the body are infected. This viraemia is responsible for the first phase of the disease while the immune system is sensitized. With the appearance of specific antibodies viraemia ceases, however, the virus further multiplies in susceptible cells of the nervous system. Encephalitis ensues at the time when specific antibodies appear in the blood. The cells preferential for virus multiplication are different in various diseases, hence, the pathology will be different in poliomyelitis, arbovirus and other infections attacking the nervous system. The perivascular localizations of the inflammatory reactions suggest that these are caused by antigen–antibody reaction occurring at places where viral antigens meet large amounts of antibody. The fact that lasting neurological disorders occur rarely in neurotropic virus infections might eventually be explained by individual differences in the degree of penetration of various immunoglobulins into the nervous system [147].

Allergic complications of viral diseases

Allergic complications seem to be less frequent in diseases of viral origin than in bacterial diseases. Nervous complications of non-neurotropic viral diseases have been the most extensively studied in this respect.

The frequency of neurological complications of viral infections shows seasonal and geographical variations. It varies from 0.4 to 1.0 in measles [50, 53, 232], from 0.01 to 0.1 in chickenpox [6, 53, 77], from 0.7 to 4.0 in smallpox [48], around 0.2 in rubella [212], per 1,000 cases; in mumps the figures are much higher, ranging between 1.3 and 33 per cent [87]. In non-neurotropic viral diseases invasion of the nervous system by the virus seems to occur more frequently than in diseases of the nervous system. In about 50 per cent of patients with uncomplicated measles EEG abnormalities were detected [76]. Others found abnormal patterns in all patients during the incubation period [180]. In mumps, neurological disorders were detected in 54 per cent of the affected patients by EEG and/or CSF examination [12]. Most probably, the invasion of the nervous system takes place already in an early stage of the infection, for encephalitic complication could not be prevented by γ-globulin administered during the incubation period of measles [202].

The possibility that the parainfectious nervous complications might have an allergic pathomechanism was first suggested by Glanzmann [78] and, subsequently, by van Bogaert [233] and Finlay [60]. Soon it became evident that the pathological changes in these diseases are similar to those found in postvaccination and serogenic encephalomyelitis that follow smallpox or rabies vaccinations or the injection of heterologous serum. Similar histological changes can be produced in laboratory animals sensitized with heterologous or homologous brain extracts [239]. The pathology of these lesions is characterized by perivenous spread and demyelination which is followed by reactive proliferation of the microglia. Pette [188] classified parainfectious and postvaccination encephalitis into the same pathogenetic group as other demyelination diseases and used the term neuroallergy to denote the common features in the pathogenesis (cf. Chapter 55, Volume 6).

A virus-induced autoallergic mechanism is postulated in the pathogenesis of nervous complications accompanied by demyelination [129, 132a]. However, this assumption, being based merely on the similarity in the histological appearance of parainfectious and experimental allergic encephalitides is to be confirmed. Although it has been demonstrated that leukocytes of patients suffering from parainfectious encephalitis [95, 174a, d, e], or disseminated encephalitis of unknown origin [9] react with antigens derived from the nervous system, it is still doubtful whether this sensitization has any pathogenetic significance, since similar alterations have deen detected in obviously non-allergic diseases associated with nervous tissue destruction [95].

The theory of virus-induced autoallergy is contradicted by the observation that the nervous complications ensue concomitantly with [4, 104, 107, 243], or prior to, the primary diseases [100] thus, the interval characteristic of allergic complications of infectious diseases is lacking [230].

A uniform pathogenesis is strongly challenged also by the lack of demyelination and reactive inflammation, both believed to be characteristic of neuro-allergic processes, in several parainfectious neurological disorders. Instead, in a number of cases the pathological picture was dominated by cerebral oedema and neuronal decay [2, 14, 23, 44].

The term encephalopathy has been proposed for this condition attributable to virus induced enhanced permeability of the cerebral capillaries, their constriction and obstruction with consequent cerebral anoxaemia [129]. It is, however, mostly impossible to distinguish these forms from encephalitis merely on the basis of the clinical picture [133]. Since demyelination is often absent in rubella-associated encephalitis [75, 162, 213], this complication is distinguished from other parainfectious encephalitides and compared with polioencephalitis developing as a consequence of direct viral impact [210]. Nevertheless, the pathogenetic role of allergy in the sense that has been considered in connection with neurotropic viral infections cannot be excluded in this case either.

Another form of encephalitis that might be connected with a non-neurotropic viral disease is *subacute sclerosing panencephalitis* (SSPE). During the last years evidence on the relation between SSPE and measles virus has been accumulating [161, 257], the most important of which are the following:

1. SSPE occurs in patients with a history of measles (or measles immunization).

2. Structures like nucleocapsid of paramyxovirus and measles antigen can be demonstrated in the diseased brain.

3. SSPE patients have high anti-measles antibody titres in their sera and cerebrospinal fluids (CSF).

4. Measles or closely related viruses have been isolated from fresh brain cultures of SSPE patients.

Though the pathogenesis of SSPE is far from being clear, on the basis of some immunological observations, the suggestion has been made that immunological processes might be involved in it. Measles antibody titres of sera of SSPE patients were much higher than those of healthy individuals after measles or measles immunization. In the CSF of SSPE patients the level of anti-measles antibodies increased during the disease and it is most probable that antibodies derived from the brain tissue itself [108]. Anti-measles antibodies in the sera and CSF of SSPE patients are of IgG and IgM type, while in healthy children having had measles, antibodies of the IgM type do not persist [32]. Some authors have found an impaired cellular responsiveness to measles and other antigens, or only against measles antigen. Therefore, it was thought that it is the impaired cellular immune function that favours the persistence of measles virus in the brain tissue [148].

Recently some epidemiological observations have been made which might be useful in understanding the pathogenesis of SSPE [43, 45]. About two thirds of SSPE patients had measles when younger than two years of age. Patients without a history of clinical measles were also found, but in these cases an intra-familial exposure to measles in early infancy was highly probable. These observations suggest that during the partial maternal immunity period the immune response to the measles infection may be incomplete, thus, permitting the virus to persist in tissues.

It was also observed that SSPE occurs at a higher rate in non-urban settings and among persons having had contact with animals, thus, an infection with an animal virus closely related to measles virus must also be taken into consideration in speculation about the aetiopathogenesis of SSPE.

SKIN TESTS IN THE DIAGNOSIS

SCHICK TEST

This intracutaneous test is used for determining susceptibility to diphtheria; it is a toxin–antitoxin neutralization test and, as such, is not a true hypersensitivity reaction. If diphtheria toxin is injected into the skin of a subject possessing no antitoxic immunity, localized delayed-type inflammatory reaction (erythema and induration) will develop at the site of injection, while the reaction will be negative if the blood contains little or no diphtheria antitoxin. The test was elaborated by Schick [206] to select from among diphtheria contacts those who required serum prophylaxis. Subsequently it was widely used to determine population immunity [258] and to estimate the efficiency of active immunization [58].

The test is made with the filtrate of a culture of a toxin-producing strain of *C. diphtheriae* grown in a liquid medium. The dosage is set by two methods: (*i*) the test dose mixed with 1/750 unit of antitoxin must not produce a local reaction in guinea pigs, while mixed with 1/1,250 unit of antitoxin it should evoke positive local inflammatory reaction. (*ii*) 1/50 of the test dose must not produce a local reaction in guinea pigs, but 1/25 of it should result in a positive intradermal test [183].

The Schick toxin contains, besides the toxin or toxoid reacting with the antitoxin, other substances of bacterial origin and contaminants from the culture medium; these may induce a delayed-type skin hypersensitivity response in some immune subjects. A control test performed with Schick toxin preheated to 70 to 85 °C for 30 min eliminates these false positive reactions.

The test dose and an adequate amount of control are usually injected in volumes of 0.1 or 0.2 ml intracutaneously, on the flexor side of the forearm. In children below the age of 10 years pseudo-reaction is seldom observed, therefore, the control injection may be omitted. The reaction is to be read first 24 to 48 h after the injection, then after 5 to 7 days. The pseudo-reaction appears within 24 to 48 h and fades rapidly, while the specific positive response attains its maximum by the 4th day and begins to fade as late as one week after the injection. Its site soon becomes pigmented, which is followed by desquamation. The reaction is considered positive if there is a local erythema at least 10 mm in diameter. Positive Schick test with negative control indicates sensitivity to the toxin, while if both tests are negative the subject is immune. If the erythema of the Schick test is larger than the control reaction and has a more protracted course, or fades with discoloration, the subject should be regarded susceptible to the toxin. The Schick test is usually negative if the serum of the test subject contains 0.005 to 0.03 IU antitoxin per ml or more. Although the majority of people with negative Schick test are protected from diphtheria, the protection may be incomplete even in subjects with higher antitoxin titres [174a].

Due to the slow development of the reaction, the Schick test is not practical for routine application. If immediate decision is needed whether or not serum therapy should be applied in a potentially infected subject, the *rapid haemagglutination* technique [224] is used which yields a result within 2 h [174b, 175].

DICK TEST

This intracutaneous test has been elaborated for the detection of antitoxic immunity to erythrogenic toxin of *Streptococcus pyogenes* and thus of immunity to scarlet fever [46]. Principally it is the same method as the Schick test. The filtrate of the culture medium of *Str. pyogenes* producing erythrogenic toxin is injected intracutaneously; inflammatory cutaneous reaction appearing in 4 to 6 h at the site of the injection indicates that the subject is susceptible to scarlet fever. Since, similarly to the Schick test, a false positive reaction may occur, control injection with heat-treated toxin is necessary.

Although the Dick test has proved to be a valuable means in elucidating numerous problems concerning scarlet fever, it is now seldom used in practice, for (*i*) standardization of the erythrogenic toxin needs tests in children; (*ii*) the reliability of the test has been called in question by several authors [155, 208]; (*iii*) the introduction of the Dick toxin may result in sensitization to streptococcal antigens which may have harmful sequelae. For the third reason some researchers regard the Dick test contraindicated [214].

SCHULTZ–CHARLTON BLANCHING TEST

This test is based on blanching of the fresh scarlatinal rash in response to the intradermal introduction of convalescent serum (or normal human serum if suitable for this purpose), or the serum of animals immunized with Dick toxin. Blanching ensues about 12–24 h after the introduction of the serum. Earlier the test was used to distinguish scarlet fever from other exanthems; nowadays it is seldom used in practice, since the reaction is only reliable if the rash is marked and if the test is applied in the early phase of the disease. Thus, it is of little value if the clinical course is mild. Moreover, it is difficult to find an adequate serum for the test because the convalescent serum of penicillin-treated patients is poor in antitoxin. Furthermore, the use of human serum involves the risk of hepatitis transmission, while non-human sera may give rise to allergic reactions. We have failed to produce blanching with commercial normal human γ-globulin.

BRUCELLIN (BURNET) TEST

In the majority of patients with brucellosis, delayed hypersensitivity to Brucella antigen develops which seems to be an important factor in the pathogenesis of the disease. Earlier attempts had been made to use killed bacterial suspensions [62], later Burnet [21] elaborated a sensitive test applying the filtrate of the 20-day broth culture of Brucella. This test material was termed brucellin by him. For culturing either *B. melitensis* (melitin), or *B. abortus* (abortin) may be used, or a mixture of *B. abortus*, *B. suis* and *B. melitensis* (polyvalent brucellin). The aim of subsequent modifications of the test have been to eliminate non-specific reactions, to prevent sensitization of the test subject with subsequent antibody production, further to improve the standardization of brucellin. Brucellins produced by different methods were named differently, e.g. brucellergen [110a], brucellin PD and brucellin PS [184], F-allergen [186a], brucergen [154], etc.

The test is performed as follows: 0.05 to 0.1 ml of brucellin is injected intracutaneously on the flexor surface of the forearm of the test subject. The test is read 24, 48 and 72 h after the injection, and it is regarded positive if a local erythema of 10 mm diameter or more develops. The intensity of the reaction may vary from mild erythema to erythema plus induration, occasionally, as the strongest reaction, necrosis may occur. The more severe forms of the local reaction may be accompanied by swelling of the regional lymph nodes and general symptoms as chill, fever and malaise. In subjects showing strong allergy to the antigen an anaphylactic-type general reaction may also occur [186a].

Positivity of the Burnet test indicates infection with Brucella. The test may be positive also in persons who have never suffered from clinical brucellosis [110b].

This is particularly frequent in people having close and frequent contact with domestic animals [93b, 186b].

In clinically manifest brucellosis positivity of the test has been found to vary between 50 and 90 per cent. The result of the test seems to be dependent upon the antigen used (positivity rate is higher with cellular antigens than with extracts), and on the phase of the disease when the test is performed. In chronic forms the reaction tends to be more intensive than in acute infections [186a]. Bekhlemishev [10] suggests that Brucella allergy can be demonstrated in patients with negative Burnet test by intravenous vaccine test, which provokes fever in part of these patients, but not in healthy persons.

In the diagnosis of brucellosis, the Burnet test is a useful complementary means to the serological reactions. The latter are mostly only positive in the acute phase and thus the intracutaneous test is applied for the demonstration of chronic cases [186a]. The test remains positive for several years after clinical recovery presumably as long as living Brucellae are present in the body. In such brucellin-positive persons relapse may occur and reinfection may cause, after a shortened incubation, a severe clinical condition [218].

Recently some authors have rejected the brucellin test, since there are some recently introduced serological reactions (e.g. mercaptoethanol agglutination, anti-globulin Coombs' test, C fixation) which yield more valuable results [15, 99].

TULARIN TEST

In subjects infected with *Francisella tularensis* delayed hypersensitivity develops, which can be readily demonstrated by intracutaneous test. Dilutions of vaccines containing killed bacterium or acetone or other extracts are used as antigen. One of the most widely used antigen is Larson's vaccine [140], which can be standardized with tularaemia serum. For intracutaneous test, 0.1 ml of the 1 : 500 or 1 : 1,000 dilutions of the lyophilized, standardized vaccine is employed. Reading and evaluation of the results are similar as made in Burnet test. The positive reaction is usually apparent by the 2nd week of the disease, but sometimes as early as at the end of the 1st week [149a]; it remains positive for 15 to 17 years or probably even longer [115]. Diagnostic evaluation of the test is made-difficult by the fact that the majority of the infections are abortive, atypical or symptomless and such infections also give rise to sustained positivity of the skin test [149b]. Consequently, persons who frequently get into contact with wild rodents show a high percentage of positive tularin test [189, 190]. Since the agglutinin titre tends to rise during infection, the agglutination test appears to be a more suitable method for the diagnosis of acute infection [149b]. Another disadvantage of the intracutaneous test is that it may reactivate the disease [87].

SKIN TEST IN MUMPS

Patients infected with mumps virus may respond with a delayed-type hypersensitivity reaction to the intracutaneous injection of inactivated mumps virus. The test was performed initially with heat inactivated virus derived from the parotid glands of injected monkeys [54], then this antigen was replaced with virus cultured in the allantoic sac of the chick embryos and inactivated by UV irradiation [100].

The test is performed with 0.1 ml of the allantoic fluid containing an adequate quantity of virus, using non-infected allantoic fluid as control. The result may be read after 24 to 36 h. The diameter of the erythema (with or without induration) is measured; if the average diameter is less than 10 mm, the test is considered negative, between 10 and 15 mm, positivity is doubtful while over 15 mm the reaction is positive. Positivity can be established on the 5th to 9th day of the disease, and 70 to 80 per cent of these convalescents remain permanently positive. Furthermore, the skin test may be positive without a well-recognizable infection; 40 to 60 per cent of adults with a negative history have positive tests, indicating that the infection may be latent, or cross-reaction with other viral antigens may occur [3, 55, 100].

The skin test of mumps is of epidemiological rather than diagnostic value. Its positivity runs roughly parallel with the results of serological (C fixation, haemagglutination inhibition) reactions, although remarkable individual variations may occur, and the value of the test in assessing the degree of immunity is inferior to the serological tests [19, 207, 235].

SKIN TEST IN CAT-SCRATCH DISEASE
MOLLARET TEST

This disease is transmitted by cat-scratch, has a protracted course, and is characterized by suppurative inflammation of the regional lymph nodes. Skin test is an important tool in the diagnosis of the disease. Debré and Lob [41] were the first to publish observations on a large clinical material. Preparation of the antigen and the performance of the test are essentially similar to those in the original Frei test used for the diagnosis of lymphogranuloma venereum.

The antigenic material is heat-treated suspension of infected lymph nodes or pus. It is advisable to employ a polyvalent antigen obtained from several patients [38b], for the pathogen may have several types [165]. 0.1 ml antigen is injected intracutaneously. The reaction is to be read on the 3rd or 4th day. The test is positive if a hyperaemic, indurated papule with a diameter of at least 6 mm is formed at the site of the injection. A small vesicle or pustule with sterile contents, which heals with a crust, may occasionally develop. Sometimes the primary reaction is accompanied by increased swelling of the lymph nodes, indicating that the test has evoked a focal reaction. Occasionally a systemic reaction may also occur.

The test is specific, infected persons always give positive reaction [38a, 41], while positivity in healthy subjects is rare. Positivity without clinical symptoms was more frequently found among family contacts and veterinaries than among control subjects [241]. The test may remain positive for many years after the illness [41, 187], thus it is of value in retrospective diagnosis. For the same reason positivity in typical cases may indicate an anamnestic reaction.

SKIN TESTS IN RICKETTSIAL INFECTIONS

Skin tests used in the diagnosis of epidemic (louse-borne) typhus have been reviewed by Wiessemann et al. [245]. Large quantities of killed *Rickettsia prowazeki* injected into the skin cause inflammatory reaction in subjects not infected previously by this Rickettsia. This response is commonly attributed to direct endotoxic effect. Smaller doses of the antigen, on the other hand, elicit a delayed-type hypersensitivity reaction in previously infected persons only.

Various other constituents of the antigen preparation, e.g. from egg, louse intestine or murine lung, may also elicit a positive reaction, however, this is an immediate-type weal and flare response.

The delayed-type skin test becomes positive by the 5th to 7th day of the disease and remains positive for years or even decades. Positivity is found in 90 per cent of subjects who have contracted the disease. In very severe cases the test is positive at the onset of the disease, then it becomes negative for several days or weeks, and positivity returns after recovery. This phenomenon is attributed to anergy which is manifested also with other antigens, e.g. tuberculin. Cutaneous allergy does not invariably develop after immunization with the killed vaccine, however, the skin test becomes positive within 7 to 10 days after administration of live, attenuated vaccine. The reaction is the same with *R. prowazeki* and *R. mooseri*, presumably because they have a common major antigen.

Skin tests performed with *Coxiella burneti* vaccine in Q fever yielded similar results [138, 236].

ALLERGIC SKIN TESTS IN OTHER ACUTE INFECTIOUS DISEASES

In addition to the above diseases, attempts have been made to elaborate cutaneous sensitivity tests for various other acute infectious diseases, e.g. for dysentery, anthrax, streptococcal and staphylococcal infections, listeriosis, measles, adenovirus infections, hepatitis and ornithosis. No critical survey of these can be made, however, for lack of sufficient data.

ALLERGIC COMPLICATIONS OF ACTIVE IMMUNIZATION PROCEDURES

The antigens incorporated in vaccines are in part of microbial or viral origin, and in part derived from the growth medium. For obtaining immunity, only the so-called protective antigens determining the pathogenicity of the microbe or virus are required. The other antigens are unnecessary or even harmful because they may interfere with the immunological effect of the protective antigen and have toxic and/or allergic side-effects.

It is a common feature of all the complications of immunization procedures that they occur only in a small proportion of the vaccinees, i.e. the complication is determined largely by individual disposition. In some cases the nature of the disposition seems to be evident: recent infectious disease in the history, cramp tendency and damages of the central nervous system, etc. In other cases, however, there is nothing to indicate such abnormalities, not even an allergic 'diathesis'. Therefore, we have to accept that no list of contraindications to vaccination can be regarded as scientifically fully justified. All the contraindications of immunization are determined by known and suspected predisposing factors.

The role of the vaccines in the manifestation of allergic complications may be variable. Antigens originating from the culture medium or the microbes, and even the protective antigens, may cause a hypersensitivity state which becomes evident on subsequent vaccinations. In subjects who have been previously infected with the same pathogen, the microbial or viral antigens in the vaccine might produce an allergic reaction already on the first occasion. In latent allergic subjects other substances of the vaccine (e.g. penicillin, egg-white) may also produce allergic reactions at the first injection. Occasionally, the vaccination may set forth an autoallergic process; finally, there are allergic complications of completely unknown pathomechanism.

In the last years, the methods of producing vaccines have been substantially improved, contaminant antigens of the culture medium have been more and more eliminated. There is reason to believe that sooner or later vaccines will only contain the protective antigen. However, the protective antigens themselves may be toxic and/or allergenic, thus, the problem of vaccination complications cannot be solved merely by purification of the vaccines.

The common allergic complications of immunization procedures will be listed in the following sections.

VACCINATIONS AGAINST VIRAL DISEASES

Smallpox and rabies vaccines are known to induce relatively numerous and severe complications of allergic nature, therefore, they deserve separate discussion. The other virus vaccines, which have been prepared by modern production methods, are much less reactogenic, or at least most of the allergic complications they may induce can be prevented by avoiding the vaccination of persons known to be allergic to the constituents of the vaccine.

Smallpox (variola) vaccination

Vaccine is prepared from the vaccinial eruptions of animals, mostly calf or sheep, or from vaccinia infected chick embryo chorio-allantoic membrane or tissue culture. Due to the very close antigenic relationship between vaccinia and variola virus, vaccination gives full protection against smallpox, provided vaccination is successful, i.e. the vaccine virus does multiply at the vaccination site. The proof of the virus multiplication is the 'take', a vesicular-pustular reaction evolving through the typical stages of vaccinia.

The frequency of smallpox vaccination complications definitely exceeds those of other vaccinations. They occur mainly after primovaccination, i.e. in an organism which is absolutely unprotected against the vaccine virus [139]. The great majority of the complications is due to the direct effect of the virus, the type and the outcome of the process being highly dependent on the general state of health and particularly on the immune function of the vaccinated person.

Of the numerous complications of smallpox vaccination only the inoculation ulcer and the neurological complications may be regarded as having allergic origin. Ulcer is a rare complication. Usually it is the consequence of a bacterial superinfection, however, in some cases secondary infection can be excluded, and after desquamation of the crust there remains an ulcer that may persist for a considerable period of time. Its allergic nature is indicated by the observation that it is more frequently encountered in subjects who have been immunized with killed vaccine (Herrlich's 'vaccine antigen') [52a].

Postvaccinal encephalitis (PVE) is one of the most dangerous complications of smallpox vaccination. The symptoms appear usually by the 9th to 13th day after vaccination. Herrlich [105] distinguished the following types according to the clinical manifestations: convulsive, paretic, meningitic, somnolent-ophthalmoplegic and bulbar forms. Mortality rate is about 30 to 50 per cent, but may reach a higher percentage in infants under one year of age. Histologically, de Vries [44] distinguished two fundamental forms: (*i*) perivenous or microglial encephalitis, and (*ii*) encephalopathy. Perivenous encephalitis occurs only in children older than 2 years, while encephalopathy is encountered in babies, owing to insufficient myelinization at this age.

The epidemiology of PVE has the following characteristics. It occurs almost exclusively after the first inoculation. Its frequency is related to the age of the vaccinee, being the lowest between 1 to 3 years and increasing afterwards. Frequency shows a regional and year-to-year variation. Epidemiological figures showing the two extremes were, e.g. the 1963 value for the U.S.A. and the 1948 figure for Belgium 1.9 and 1,444 PVE cases, respectively, per one million vaccinations [104, 170]. The prevalence of PVE in Hungary in 1963 as calculated from a total of 140,409 primovaccinated children attained 1 : 35,000 in the age group of 1–3 years, whereas in the age group of 4–14 years it was 1 : 7,600 [57].

The aetiology of PVE has been debated for a long time. Some authors have attributed this complication to the direct effect of the vaccinia virus, while others claim that it is the result of activation of a latent viral infection. A relationship has been looked for between PVE and the toxic effects of the virus, nutritional conditions, and even the patient's blood group. However, it appears more plausible that PVE has an allergic pathomechanism. The sequence of events appears to be initiated primarily by the inoculated virus, since the reaction occurs only in subjects who are not protected against the vaccinia virus, and it can be prevented, or at least substantially mitigated, by prophylactic injection of immunoglobulin containing anti-vaccinia antibodies or of killed vaccine [169, 204]. The mode of action of the virus is nevertheless unknown. This, however, holds not only for PVE but for all central nervous system complications induced by viral infections, since PVE is certainly one of the parainfectious encephalitides.

The great majority of smallpox vaccination complications—although not PVE—could be prevented if contraindications to vaccination were rigorously respected [170]. The following precautions have proved to reduce the incidence of PVE considerably. Primovaccination should be carried out between 1 and 3 years of age. Older children, particularly those over 6 years of age should be primovaccinated with special care, possibly with a simultaneous injection of

24

anti-vaccinia immune globulin. Children with present or past neurological disorders, with neurological sequelae, or with convulsions in the history should not be vaccinated. Finally, it is advisable to prepare the vaccine from a vaccinia virus strain known to induce relatively mild vaccination reaction and few neurological complications.

Rabies vaccination

Human rabies vaccines contain completely or partially inactivated fixed virus. Vaccines in wide use have in fact relatively poor immunizing power, therefore, for postexposure prophylaxis a large number of injections (ranging from 6 to 21) at daily intervals followed by one or several boosters are necessary for establishing protection. In most countries antirabies serum of animal origin is given in addition to the vaccine when exposure to rabies is very likely or have been proved [68]. In the case of active-passive prophylaxis the number of boosters should be raised since passive immunization interferes with active immunization process. Both the numerous injections of vaccines with high concentration of animal tissue and the passive immunization with foreign sera carry with them the risk of allergic reactions. Since rabies is a fatal illness, there is no contraindication to vaccination when infection is very likely to have occurred. On the other hand, because of the serious risk of complications unnecessary vaccinations should be avoided, i.e. the necessity of the immunization must be decided on the likelihood of the infection (type and site of the injury, the state of health of the biting animal). The WHO has published a guide for postexposure prophylaxis [253], which has been adopted by different countries with more or less modifications.

There are two main types of rabies vaccine currently widely used: (*i*) nervous tissue vaccines (NTV) prepared from the brain of adult animals (Semple, Fermi, Hempt vaccine) and from the brain of suckling animals; and (*ii*) duck embryo vaccines (DEV).

Local allergy due to the foreign protein in the vaccines is a frequent complication, but of lesser significance. It is thought to be an Arthus-type phenomenon, and is characterized by indurated erythema appearing at the site of the inoculation by the 6th to 11th day after the first injection. It may be accompanied by systemic symptoms (low-grade fever, and, occasionally, shock) but usually disappears within 1 or 2 days.

Severe complications after rabies vaccination are those manifested in the *central nervous system*, like post-rabies vaccination encephalomyelitis. The symptoms usually appear 10 to 17 days after the first injection. Encephalitis, Landry's ascending myelitis, dorsolumbar myelitis, or peripheral neuritis are the most frequent clinical manifestations. It is much more frequent in adults than in children. Mortality depends on the type of complication; on the average, it is about 10 per cent. Histological examination reveals perivenous demyelinating encephalitis. These complications have been considered to be of allergic nature the allergen being associated with the myelin of the neural tissue component of the vaccine. There are several features which are remarkably similar in neurological disorders due to rabies vaccination and in experimental allergic encephalomyelitis. These similarities have been summarized by Jervis [114] as follows: (*i*) incubation time is identical; (*ii*) same histological changes; (*iii*) C-fixing antibodies are present in the sera of the majority of patients and experimental animals; (*iv*) pathological features of PVE in animals vaccinated against rabies and of the experimental allergic encephalomyelitis are very much alike. The allergic character of the neurological complications after rabies vaccination is also indicated by the observation that their incidence shows linear relationship with the number of subsequent vaccine injections [5].

Most of the data on the frequency of neurological complications refer to NTV produced in adult animal brain. Figures show great variations in different countries, and even year-to-year variations may be substantial. The two extremes ever reported are 86 and 2,367 per 1 million vaccines [248]. Occurrence in Hungary was estimated at 1 per 5,000 [135]. After DEV much less neurological complications were observed (about 1 for 25,000 vaccinations or less) [193].

Vaccines produced in suckling mouse brain with low myelin content had been declared to cause no neuroallergic accidents at all [71]. Further observations however disproved this statement [1].

If neurological complication occurs during the postexposure vaccination period, injection of the same type of vaccine has to be immediately discontinued and the vaccination course completed with another type of vaccine (DEV instead of NTV).

Recently tissue culture vaccines prepared in cells of animal and of human origin have been developed [130, 132*b*]. It is hoped that these vaccines, containing no neural tissue, will eliminate the risk of neurological complication of rabies vaccination. Although the fact that vaccines produced in adult animal brain have been used for almost 100 years makes any changes extremely difficult, it is evident that these highly reactogenic vaccines should be abandoned in the near future.

Immunization with vaccines produced in embryonated egg and in tissue culture

Egg-vaccines contain either live or inactivated virus or Rickettsia. Among them the most widely used ones are yellow-fever (17D), influenza, mumps, typhus and rabies (DEV) vaccines. Persons allergic to egg-white often developed severe allergic reactions to egg vaccines in the early period of the production of such vaccines. Improvement of the vaccine purification methods, however, has significantly reduced this problem. Some observations have nevertheless indicated that egg-vaccines may enhance hypersensitivity to egg-white, as it was shown in subjects who had been vaccinated with yellow-fever 17D vaccine and later with duck-embryo rabies vaccine. In these subjects, who had not developed any allergic reaction to yellow-fever vaccination, rabies vaccine evoked severe gastrointestinal allergic symptoms. Since subjects previously not vaccinated against yellow-fever did not develop any reaction to the same DEV, there is a good reason to believe that previous yellow-fever vaccination had augmented the subjects' allergy to egg protein [35].

It has also been shown that bronchospasm of asthmatic patients in response to acetylcholine is significantly enhanced on the day following vaccination against influenza [7].

Tissue culture vaccines have been extensively used against poliomyelitis, measles, rubella and mumps. They contain either live or inactivated virus.

Numerous observations have proved the safety of tissue culture vaccines from the point of view of allergic complications. For instance, children with marked egg-white allergy tolerated tissue culture measles vaccine without the slightest reaction [119], moreover, extensive epidemiological studies have shown that the Salk-type poliomyelitis vaccine does not induce any undesirable reaction [67]. Some exceptions to the rule, however, have been described. Inactivated measles vaccine turned out to possess remarkable sensitizing effect to subsequent homologous viral infection (cf. p. 12); a similar phenomenon was observed in subjects vaccinated with respiratory-syncitial (RS) virus vaccine and then superinfected by RS virus [185]. Recently some authors detected bovine serum residue in licensed viral vaccines. Because of the possibility of bringing about allergic reactions, tissue culture vaccines should be tested for animal serum content by rigorous laboratory control [14a, 57a].

VACCINATIONS AGAINST BACTERIAL DISEASES

Diphtheria immunization

The immunizing substance is diphtheria toxoid, i.e. toxin detoxified with formalin and heat. Vaccines currently in use are more or less purified products containing aluminium gel adjuvants (hydroxide or phosphate) for enhancing immunogenic power. Immunization of children is generally carried out with combined vaccines (diphtheria-pertussis-tetanus or diphtheria-tetanus).

Natural infection with *C. diphtheriae* and repeated immunization procedures may sensitize the organism to the vaccine. Allergy may develop against the toxoid or other products of *C. diphtheriae* [182]. In sensitized subjects, the vaccination may cause a painful local reaction with gross induration and, also, fever, nausea, headache and muscle pain. Neuritis is a rare complication, its allergic pathomechanism is indicated by the fact that it appears mainly in subjects who have been repeatedly vaccinated against diphtheria. It ensues by the 7th to 10th post-vaccination day, and may be associated with angioedema of the skin [134]. Some authors have claimed that the symptoms, which are similar to the nervous system complications of diphtheria, are the result of some retained toxicity of the materials used for vaccination [234]. The probability of sensitization increases with age, vaccinations in older children and adults being more often followed by allergic reactions. The persons thus sensitized possess at the same time satisfactory antitoxic immunity [111], consequently, they should by no means be immunized. Hypersensitivity can be detected by the Moloney test: on the intradermal injection of 0.1 ml of 1/100 diluted unpurified formoltoxoid susceptible persons develop an infiltration at the site of injection within 24 to 48 h. The frequency of allergic complications is reduced by better purification of the vaccine, nevertheless, the reactions resulting from specific sensitization to the toxoid cannot be eliminated in this way [181].

This problem has, however, been almost completely solved by the introduction of the modern vaccination practice in most of the countries. The vaccinations are carried out in infancy and at school-age; moreover, the toxoid content of the vaccines has been reduced to the minimum necessary to achieve protection.

Tetanus immunization

The immunizing substance is tetanus toxoid, i.e. toxin detoxified with formalin and heat. Most of the presently available vaccines contain purified toxoid, and aluminium salt as adjuvant. It was believed for a long time that tetanus toxoid did not produce allergic reactions, although occasionally fatal anaphylactic shock or serum sickness ensuing within a few minutes after the injection has been observed. Since these reactions were attributed to the peptone content of the vaccine, it was thought that with purification of the toxoid such fatalities could be prevented. Since sensitization against the tetanus toxoid by natural infection had not to be reckoned with, it was believed that tetanus vaccination could be administered repeatedly at any time when risk of tetanus was suspected. The wide use of repeated vaccinations, however, resulted in an increased incidence of local or systemic reaction [52c, 131a, 151, 217a, 219a] with occasional fatal outcome [197, 201]. Hypersensitivity can be demonstrated by cutaneous tests [201, 215]. The allergic responses are in part of the Arthus-type, and in part of the tuberculin-type [220]. There is a positive correlation between the degree of anti-toxic immunity and the severity of the reaction following booster injections. Thus, vaccination of allergic persons is unnecessary from the aspect of immunity; it is undesirable because of the risk of serious complications [145]. Since highly purified vaccines may also give rise to allergic reactions, the number of booster injections should be reduced [172].

Pertussis vaccination

The immunizing agent is *Bordetella pertussis* killed and detoxified with heat and merthiolate or formalin. Vaccination against pertussis is usually carried out with adjuvant-containing or plain combined vaccine (diphtheria-pertussis-tetanus).

The reactivity of the vaccine is mainly attributed to the various toxic components of the bacterium, e.g., heat-susceptible and heat-resistant toxin, histamine-sensitizing factor, etc. Most probably, the complications are the result of the cumulative effect of direct toxicity and allergic components. The participation of allergic factors is indicated by the following observations. (*i*) A painful indurated erythema may appear at the site of the injection, already on the first vaccination. It has been encountered more frequently in old persons and in subjects who have already been vaccinated several times [29]. (*ii*) In subjects vaccinated against pertussis immediate-type skin reaction, can be elicited by purified agglutinin [64]. (*iii*) After booster injections, occasional angioedema, anaphylactic shock and asthmatic attack were reported [90], and the frequency of urticaria was found to be closely related to the number of previous vaccinations [92]. (*iv*) In experiments on mice and rats a significant correlation was demonstrated between the histamine sensitizing factor of *B. pertussis* and the anaphylactic tendency of the animal. The pertussis vaccine has been shown to cause partial blockade of the adenyl-cyclase of β-adrenergic receptors, accounting for the occasional occurrence of anaphylactic shock and bronchospasm even after introduction of small doses of antigen [127].

It has also been reported that pertussis vaccination may evoke, within a few minutes, but not later than after 24 h, severe, sometimes fatal, shock [47, 65, 222]. Since shock may even occur after the first injection, it seems attributable to both primary sensitization to *B. pertussis* and the direct toxic effect of the vaccine.

A serious complication of pertussis vaccination is encephalopathy the main symptoms of which are convulsions. They appear usually within a few minutes — but not more than 3 days — after vaccination. The complication may disappear leaving no apparent residue although, in some instances, severe irreversible damages to the CNS have been noted. The frequency of this complication shows a geographical variation and depends on the kind of the vaccine; the highest incidence was recorded in Sweden, 1 : 50,000 [153]. For other countries, e.g. the Netherlands, the corresponding figures are much lower [91]. In the majority of cases it seems to be the result of direct toxic effects of the vaccine, since it occurs the most frequently after the first injection [52b]. Its pathogenesis is not uniform and allergic components may, although rarely, be involved. This is demonstrated by the case of a child who was immunized actively while he was ill with pertussis, and developed encephalitis two weeks later. After each subsequent pertussis vaccination, his encephalitis invariably recurred but with gradually shortened incubations; finally, after an intracutaneous test performed with pertussis vaccine the child developed severe palsy and soon died [118].

Demyelinating encephalitis has also been observed after pertussis vaccination [222].

Typhoid, paratyphoid fever and cholera vaccination

Immunization is performed with plain or adjuvated complete bacterial suspensions or extract vaccines. Unfortunately, attempts to separate the protective components from the toxic ones have not been successful, and the allergizing effect seems to be closely related to the latter components [160].

The side-effects are dose dependent, nevertheless, the method of preparation and the adjuvant may also be of significance [116]. They are due to a complex effect of direct toxic impacts and allergic factors. Vaccination may be followed by local and systemic reactions lasting for 1 to 3 days, e.g. painful erythematous induration, fever, malaise, headache and vomiting. In the case of typhoid and parathyphoid vaccinations these reactions seem to be due predominantly to the direct toxic effects of the vaccine; this is indicated by the fact that complications have been observed more frequently after the first than after the second injection [8, 98, 117].

In similar side-effects following cholera vaccinations allergic components seem to play a more important part, for the complications tend to occur more frequently and are more serious in older subjects and in patients with repeated vaccinations in their history. Such persons are also more likely to develop delayed-type vaccination reactions, characterized by the reappearance of the systemic and local reactions 4 to 6 days after the disappearance of the normal primary reaction [11]. Previously, nervous system complications of typhoid fever and TABT vaccinations were published [248]; now it seems that these must have been due to the impurity of the vaccine. A recent WHO report on 800,000 vaccinations failed to disclose such side-effects [117].

REFERENCES

1. Abdussalam, M. and Bögel, K.: *Pan Amer. Health Org. WHO (Wash.)* **266**, 54 (1971).
2. Adams, J. M., Baird, C. and Filloy, L.: *J. Amer. med. Ass.* **195**, 290 (1966).
3. Angle, R. M. and Santa-Fe, N. M.: *J. Amer. med. Ass.* **177**, 650 (1961).
4. Appelbaum, E., Dolgopol, V. B. and Dolgin, J.: *Amer. J. Dis. Child.* **77**, 25 (1949).
5. Appelbaum, E., Greenberg, M. and Nelson, J.: *J. Amer. med. Ass.* **151**, 188 (1953).
6. Appelbaum, E., Rachelson, H. M. and Dolgopol, V. B.: *Amer. J. Med.* **15**, 223 (1953).
7. Arand, S. C., Itkin, I. H. and Kond, L. S.: *J. Allergy* **42**, 187 (1968).
8. Ashcroft, M. T., Morrison, J. R. and Nicholson, C. C.: *Amer. J. Hyg.* **79**, 196 (1964).
9. Behan, P. O. and Geschwind, N.: *Lancet* ii 1009 (1968).
10. Bekhlemishev, N. D.: In *Die Bruzellose des Menschen*. Ed. by Parnas, J., Krüger W. and Töppich, E. VEB Verlag, Berlin 1966, p. 297.
11. Benenson, A. S., Joseph, P. R. and Oseasohn, R. O.: *Bull. Wld. Hlth. Org.* **38**, 347 (1968).
12. Bengtsson, E. and Örndahl, J.: *Acta med. scand.* **149**, 381 (1954).
13. Berge, T. O., Gleiser, C. A., Gochenour, W. S., Miesse, M. L. and Tigert, W. D.: *J. Immunol.* **87**, 509 (1961).
14. Blair, A. W., Jamieson, W. M. and Smith, G. M.: *Brit. Med. J.* **2**, 981 (1965).
14a. Bonin, O., Schmidt, I. and Ehrengut, W.: *J. Biol. Stand.* **1**, 187 (1973).
15. Bradstreet, C. M. P., Tannahill, A. J., Pollock, T. M. and Mogford, H. E.: *Lancet* ii, 6531 (1970).
16. Breese, B. B. and Disney, F. A.: *New Engl. J. Med.* **259**, 57 (1958).
17. Brockman, H., Brill, J. and Frendzell, J.: *Klin. Wschr.* **16**, 502 (1937).
18. Brody, M. and Sorley, R. G.: *N. Y. St. J. Med.* **47**, 1016 (1947).
19. Brunel, P. A., Brickman, A., O'Hare, D. and Steinberg, G.: *New Engl. J. Med.* **279**, 1357 (1968).
20. Budai, J., Farkas, E., Nyerges, G. and Csapó, J.: *Acta paediat. Acad. Sci. hung.* **4**, 411 (1963).
21. Burnet, E.: *C. R. Acad. Sci.* **174**, 421 (1922).
21a. Burnet, F. M.: *Lancet* ii, 610 (1968).
22. Buser, F.: *New Engl. J. Med.* **277**, 250 (1967).
23. Castleman, B.: *New Engl. J. Med.* **276**, 47 (1967).
24. Catanzaro, F. J., Rammelkamp, C. H. and Chamowitz, R.: *New Engl. J. Med.* **259**, 51 (1958).
25. Catanzaro, F. J., Stetson, C. A., Morris, A. J., Chamotitz, R., Rammelkamp, C. H., Stolzer, B. L. and Perr, W. D.: *Amer. J. Med.* **17**, 749 (1954).
26a. Cavelti, P.: *Proc. Soc. Exp. Biol. (N. Y.)* **60**, 639 (1945).
26b. id., *Arch. Path.* **44**, 1 (1947).
26c. id., *Schweiz. med. Wschr.* **78**, 83 (1948).
27a. Christ, P.: *Z. Rheumaforsch.* **12**, 141 (1953).
27b. id., *Ergebn. inn. Med. Kinderheilk.* **11**, 379 (1959).
28a. Coburn, A. F. and Pauly, R. H.: *J. exp. Med.* **56**, 609 (1932).
28b. ibid., **56**, 651 (1932).
29. Cockburn, W. H.: *Bull. Wld. Hlth. Org.* **19**, 109 (1958).
30. Cole, G. A., Nathanson, N. and Gilden, J.: *Fed. Proc.* **30**, 1831 (1971).
31. Collins, D. N., Weigand, H. and Hotchins, J.: *J. Immunol.* **87**, 682 (1961).
32. Conolly, J. H., Haire, M. and Hadden, D.: *Brit. med. J.* **1**, 23 (1971).
33. Cooke, J. V.: *Amer. J. Dis. Child.* **34**, 969 (1927).
34. Cooper, N. R. and Fogel, B.: *J. Pediat.* **70**, 982 (1967).
35. Cowdrey, S. C.: *New Engl. J. Med.* **274**, 1311 (1966).
36. Cuppari, G., Quagliota, F., Ieri, A. and Taranta, A.: *J. Lab. clin. Med.* **80**, 165 (1972).
37. Czoniczer, G.: In *Allergie und Allergische Erkrankungen*. Vol. II. Ed. by Rajka, E. Akadémiai Kiadó, Budapest 1959, p. 741.
38a. Daniels, W. B. and McMurray, F. G.: *J. Amer. med. Ass.* **154**, 1247 (1954).
38b. id., *Ann. intern. Med.* **37**, 697 (1955).

30

39. Davies, A. M., Laufer, A., Gery, I. and Rosenmann, E.: *Arch. Path.* **78**, 369 (1964).
40. Debré, R., Bonnet, H. and Broca, R.: *C. R. Soc. Biol.* **89**, 70 (1923).
41. Debré, R. and Lob, J. C.: *Acta paediat. scand.* **43**, Suppl. 96, 1 (1954).
42. Denny, F. W. and Wannamaker, L. W.: *J. Amer. med. Ass.* **143**, 151 (1950).
43. Detels, R., Brody, J. A., McNew, J. and Edgar, A.: *Lancet* **ii**, 11 (1973).
44. de Vries, E.: *Postvaccinal Perivenous Encephalitis.* Elsevier, Amsterdam 1966.
45. Dick, G.: *Brit. med. J.* **3**, 359 (1973).
46. Dick, G. F. and Dick, G. H.: *J. Amer. med. Ass.* **82**, 265 (1924).
47. Dick, G. W. A.: *Symp. Series in Immunbiol. Standard.* Karger, Basel **7**, 2 (1967).
48. Dixon, J. A.: *Smallpox.* Churchill, London 1962, p. 96.
49. Dóbiás, Gy., Balló, T., Bertalan, T. and Loránt, O.: *Magy. Belorv. Arch.* **18**, 313 (1965).
50. Editorial: *Brit. med. J.* **2**, 64 (1966).
51. Edsall, G., Elliot, M. W., Peebles, Th. C., Levine, L. and Eldred, M. C.: *J. Amer. med. Ass.* **202**, 1719 (1967).
52a. Ehrengut, W.: *Impffibel*, Schattauer, Stuttgart 1964, p. 134.
52b. id., *Mschr. Kinderheilk.* **117**, 77 (1969).
52c. id., Dtsch. med. Wschr. **98**, 517 (1973).
53. Encephalitis Surveillance, 1965: *Annual Summary, Communicable Disease Center*, U.S.A. Dept. of Health and Welfare. Washington 1966.
54. Enders, J. F., Kane, L. W., Maris, E. P. and Stokes, J.: *J. exp. Med.* **84**, 341 (1946).
55. Enders, J. F., McCarthy, K., Mitus, A. and Cheatham, W. J.: *New Engl. J. Med.* **261**, 875 (1959).
56. Enders, J. F. and Peebles, T. C.: *Proc. Soc. exp. Biol. (N.Y.)* **86**, 277 (1954).
57. Erdős, L.: Personal communication (1967).
57a. Erdős, L., Láng, Cs., Jaszovszky, I. and Nyerges, G.: *J. biol. Stand.* **3**, 77 (1975).
58. Faragó, F.: *Diphtheria, scarlatina és pertussis védőoltás.* (Vaccination against Diphteria, Scarlet fever and Pertussis.) Magyar Orvosi Könyvkiadó Társulat, Budapest 1947, p. 68.
59. Fenner, F.: *The Biology of Animal Viruses.* Vol. II. Academic Press, New York 1968, p. 503.
60. Finlay, K. H.: *Arch. Neurol. Psychiat. (Chic.)* **39**, 1047 (1938).
61. Fireman, P., Friday, G. and Kumate, J.: *Pediatrics* **43**, 264 (1969).
62. Fleischner, E. C. and Meyer, K. F.: *Amer. J. Dis. Child.* **16**, 268 (1918).
63. Flick, J. A. and Pincus, W. B.: *J. exp. Med.* **117**, 633 (1963).
64. Flosdorf, E. W., Felton, H. M., Bondi, A. and McGuiness, A. C.: *Amer. J. med. Sci.* **206**, 422 (1943).
65. Forrester, R. M.: *Brit. med. J.* **2**, 232 (1965).
66. Foshay, L. and Mayer, O. B.: *J. Amer. med. Ass.* **106**, 2141 (1936).
67. Francis, T., Korns, R. F., Voight, R. B., Boisen, M., Hemphill, F. M., Napier, J. A. and Tolchinski, E.: *Amer. J. publ. Hlth.* **45**, Appendix (May) (1955).
68. Freedman, S. O.: In *Clinical Immunology.* Ed. by Freedman, S. O. Harper and Row, New York 1971, p. 569.
69. Friedman, R. M. and Baron, S.: *J. Immunol.* **87**, 379 (1961).
70. Friedman, R. M., Baron, S., Buckler, C. E. and Steinmüller, R. I.: *J. exp. Med.* **116**, 347 (1962).
71. Fuenzalida, E., Palacios, R. and Borgono, M.: *Symp. Series in Immunobiol. Standard*, Karger, Basel **1** (1966).
72. Fulginiti, V. A., Arthur, J. H., Pearlman, D. S. and Kempe, C. H.: *Amer. J. Dis. Child.* **115**, 671 (1968).
73. Fulginiti, V. A., Eller, J. J., Downie, A. W. and Kempe, C. H.: *J. Amer. med. Ass.* **202**, 1075 (1967).
74. Gazenfeld, E., Rosenmann, E., Davies, A. M. and Laufer, A.: *Immunology* **10**, 193 (1966).
75. Gianelli, F.: *G. Mal. infett. parass.* **20**, 170 (1968).
76. Gibbs, F. A., Gibbs, E. L., Carpenter, P. R. and Spies, H. W.: *J. Amer. med. Ass.* **171**, 1050 (1959).
77. Gibel, H., Kramer, B. and Naji, A. F.: *Amer. J. Dis. Child.* **99**, 669 (1960).
78. Glanzmann, E.: *Schweiz. med. Wschr.* **57**, 145 (1927).

79. Gleiser, C. A., Gochenour, W. S., Berge, T. O. and Tigert, W. D.: *J. Immunol.* **87,** 504 (1961).
80. Glynn, L. E.: In *Clinical Aspects of Immunology.* 2nd ed. Ed. by Gell, P. G. H. and Coombs, R. R. A. Blackwell, Oxford 1968, p. 831.
81. Goldstein, J., Halpern, B. and Robert, L.: *Nature* **213,** 44 (1967).
82. Good, R. A., Bridges, R. A. and Condig, R. M.: *Bact. Rev.* **24,** 115 (1960).
83. Goodpasture, E. W.: *Amer. J. Path.* **13,** 175 (1937).
84. Goodpasture, E. W. and Anderson, K.: *Amer. J. Path.* **13,** 149 (1937).
85. Grimble, J. and Lessof, M. A.: *Brit. med. J.* **2,** 263 (1965).
86a. Groer, F.: *Klin. Wschr.* **6,** 97 (1927).
86b. ibid., **8,** 774 (1929).
87. Grunke, W.: *Klinik der einheimischen Infektionskrankheiten.* VEB Thieme, Leipzig 1956, p. 559.
88. Haas, V. H., Stewart, S. E. and Briggs, G. M.: *Virology* **3,** 12 (1957).
89. Halbert, S. P., Brichen, P. and Dahle, E.: *J. exp. Med.* **113,** 759 (1961).
90. Halpern, S. R. and Halpern, D.: *J. Pediat.* **47,** 60 (1955).
91. Hannik, Ch. A.: *Symp. Series in Immunobiol.Standard.* Karger, Basel **13,** 161 (1970).
92. Hansen, F.: In *Schutzimpfungen,* Ed. by Spiess, H. VEB Thieme, Leipzig 1966, p. 63.
93a. Harris, H. J.: *Brucellosis (Undulant Fever) Clinical and Subclinical.* Hoeber, New York 1950, p. 98.
93b. ibid., p. 341.
94. Harris, R. W., Isacson, P. and Karzon, D. T.: *J. Pediat.* **74,** 552 (1969).
95. Hashem, N. and Barr, L. M.: *Lancet* ii, 1029 (1963).
96. Hawkins, D.: In *Clinical Immunology.* Ed. by Freedman, S. O. Harper and Row, New York 1971, p. 185.
97. Heilman, J.: *J. exp. Med.* **107,** 319 (1958).
98. Hejfec, L. B., Salmin, L. W., Leitman, M. Z., Kuzmunova, M. L., Vasileva, A. V. and Levina, L. A.: *Bull. Wld. Hlth. Org.* **34,** 321 (1966).
99. Henderson, K.: *Lancet* i, 518 (1971).
100. Henle, G., Henle, W., Burgon, J. S., Bashe, W. J. and Stokes, J.: *J. Immunol.* **66,** 535 (1950).
101. Hennessen, W. and Mauler, R.: *Lancet* i, 902 (1967).
102. Henry, K.: *Clin. exp. Immunol.* **3,** 509 (1968).
103. Herbert, W. J. and Wilkinson, P. C. (Eds): *A Dictionary of Immunology.* Blackwell, Oxford 1971.
104. Herrlich, A.: *Münch. Med. Wschr.* **94,** 2371 (1952).
105. Herrlich, A., Ehrengut, W. und Schleussing, H.: In *Handbuch der Schutzimpfungen.* Ed. by Herrlich, A. Springer, Berlin 1965, p. 212.
106. Hillemand, J.: *Presse méd.* **71,** 2143 (1963).
107. Holliday, B. P.: *J. Pediat.* **36,** 185 (1950).
108. Horta-Barboza, L., Krebs, H., Ley, A., Chen Ta-Chuan: *Pediatrics* **47,** 782 (1971).
109a. Höring, F. O.: *Acta allerg.* **6,** Suppl. 3, 158 (1953).
109b. id., *Berl. med. Rundsch.* **12,** 42 (1961).
109c. id., In *Infektionskrankheiten.* Vol. II. Ed. by Gsell, O. and Mohr, W. Springer, Berlin 1968, p. 555.
110a. Huddleson, I. F.: *Brucellosis in Man and Animals.* Commonwealth Found. New York 1939, p. 120.
110b. id., *Amer. J. publ. Hlth.* **30,** 944 (1940).
111. James, G. W. A., Longshore, J. and Hendry, J. L.: *Amer. J. Hyg.* **53,** 178 (1954).
112. Janneway, C.: *J. Pediat.* **72,** 885 (1968).
113. Janneway, C. A., Moll, G. H., Armstrong, S. H., Wallace, W. M., Hallman, N. and Barness, L. A.: *Trans. Ass. Amer. Physiol.* **61,** 108 (1948).
114. Jervis, G. A.: *Bull. Wld. Hlth. Org.* **10,** 837 (1954).
115. Jirovec, O.: *Zbl. Bakt. I Abt. Orig.* **168,** 591 (1957).
116. Joó, I.: *Pan Amer. Health Org. (Wash.)* **226,** 329 (1971).
117. Yougoslav Typhoid Commission: *Bull. Wld. Hlth. Org.* **30,** 623 (1964).
118. Kadowski, J. I., Nihira, M. and Nakao, T.: *Pediatrics* **45,** 508 (1970).
119. Kamin, P. B., Fein, B. T. and Britton, H. A.: *J. Amer. med. Ass.* **193,** 1125 (1965).
120a. Kaplan, M. H.: *N. Y. Acad. Sci.* **86,** 974 (1960).

120b. id., *J. Immunol.* **90**, 595 (1963).
120c. id., *Progr. Allergy* **13**, 408 (1969).
121. Kaplan, M. H. and Craig, J. M.: *J. Immunol.* **90**, 725 (1963).
122. Kaplan, M. H. and Dallenbach, F. D.: *J. exp. Med.* **113**, 1 (1961).
123. Kaplan, M. H. and Frengley, J. D.: *Amer. J. Cardiol.* **24**, 459 (1969).
124. Kaplan, M. H. and Meyeserian, M.: *Lancet* **i**, 706 (1962).
125. Kaplan, M. H., Meyeserian, M. and Kushner, I.: *J. exp. Med.* **113**, 17 (1961).
126. Kaplan, M. H. and Rakita, L.: In *Immunological Diseases*. 2nd ed. Vol. II. Ed. by
     Samter, M. Little-Brown, Boston 1971, p. 1367.
127. Keller, K. F. and Fishel, C. W.: *J. Bact.* **94**, 804 (1967).
128. Kempe, H.: *Pediatrics* **26**, 169 (1960).
129. Kennedy, C. and Wanglee, P.: *Pediat. Clin. N. Amer.* **14**, 809 (1967).
129a. Kiczka, W., Szkaradkiewicz, A. and Kryska, A.: *VIth International Congress
     of Infectious and Parasitic Diseases. Warszawa* 1974, p. 216.
130. Kissling, R. E. and Reese, D. R.: *J. Immunol.* **91**, 362 (1963).
131. Klein, P.: *Verh. dtsch. Ges. Kreisl.-Forsch.* **20**, 176 (1954).
131a. Kleinmann, P. K. and Weksler, M. E.: *J. Pediat.* **83**, 827 (1973).
132a. Koprowski, H.: *Amer. J. Dis. Child.* **103**, 273 (1962).
132b. id., In *Rabies*. Ed. by Nagano, Y. and Davenport, F. M. University Tokyo 1971,
     p. 111.
133. Kovács, F., Baranyai, E., Tóth, L., Lénárt, J., Molnár, L. and Vukmirovits, Gy.:
     Orv. Hetil. **111**, 369 (1970).
134. Kovács, F., Dudás, P. and Kovács, K.: *Gyermekgyógyászat* **19**, 518 (1968).
135. Kovács, F., Vidor, É. and Bodor, Gy.: *Orv. Hetil.* **109**, 2264 (1968).
136. Köttgen, V.: In *Handbuch der Kinderheilkunde*. Ed. by Opitz, H. and Schmidt,
     F. Springer, Berlin 1966, p. 156.
136a. Kumar, R., Malaviya, A. E., Murthy, R. G. S., Venkatarman, M. and Moha-
     patra, L. N.: *Infection and Immunity* **10**, 1219 (1974).
137. Küpper, K., Langer, E. and Klei, P.: *Virchows Arch. path. Anat.* **334**, 342 (1961).
138. Lackman, D. B., Bell, E. J., Bell, J. F. and Pickens, E. G.: *Amer. J. publ. Hlth.*
     52, 87 (1962).
139. Lane, J. M., Ruben, F. L., Neff, J. M. and Millar, J. D.: *New Engl. J. Med.* **281**,
     1201 (1969).
140. Larson, C. L.: *Publ. Hlth. Rep.* **60**, 725 (1945).
141. Lawrence, H. S.: *J. Immunol.* **68**, 159 (1952).
142. Lennon, R. G. and Isacson, P.: *J. Pediat.* **71**, 525 (1967).
143. Lennon, R. G., Isacson, P., Rosales, T., Elsea, W. R. and Karzon, D. G.: *J.
     Amer. med. Ass.* **200**, 275 (1967).
144a. Lerner, A. M., Klein, J. O., Cherry, J. D. and Finland, M.: *New Engl. J. Med.*
     269, 678 (1963).
144b. ibid, **269**, 736 (1963).
145. Levine, L.: *Amer. J. Hyg.* **73**, 20 (1961).
146. Levy, H. B. and Haas, V. B.: *Virology* **5**, 401 (1958).
147. Lipton, M. M., Steigman, A. J. and Dizon, F. C.: *J. infect. Dis.* **115**, 356 (1965).
147a. Lisak, R. P., Behan, P. O., Zweiman, B. and Shetty, T.: *Neurology* **24**, 560 (1974).
148. Lischner, H. W., Sherma, M. K., Grover, W. D.: *New Engl. J. Med.* **286**, 786
     (1972).
149a. Ljung, O.: *Acta med. scand.* **160**, 135 (1958).
149b. ibid., **163**, 243 (1959).
150. Lorenz, E. and Rossipal, E.: *Mschr. Kinderheilk.* **113**, 161 (1965).
151. Lorenz, K. and Geidel, H.: *Z. Rheumaforsch.* **25**, 335 (1966).
152. Lundstedt, C.: *Acta path. microbiol. Scand.* **75**, 139 (1969).
153. Malmgren, B., Vahlquist, B. and Zeiterström, R.: *Brit. med. J.* **2**, 180 (1960).
153a. Mann, P. G. and Richens, E.: *J. clin. Path.* **26**, 386 (1973).
154. Markos, Gy., Nagy, G. and Szathmáry, J.: *Orv. Hetil.* **111**, 2544 (1970).
155. Marth, H.: *Berl. Med.* **8**, 542 (1957).
156. Massel, F. B., Honikman, L. H. and Amezova, J.: *J. Amer. med. Ass.* **207**, 1115
     (1969).
157. Mayer, J. B.: In *Infektionskrankheiten*. Vol. I. Ed. by Gsell, O. and Mohr, W.
     Springer, Berlin 1968, p. 454.

158. McFarland, R. B.: *New Engl. J. Med.* **258**, 1277 (1958).
159. McNair Scott, P. F. and Bonnano, D. E.: *New Engl. J. Med.* **277**, 248 (1967).
160. Melikova, E. N. and Lesnjak, S. V.: *Bull. Wld. Hlth. Org.* **40**, 395 (1969).
161. Meulen, V. Ter., Katz, M. and Müller, D.: *Current Topics in Microbiol. Immunol.* **57**, 1 (1972).
162. Miller, H. G., Stanton, J. B. and Gibbons, J. L.: *Quart. J. Med.* **25**, 427 (1956).
163. Mims, C. A.: *Bact. Rev.* **30**, 739 (1967).
164. Mims, C. A. and Tosolini, F. A.: *Brit. J. exp. Path.* **50**, 584 (1969).
165. Mollaret, P., Reilly, J., Bastin, R. and Tournier, P.: *Presse méd.* **59**, 681 (1951).
166. Murphy, S. E.: *Medicine* **39**, 619 (1960).
167. Murphy, S. E. and Swift, H. F.: *J. exp. Med.* **89**, 687 (1949).
168. Nader, P. R., Horwitz, M. S. and Rousseau, J.: *J. Pediat.* **72**, 22 (1968).
169. Nanning, W.: *Bull. Wld. Hlth. Org.* **27**, 317 (1962).
170. Neff, J. M., Lane, J. M., Pert, J. H., Moore, R., Millar, J. D. and Henderson, D. A.: *New Engl. J. Med.* **276**, 1 (1967).
171. Nelson, J. D., Sandusky, G. and Peck, F. B.: *J. Amer. med. Ass.* **198**, 653 (1966).
172. Nielsen, P. A., Ablodi, F. B., Querry, M. V., Gussoni, C. and Cooper, M. S.: *J. Immunol.* **98**, 1248 (1967).
173. Niggemeyer, H.: *Dtsch. med. Wschr.* **87**, 95 (1962).
174a. Nyerges, G.: *Pédiatrie (Lyon)* **23**, 405 (1968).
174b. id., *Gyermekgyógyászat* **20**, 44 (1969).
174c. Nyerges, G., Garami, E. and Kukán, E.: *Acta paed. Acad. Sci. hung.* **16**, 111 (1975).
174d. Nyerges, G. and Káli, G.: *Acta paed. Acad. Sci. hung.* **16**, 225 (1975).
174e. Nyerges, G., Nyerges, Gy., Molnár, L. and Kovács, F.: *Acta allergol.* **29**, 433 (1974).
175. Nyerges, G., Nyerges, G., Surján, M., Budai, J. and Csapó, J.: *Acta paediat. Acad. Sci. hung.* **4**, 399 (1963).
175a. Nyerges, G. and Telegdy, L.: *Infection* **3**, 213 (1975).
176. Olderhausen, H. F.: In *Injektionskrankheiten*. Vol. II. Ed. by Gsell, O. and Mohr, W. Springer, Berlin 1968, p. 500.
177a. Oldstone, M. B. A. and Dixon, F. J.: *J. exp. Med.* **129**, 483 (1969).
177b. id., In *Immunopathology. VIth International Symposium*, Ed. by Miescher, P. A, Schwabe, Basel 1970, p. 391.
177c. id., *Virology* **42**, 805 (1970).
177d. id., *J. exp. Med.* **131**, 1 (1970).
178. O'Meara, R. A. Q.: *Mschr. Kinderheilk.* **98**, 57 (1950).
179. Osváth, P., Cseh, Gy. and Simon, L.: *Arch. Kinderheilk.* **166**, 152 (1962).
180. Pampiglione, G.: *Brit. msd. J.* **2**, 1296 (1964).
181. Pappenheimer, A. M., Edsall, G., Lawrence, H. S. and Bandon, H. J.: *Amer. J. Hyg.* **52**, 353 (1950).
182. Pappenheimer, A. M. and Lawrence, H. S.: *Amer. J. Hyg.* **47**, 233 (1948).
183. Parish, H. J. and Cannon, D. A.: *Antisera, Toxoid, Vaccines and Tuberculins in Prophylaxis and Treatment*. Livingstone, Edinburgh 1962, p. 104.
184. Parnas, J., Krüger, W. and Töppich, E.: *Die Bruzellose des Menschen*. VEB Verlag, Berlin 1966, p. 127.
185. Parrot, R. H., Kim, H. W., Arrobio, J. O., Canchola, J. G., Brandt, C. D., DeMeio, J. L., Jensen, K. E. and Chanock, R. M.: *Pan Amer. Hlth. Org.* WHO, New York 1967, p. 35.
186a. Pavlák, R.: *Z. ges. inn. Med.* **17**, 305 (1962).
186b. id., *Z. ges. Hyg.* **13**, 533 (1967).
187. Petermann, M. G.: *J. Pediat.* **44**, 563 (1954).
188. Pette, E.: *Die akut entzündlichen Erkrankungen des Rückenmarks*. Thieme, Leipzig 1942, p. 426.
189. Philip, R. N., Casper, E. A. and Lackman, D. B.: *J. infect. Dis.* **117**, 393 (1967).
190. Philip, R. N., Huntley, B., Lackman, D. B. and Comstock, C. W.: *J. infect. Dis.* **110**, 220 (1962).
191. Pincus, W. B. and Flick, J. A.: *J. infect. Dis.* **113**, 13 (1963).
192a. Pirquet, Cl. v.: *Dtsche. med. Wschr.* **33**, 1908 (1927).
192b. id., *Arch. intern. Med.* **7**, 259 (1911).

192c. ibid., **7**, 383 (1911).
192d. id., *Z. Kinderheilk.* **6**, 1 (1913).
193. Plotkin, S. A. and Clark, H. F.: *J. infect. Dis.* **123**, 227 (1971).
194. Preisich, C.: *Orv. Hetil.* **48**, 849 (1907).
195. Rammelkamp, C. H.: *Circulation* **17**, 842 (1958).
196. Rammelkamp, C. H., Denny, F. W. and Wannamaker, L. W.: *Rheumatic Fever.* Thomas, Minneapolis 1952, p. 72.
197. Regamey, R. H.: *Ergebn. Mikrobiol.* **32**, 270 (1959).
198. Regamey, R. H. and Paccaud, M. F.: In *Infektionskrankheiten.* Vol. I. Ed. by Gsell, O. and Mohr, W. Springer, Berlin 1968, p. 1061.
199a. Reiter, H.: *Dtsch. med. Wschr.* **41**, 1535 (1916).
199b. ibid., **82**, 1336 (1957).
200. Reitz, B. A., Prager, D. J. and Feigen, G. A.: *J. exp. Med.* **128**, 1401 (1969).
201. Réthy, L. and Losonczy, Gy.: *Ann. Immunol. Hung.* **2**, 65 (1959).
202. Riley, H. D.: *Amer. J. Dis. Child.* **95**, 270 (1958).
203. Robinson, W.: *Arch. Pediat.* **61**, 6 (1944).
204. Rohde, W.: *Arch. Hyg. Bact.* **149**, 547 (1965).
205. Rotbard, S., Watson, R. F., Swift, H. F. and Wilson, A. T.: *Arch. intern. Med.* **92**, 229 (1948).
206. Schick, B.: *Münch. med. Wschr.* **60**, 2608 (1913).
207. Schlüter, K.: *Arch. Kinderheilk.* **171**, 26 (1964).
208. Scholten, H.: *Z. klin. Med.* **193**, 640 (1944).
209. Seckel, H. P. G,: *Jb. Kinderheilk.* **145**/9, 7 (1935).
210. Seitelberger, F. and Zischinsky, H.: *Münch. med. Wschr.* **104**, 1681 (1962).
211. Sergiev, P. G., Ryarantseva, N. E. and Shroit, I. G.: *Acta. virol.* **4**, 265 (1960).
212. Sherman, F. E., Michael, R. H. and Kenny, F. M.: *J. Amer. med. Ass.* **192**, 675 (1965).
213. Siegel, A. C., Johnson, E. E. and Stollermann, G. H.: *New. Engl. J. Med.* **265**, 559 (1961).
214. Silver, H. K., Kempe, C. H. and Bruyn, H. B.: *Handbook of Pediatrics*, Lange, Los Altos 1967, p. 102.
215. Smith, J. G. W.: *Brit. med. Bull.* **25**, 177 (1969).
216. Smithwick, E. M. and Berkovich, S.: *Proc. Soc. exp. Biol.* (*N. Y.*) **123**, 276 (1966).
217. Spagnuolo, M., Pasternack, B. and Taranta, A.: *New Engl. J. Med.* **285**, 641 (1971).
217a. Spiess, H.: *Dtsch. med. Wschr.* **98**, 517 (1973).
218. Spink, W. W.: *Lancet* ii, 161 (1964).
219. Steffen, C.: *Acta. neuroveg.* **15**, 154 (1957).
219a. Staak, M. and Wirth, E.: *Dtsch. med. Wschr.* **98**, 110 (1973).
220. Steigmann, A. J.: *J. Pediat.* **72**, 753 (1968).
221. Stetson, C. A.: In *Streptococcus Infection.* Ed. by McCarty, M. Columbia University Press, New York 1954, p. 208.
222. Ström, J.: *Brit. med. J.* **2**, 1184 (1960).
223. Surgina, D. W. R., Bank, L. J. and Ackerman, A. B.: *New Engl. J. Med.* **283**, 1139 (1970).
224. Surján, M. and Nyerges, G.: *Z. Immun.-Forsch.* **124**, 401 (1962).
225. Swift, H. F., Wilson, M. G. and Todd, E. W.: *Amer. J. Dis. Child.* **37**, 98 (1929).
226. Székely, Á.: *Acta pediat. Acad. Sci. hung.* **12**, 173 (1971).
227. Szontagh, P.: *Jb. Kinderheilk.* **76**, 654 (1912).
228. Tagg, J. R.: Ph. D. thesis. Monash Univ. Melbourne (1972).
229. Tagg, J. R. and McGiven, A. R.: *Lancet* ii, 686 (1972).
230. Thalhammer, O.: *Neue Öst. Kinderheilk.* **3**, 57 (1958).
231. Torres, C. M.: cited by Allison, A. C.: *Brit. med. Bull.* **23**, 60 (1967).
232. Tyler, H. R.: *Medicine* **36**, 147 (1957).
233. van Bogaert, L.: *Rev. Neurology* **1**, 150 (1933).
234. van Ramshorst, J. D. and Ehrengut, D.: In *Handbuch der Schutzimpfungen.* Ed. by Herrlich, A. Springer, Berlin 1965, p. 394.
235. Vincens, C. N., Nobrega, F. T., Joseph, J. M. and Meyer, M. B.: *Amer. J. Epidemiol.* **84**, 371 (1966).

236. Vivona, S., Lowenthal, J. P., Berman, S., Benenson, A. S. and Smadel, J. E.: *Amer. J. Hyg.* **79**, 143 (1964).
237. Volkert, M. and Lundstedt, C.: In *Immunopathology. VI. International Symposium.* Ed. by Miescher, P. A. Schwabe, Basel 1970, p. 399.
238a. Vorlaender, K. O.: *Klin. Wschr.* **31**, 748 (1953).
238b. id., In *Immunpathologie in Klinik und Forschung.* Ed. by Miescher, P. and Vorlaender, K. O. Thieme, Stuttgart 1961, p. 447.
239. Waksman, B. H.: *Int. Arch. Allergy* **14**, Suppl. 1 (1959).
240. Walter, G.: In *Infektionskrankheiten.* Vol. II. Ed. by Gsell, O. and Mohr, W. Springer, Berlin 1968, p. 692.
241. Warwick, W. J. and Good, R. A.: *Amer. J. Dis. Child.* **100**, 241 (1960).
242. Webb, H. E. and Gordon Smith, C. E.: *Brit. med. J.* **2**, 569 (1964).
243. Weisse, K., Krücke, W. and Siegert, R. Z.: *Z. Kinderheilk.* **73**, 23 (1953).
244. Wenner, H. A. and Yong Lon, T.: *Progr. med. Virol.* **5**, 219 (1963).
245. Wiessemann, C. L., Batawi, El. Y., Wood, W. H. and Noriega, L.: *J. Immunol.* **98**, 194 (1967).
246. Wilhelm, G. and Dippel, J.: *Zbl. Bakt. I. Abt. Orig.* **214**, 383 (1970).
247. Wilhelm, G. and Hassan, El, A.: *Mschr. Kinderheilk.* **115**, 324 (1967).
248. Wilson, G. S.: *The Hazards of Immunization.* Athlone, London 1967, p. 184.
249. Winbald, St., Malmros, H. and Vorlaender, O.: *Acta. med. scand.* **196**, Suppl. 533 (1947).
250. Winterhoff, D. and Gotthardt, K.: *Z. Immun.-Forsch.* **144**, 167 (1972).
251. Virus Associated Immunopathology: Animal Models and Implications for Human Disease: *Bull. Wld. Hlth. Org.* **47**, 257 (1972).
252. *Wld. Hlth. Org. techn. Rep.* Ser. No. 126. WHO, Geneva 1957.
253. *Wld. Hlth. Org. techn. Rep.* Ser. No. 321. WHO, Geneva 1966.
254. Yuceoglu, A. M., Berkovich, S. and Chin, J.: *J. Pediat.* **74**, 291 (1969).
255a. Zabriskie, J. B.: *Clin. exp. Immunol.* **7**, 147 (1970).
255b. id., *Zbl. Bakt. I. Abt. Orig.* **214**, 339 (1970).
256. Zabriskie, J. B. and Freimer, E. H.: *J. exp. Med.* **124**, 661 (1966).
257. Zeman, W. and Kolar, O.: *Neurology (Minneap.)* **18**, 1 (1968).
258. Zingher, A.: *Amer. J. Dis. Child.* **25**, 392 (1923).

CHAPTER 72

ALLERGY AND IMMUNITY IN TUBERCULOSIS

by

I. FÖLDES

Interest in the allergo-immunological phenomena of tuberculosis somewhat faltered in the fifties and early sixties of our century, which might be attributed to the spectacular achievements of chemotherapy and surgical management of this disease. More recently, however, research workers and clinicians of this field have turned with renewed interest to the developments of immunology.

BASIC PHENOMENA

It was recognized long ago that individuals with a healed focal tuberculous process (e.g. cervical lymphoma) rarely developed pulmonary tuberculosis. It was supposed that the local process induced an immunity, which protected the organism against progressive tuberculosis. Anti-tuberculous immunity became accessible for experimental investigation by the discovery of *M. tuberculosis* in 1882.

KOCH'S PHENOMENON

In 1891 Robert Koch described that the response of the organism to super-infection with *M. tuberculosis* was different from that to the primary infection. The essence of the phenomenon, now termed Koch's phenomenon, is as follows. If healthy guinea pigs are inoculated with tuberculosis subcutaneously, a small local damage develops which apparently heals in a few days. However, after 10 to 14 days an inflamed nodule appears at the site of the injection, which later penetrates the skin and thus the developing ulcer persists until the animal dies. This process is accompanied by specific inflammatory changes in the regional lymph nodes showing no healing tendency. If, however, a previously infected guinea pig is inoculated with tuberculosis in the same way, then strong infiltration develops within 1 or 2 days, which is followed by necrosis, and ulceration at the site of superinfection. The ulcer heals rapidly and regional lymph nodes do not participate in the process. Thus, Koch's phenomenon clearly shows that the reactions of the organism have been changed by the first infection. The changed reaction indicates the development of immunity (lack of spread of the process) on the one hand, and hyperergy (marked, rapidly developing infiltration) on the other.

TUBERCULIN REACTION

Another indicator of the altered reactivity in tuberculosis is the tuberculin reaction. While in healthy individuals parenteral introduction of an appropriate tuberculin dose does not cause morphologically demonstrable changes, individuals once naturally infected by, or vaccinated against, *M. tuberculosis* respond to the same tuberculin doses with local reactions, focal reactions (exacerbation of existing tuberculous foci) and general reactions (fever, malaise). Besides the tuberculin tests, diagnostical tests can be performed with killed *M. tuberculosis* or live bacteria of attenuated virulence (BCG). Since the results of these tests may not run parallel with those of the tuberculin reactions, they are used in practice scarcely, mainly in addition to the tuberculin test.

NATURAL RESISTANCE
(NATIVE IMMUNITY)

If a previously non-infected experimental animal is infected with virulent *M. tuberculosis*, the resulting reaction depends, besides the size of the inoculum also on the species. Goats and rats, e.g., are very resistant even to large doses, whereas Syrian hamsters and guinea pigs, being very susceptible, develop lethal tuberculosis even if injected with very small doses. Thus, the natural resistance against tuberculosis is an inherited, species-specific property, which, however, shows considerable individual variations and is influenced by numerous factors (see below).

ACQUIRED IMMUNITY

Koch's phenomenon as well as the changed reactivity of the organism following vaccination with BCG or other effective vaccines have shown that infection with *M. tuberculosis* is followed by the development of a certain degree of acquired immunity. This is, in contrast to natural resistance, primarily not species-specific, but characteristic of the individual.

Study of the Koch's phenomenon and of the tuberculin reaction, furthermore, experimental investigation of natural resistance (native immunity) and acquired immunity are the basic methods to explore the mechanisms of allergy and immunity in tuberculosis.

ALLERGY IN TUBERCULOSIS (DELAYED, OR TUBERCULIN-TYPE, OR CELL-MEDIATED HYPERSENSITIVITY)

TUBERCULIN REACTION

The specific sensitivity of animals and human organisms previously exposed to *M. tuberculosis* can be demonstrated by injecting tuberculin or proteins extracted from *M. tuberculosis*. The tuberculin reaction depends upon the dose and quality of tuberculin, the mode of administration, the individual characteristics and degree of sensitization of the recipient, and upon numerous other factors. To demonstrate specific sensitivity tuberculin is usually injected intradermally or the skin is exposed to tuberculoprotein patch test. The developing local reaction is characterized by circumscribed erythema and induration. The reaction needs 24, 48 or 72 h to reach its maximum. As a more severe reaction, central necrosis may develop which may occasionally be haemorrhagic. After reaching its peak, the reaction gradually fades.

Brief historical review

The local and systemic tuberculin reactions were described by Robert Koch. He proposed tuberculin as a specific therapy of tuberculosis [76]. Although clinical experience failed to fulfil Koch's therapeutic expectations, local tuberculin reaction as an index of tuberculous infection or of antituberculous immunization has remained a valuable diagnostic tool. A standard intracutaneous test technique has been developed by Mantoux [91] and a percutaneous test technique by von Pirquet [111]. Von Pirquet was the first to regard tuberculin reaction as an allergic phenomenon although unlike in other immunological reactions (anaphylaxis, Arthus phenomenon, serum sickness), humoral antibodies could not consistently be demonstrated in tuberculin sensitized animals and attempts to transfer tuberculin sensitivity with serum failed. For this reason tuberculin reaction was considered a unique immunological phenomenon, until it became evident that pneumococci [68], streptococci [149], fungi, viruses, and even purified protein can elicit a similar delayed-type reaction. At present it is reasonable to suppose that contact sensitivity [79, 80], homograft rejection [95a, b] and certain experimental auto-allergic diseases are based on immunological reactions similar to the tuberculin reaction. The tuberculin-type reaction is the most widely occurring immunological event in animal and human pathology known as cellular, or cell-mediated hypersensitivity or delayed-type allergy. In the literature of tuberculosis the term allergy indicates hypersensitivity against tuberculin.

Tuberculins

Koch's old tuberculin (OT) is prepared from 6- to 8-week-old, 5 per cent glycerol containing broth cultures of *M. tuberculosis*. The culture is boiled, then filtered and the medium is concentrated to one-tenth of its original volume. The brown liquid thus obtained is a concentrate of some components of the bacterium and of the medium, in which the active substance, tuberculin, is protein in nature [86]. Its molecular weight may vary between 8,000 and 64,000, depending on the bacterial strain, the composition of the medium and the mode of preparation. OT is a chemically poorly defined substance. It contains, in addition to protein, remnants of bacterial cells, polysaccharides, nucleic acids and components of the medium. Therefore, efforts have been made to purify the active constituent in order to achieve well-reproducible reactions. For this purpose ultrafiltration, precipitation with trichloroacetic acid and ammonium sulphate, or a combination of these has been applied, supplemented by dialysis and centrifugation.

The most widely used purified tuberculin preparations are PPD-S (purified protein derivative) produced by Seibert [122]; *gereinigtes Tuberkulin* Hoechst (GT); purified tuberculins produced by the Statens Seruminstitut (Copenhagen), marked RT; purified tuberculin produced by precipitation with trichloroacetic acid [73].

Tuberculin is usually assayed and standardized by injecting sensitized guinea pigs intradermally. This assay, being a biological one, has many sources of error [59]. The amount of tuberculin is expressed in tuberculin units (TU). In general 1 TU PPD-S contains 0.00002 mg protein.

Tuberculins (generally called sensitins) can be obtained not only from *M. tuberculosis* or *M. bovis*, but also from other mycobacterial species.

Tuberculin tests

Tuberculin reaction can be elicited in many, though not all, organs and tissues of the sensitized organism. However, its intensity is not identical, even if the same tuberculin dose is administered; it depends, besides the grade of sensitization, on many other factors, such as blood, lymph and nervous supply, absorption properties, tissue characteristics, etc. In practice, the intracutaneous test is applied most frequently. The tuberculin tests most widely used are as follows:

Mantoux test. Intracutaneous injection of 0.1 ml diluted tuberculin until a small bleb is raised in the skin. The advantage of the intracutaneous injection is that the amount of the introduced tuberculin can be measured with sufficient accuracy and the result can be expressed quantitatively (in mm).

Von Pirquet's test. Tuberculin is dripped to the cleansed skin, which is then scarified through the drop, without causing bleeding. The test is technically simple, but the amount of tuberculin introduced cannot be measured.

Trambusti's reaction. Essentially, this is a percutaneous prick test. The skin is punctured with the injection needle through a drop of tuberculin.

Multiple-puncture test (Heaf). Several prick tests can be accomplished simultaneously with an automatic multiple-puncture apparatus. This has 6 needles which penetrate the skin to a depth of 2–3 mm.

Ointment and patch tests. (Moro's inunction test, Vollmer's patch test, etc.) These are carried out by the inunction of an ointment containing tuberculin into the skin and by using tuberculin impregnated gauze, respectively. The advantage of these tests is that they can be carried out in masses. However, the amount of the introduced tuberculin cannot be measured.

Ophthalmo-reaction (Calmette). Diluted tuberculin is dropped into the conjunctival sac of one eye. In case of a positive reaction conjunctivitis develops. Since the reaction may induce exacerbation of latent eye disease, it must not be applied except under very strict indication.

Local, focal and general reactions

At the site of tuberculin injection, as mentioned above, a local reaction develops (see p. 39). In addition to this, particularly in case of intravenous administration, focal and systemic reactions may develop.

Focal reaction means an exacerbation of active tuberculous foci or fresh skin tests, i.e. inflammatory vasodilation, oedema, and haemorrhage in these areas [76, 136]. A similar reaction occurs if tuberculin is given locally into tuberculous foci. The exact mechanism of the focal reaction is not known. It might correspond to a local Shwartzman reaction [128].

The so-called re-test reaction may also be related to the focal reactions. Von Pirquet observed that at the site of a primary tuberculin reaction re-testing might strongly accelerate the development of the allergic reaction. It was shown by crossed re-testing of two protein antigens in guinea pigs that the accelerated reactivity was specific [4].

As to the mechanism of focal reactions it was presumed that tuberculous tissues bind increased amounts of tuberculin. The introduction of radioactive tracer techniques rendered this problem accessible for investigation. The presumptions seemed to be supported by investigations carried out with ^{32}P-labelled BCG in guinea pigs [130] and children [129]. In tuberculin-positive individuals the labelled bacteria injected intradermally remained at the site of introduction for a longer time than in tuberculin-negative subjects. However, a similar difference could not be demonstrated by other workers [46b, 48, 96a, b, c] administering, e.g. purified ^{131}I-labelled tuberculin to infected and healthy animals.

The general (systemic) tuberculin reaction was first described by Koch. Its well-known clinical picture may develop in tuberculin-sensitized individuals after the intravenous or subcutaneous introduction of tuberculin and in intensely sensitized subjects even after intracutaneous exposure. It may also occur in laboratory workers 3 to 4 h following tuberculin inhalation. Depending on the severity of the reaction, headache, myalgia, flush, general malaise, chills and fever may appear. In extraordinarily severe cases tuberculin shock, occasionally fatal in outcome, may develop. The reaction is not specific in the sense that similar reaction can be elicited by all those antigens that are able to induce delayed-type allergic reactions.

In sensitized small laboratory animals 2 to 4 h following injection of tuberculin, fever appears concomitant with peripheral vasodilatation. The animals hardly move and eat poorly. The peripheral lymphocyte, monocyte and platelet counts strongly diminish. The majority of cells which had disappeared from circulation were found accumulated in the lungs, liver and, to a lesser degree, in other organs. The mechanism of development of tuberculin fever is not clarified either. The possibility of a role of contaminating endotoxin has been ruled out by accurate investigations [6, 14, 60, 67, 131]. The role of humoral anti-tuberculin antibodies can also be excluded since the release of considerable amounts of histamine could not be demonstrated in tuberculin fever and the fever could not be prevented by anti-histamine drugs. Since not only tuberculin allergy but also tuberculin fever can be passively transferred with cells to non-sensitized animals it was postulated that the sensitized cells were responsible for the liberation of an endogenic pyrogenic substance. Such a substance, however, could not be isolated yet.

Increasing the dose of tuberculin beyond that sufficient to achieve a maximal fever is followed, instead of fever, by hypothermia and tuberculin shock with decreasing blood pressure, lassitude, hypokinesia, muscular weakness and dizziness, and ruffled fur in experimental animals. The shock may be fatal in outcome. This clinical picture is accompanied by characteristic pathological changes. Macroscopically, serous or slightly haemorrhagic effusions in the body cavities and swollen, oedematous lymph nodes and thymus are seen. In the lungs, liver, spleen, lymph nodes, and in the thymus, punctate, sometimes larger haemorrhages occur. Haemorrhages, not characteristic in appearance [112], develop also at the sites of previous skin tests and tuberculous lesions. In the lungs congestion, hepatization, in the liver hyperaemia and round-cell infiltration, in the enlarged spleen decrease in the number and volume of follicles may occur. Histological examination of the lungs of rabbits succumbed in tuberculin shock revealed a high-grade lymphocytic and polymorphonuclear infiltration. The infiltrating cells filling the veins and venules produce thrombus-like formations in many places[120].

The mechanism of the development of tuberculin shock has not been clarified either. It is possible that delayed-type allergy and tuberculin shock are processes of different pathomechanism. This is supported by the facts that (*i*) in the course of the systemic delayed-type reaction induced by purified tuberculo-protein shock does not develop, no matter how large the dose is; (*ii*) the polysaccharides of *M. tuberculosis* are able to induce tuberculin shock but do not induce delayed-type skin reactions. Nevertheless, the fact that the allergy manifesting in tuberculin shock can be passively transferred with peritoneal exudate cells of sensitized animals into other animals indicates that tuberculin shock and delayed-type hypersensitivity are closely related phenomena.

Morphology

While the literary data concerning the macroscopic morphological features (erythema, induration) of tuberculin reaction are generally consistent, reports on the histological picture are contradictory. It is not disputed that the macroscopically evident induration is due to inflammatory cell accumulation. Opinions differ, however, as to the type of cells, and in particular, as to the order of the appearance of different cells at the site of reaction. Formerly, the inflammatory reaction was believed to be non-specific, with the preponderance of polymorphonuclears. It has, however, been shown that in the earliest and mildest tuberculin reactions the infiltration consists almost exclusively of mononuclears. Lymphocytes accumulate in the venules and, later, in perivenular cuffs.

Polymorphonuclear infiltration occurs only secondarily, when necrosis has developed [35a, b, 54, 55, 81]. It has been revealed by experiments with tritiated thymidine that mitoses are frequent in the perivascular cuffs, moreover, that in the tuberculin reaction (and in other delayed-type allergic reactions) the majority of cells reach the site of reaction from circulating blood, and then proliferate locally. The majority of the initially small mononuclear cells are transformed into larger cells, i.e. histiocytes within 24 to 48 h [126, 141]. Cellular reactions, similar to those described in the skin, can be observed if the reaction is elicited in other parts of the organism. However, organ-specific features cannot be disregarded (e.g. in the avascular cornea the reaction starts only when the mononuclear cells have reached the site of reaction from the capillaries and venules of the vascular limbus corneae).

In summary, the tuberculin reaction is characterized by marked accumulation of cells. The cells have been described to be lymphocytes, lymphoblasts, monocytes and mononuclear cells. They are mainly haematogenic and leave the vascular bed through the venules to proliferate locally. The cellular reaction described here is characteristic not only of the tuberculin reaction, but of delayed-type hypersensitivity reactions in general.

Desensitization

In man, hypersensitivity to tuberculin persists for years, often life-long even after clinical recovery. Even BCG vaccination, a weaker immunogenic effect than natural infection, may be followed by cutaneous allergy lasting for years. Tuberculin allergy can be reduced or suspended, but not abolished, by repeated parenteral injection of tuberculin. In desensitized subjects giving no cutaneous reaction reinfection or vaccination is followed by an accelerated tuberculin sensitization (infra-allergy). The mechanism of this phenomenon is not known in detail.

Desensitization is initiated with small doses causing no symptoms; later the dose is gradually increased until the skin reaction cannot be elicited any more. According to our own examinations, in the course of tuberculin desensitization, before the disappearance of skin reaction the so-called phasic phenomena described by Wvedenskij can be observed [47].

The phenomenon of desensitization has been particularly investigated from the point of view whether anti-tuberculous immunity is influenced by desensitization. From such studies an answer was expected to the crucial question of the correlation between allergy and immunity (see p. 65).

Factors influencing tuberculin reaction

Factors influencing the development, intensity and time course of tuberculin allergy have been extensively studied both in clinical practice and experimentally.

Nature and dose of the antigen. The quality and the dose of the antigen are decisive factors in tuberculin allergy. In the earliest studies living bacteria were used for sensitization. In guinea pigs and rabbits, under the effect of large doses of virulent bacteria, skin allergy develops within a few days. After administration of a large dose of less virulent bacteria (*M. avium*, BCG, etc.) or a small dose of virulent bacteria the time of sensitization is longer but usually does not exceed 14 days. On the effect of small doses of living bacteria of low virulence, allergy develops still slower. It is of interest that tuberculin allergy can also be elicited with killed bacteria and the allergy elicited in this way may also persist for a long time. Consequently, the presence of living bacteria in the organism cannot be considered to be a prerequisite of tuberculin allergy and, presumably, long-lasting sensitivity may be present without continuous antigen diffusion from active tuberculous foci.

For experimental purposes it is most appropriate to induce tuberculin allergy with complete Freund's adjuvant, i.e. a water-in-oil emulsion adjuvant, in which killed, dried mycobacteria are suspended in the oil phase. With the aid of this technique reliable tuberculin allergy, without any additional complicating disease, can be induced even in species (e.g. rat, mouse) in which other techniques have failed [42].

Technique of sensitization. Tuberculin allergy can be induced by any type of (intracutaneous, subcutaneous, intramuscular, intraperitoneal or intraorganic) parenteral introduction of proper antigens. In man tuberculin allergy develops even after alimentary infection, i.e. oral antigen stimuli can also cause allergy. This has been corroborated by animal experiments. The intracutaneous introduction and particularly the injection into the foot-pad have proved to be the most effective methods. This seems to be explainable by the fact that the skin, and particularly the foot-pad, is very rich in lymph vessels through which the antigen can easily reach the lymph nodes, i.e. the seat of cells responsible for the delayed-type immunological reaction (see below). Supposedly, the same mechanism can explain the clinical experience that the tuberculin allergy accompanying the tuberculosis of lymph nodes, of bones and of the skin is in general much stronger than that in pulmonary tuberculosis.

Age and species differences. It is difficult, though not impossible, to induce delayed-type allergy in newborns. The induction of tuberculin allergy is the easiest in young, healthy individuals, while the reactivity declines in old age [24]. Among the laboratory animal species the guinea pig is easiest to sensitize, and it is followed by the rabbit. Mice and rats were regarded formerly as refractory, however, with suitable techniques sensitization can convincingly be demonstrated even in these species [42]. Tuberculin allergy also develops in large domestic

44

animals (cattle, horse, etc.), and this can well be utilized in screening tests. It has proved to be an indispensable technique in the animal hygiene.

Co-existent antibodies. The role of humoral antibodies in the immunology of tuberculosis will be treated in detail below, here merely their relation to the delayed-type reactions is discussed. There is no correlation between the serum antibody level demonstrable against the antigens of *M. tuberculosis* and the tuberculin allergy, furthermore, the allergy can exist both in the presence and absence of serum antibodies [5, 7, 8, 9, 14, 17b, 19, 27, 36, 43, 44, 50, 75, 109, 148]. For example, in agammaglobulinaemia, besides the lack of humoral antibodies, the tuberculin reaction may be normal [27]. On the other hand, e.g. in postnatally thymectomized animals small lymphocytes strongly decrease in number and delayed-type hypersensitivity does not develop while their globulin level and plasma cell content are normal [3]. By X-ray irradiation of sufficient dose antibody formation can be reduced without affecting delayed-type reactions [137].

All these, however, do not mean that pre-existing antibodies have absolutely no effect on the delayed-type allergy. With the injection of BCG or tuberculo-proteins antibody formation can be induced and this can remarkably reduce the delayed-type response elicited subsequently [1, 2, 17a,b.] But elucidation of the problems of the correlation of cell-mediated immunity and pre-existing antibodies [20, 69, 107] requires further studies.

Local factors, drugs, chemicals. It is evident that delayed-type allergy can be influenced by different substances in a variety of ways. They may have a direct or indirect action on the cells that play a part in the immunological reaction; they may influence the permeability of blood and lymph vessels, and in this way they can affect the absorption of the antigen and the appearance of cells at the site of the reaction. Stimuli reaching the nervous system may have similar effects.

Studying the effect of *local vascular factors* Pepys [108] found that local vascular stasis (CO_2, heat, testing in tourniquet) increase the intensity of tuberculin reaction by impeding the disappearance of antigen from the site of injection. On the contrary, local influences which, through increased lymphatic drainage, e.g. in inflamed, oedematous skin [121], result in rapid disappearance of antigen from the site of injection, diminish the intensity of the tuberculin reaction. For example, local injection of histamine, intense irradiation with visible or UV light etc., have such an effect, but the inhibited, delayed-type reactions in pregnancy, during delivery, in the premenstrual period, in some febrile and infectious diseases and in starvation and cachexia may also be explained by this mechanism.

Local vasoconstriction also reduces the intensity of the reaction. For example, the inhibitory effect of antihistamines is based on this and not on antihistamine activity. Hyaluronidase diminishes the intensity of the reaction by increasing its area. Also, the actual functional state of the central nervous system has a substantial effect on delayed-type sensitivity [83, 84].

The intensity of tuberculin reaction is markedly modified by influences which induce *ablation or depletion of cells* responsible for, or participating in, the reaction. All factors reducing remarkably the number of circulating lymphocytes, also decrease the intensity of tuberculin reaction and of other delayed-type hypersensitivity reactions. The effects of cortisone (see below), X-ray irradiation, nitrogen mustard, anti-lymphocyte serum [65], etc., are all based on this mechanism. Thymectomy performed early in life also reduces delayed-type hypersensitivity to all kinds of antigen by reducing the lymphocyte count.

Antimetabolites, particularly mercaptopurine, decrease delayed-type hypersensitivity apparently via inhibition of nucleic acid and protein synthesis.

Hormones. Cortisone and ACTH, given systematically, markedly decrease tuberculin reaction both in man and in experimental animals. This effect is the most pronounced on the development of necrosis; induration and, especially, erythema are impeded to a lesser degree [29b, 87, 106, 139]. Histologically, the mononuclear cellular response is reduced, the number of polymorphonuclears does not change considerably. Thus, it seems likely that cortisone and ACTH diminish the delayed-type reaction through the effect exerted upon the mononuclear cells. This explanation is supported by the fact that cortisone and ACTH inhibit delayed-type reactions even in such small doses that do not influence histamine hyperaemia, anaphylaxis or the Arthus reaction. Furthermore, cortisone given systematically induces a strong lymphopenia. Cortisone administered locally also inhibits tuberculin reaction, while such an effect of ACTH is not known.

In *hypothyroidism* the tuberculin allergy is weak, and can be reestablished by the administration of thyroid hormone [70]. In contrast, in slight hyperthyroidism elicited by the administration of thyroxine in guinea pigs the tuberculin reaction is more expressed. Considering that (*i*) the effect of thyroxine can be suspended by partial pancreatectomy, which alone does not influence the delayed-type reaction, (*ii*) insulin alone increases allergy and (*iii*) the thyroxine effect in partially pancreatectomized guinea pig can be restored by insulin, it can be concluded that thyroxine enhances allergy by inducing hyperinsulinism. This is in accordance with the fact that delayed-type reactions are in general weaker in diabetics than in the general population [25].

Lurie et al. [88, 89], investigating the effect of *oestrogens*, progesterone and chorionic gonadotropin on rabbits, succeeded in reducing cutaneous allergy with oestrogen and chorionic gonadotropin. The former caused atrophy of the thymus, decreased the number of circulating lymphocytes and inhibited the spread of *M. tuberculosis* but did not inhibit the Rich phenomenon in tissue culture: the latter promoted bacterial spread. Since the same hormones proved to be ineffective in ovariectomized animals, it seems to be reasonable to suppose that the above phenomena were due to progesterone effect. Progesterone and oestrogen given together also decreased cutaneous allergy.

Other diseases. It is a clinical observation of long standing that in *measles* tuberculin allergy strongly diminishes suddenly 2 to 3 days before the development of exanthema and is restored with similar rapidity 6 to 8 days after it. It has been postulated that (*i*) the measles virus acting directly on lymphoid cells induces a decrease in their reactivity; and (*ii*) the immune apparatus becomes exhausted on account of the immunological reaction against the virus.

In other infectious diseases, e.g. in *mumps, infectious mononucleosis, poliomyelitis, chickenpox* [12, 101, 103], the tuberculin reaction may be reduced but to a lesser degree. In *influenza* this effect is in general considerable [16].

The tuberculin-type reactions are strongly reduced in certain diseases of the lymphoreticular system, such as lymphogranulomatosis and sarcoidosis. Often, these patients do not reject skin homografts [56, 71, 72]. At the same time their antibody formation is normal and histamine induces the usual skin reaction.

As to delayed-type hypersensitivity in *carcinoma,* the available data are rather contradictory; in reticulosarcoma and lymphosarcoma it shows a slight decrease while in *leukaemia* (even in lymphatic leukaemia !) it is more or less preserved; in *rheumatoid arthritis* and in systemic lupus erythematosus it is often exaggerated.

Passive transfer of tuberculin allergy

In contrast to the immunological response mediated by humoral antibodies, passive transfer of tuberculin allergy and other delayed-type sensitivities into normal individuals had failed until 1942 when Landsteiner and Chase succeeded in transferring contact allergy with living cells of sensitized animals [80]. Subsequently Chase reported on the passive transfer of tuberculin allergy [26]. It may be noted that tuberculin fever was successfully transferred into healthy guinea pigs with full blood transfusion (but not with serum) as early as in 1913 [93]. The procedure was as follows: in strongly sensitized guinea pigs peritoneal exudation was induced with intraperitoneally administered paraffin oil. Subsequently, the washed peritoneal exudate cells were given intravenously to normal guinea pigs. After a latency of 20–36 h positive skin tests could be evoked by the corresponding antigen. Transfer with cells from the spleen was as effective as with cells from lymph nodes or with those from the thoracic duct, while it failed with other cells. The allergy transferred passively was of short duration, the transfer was only successful if living cells were used [26, 80].

The first successful experiments were soon confirmed by many investigators [63a, b, 74, 78, 82a, 97a, b, c, 127]. Many variations in the technique of passive transfer have been described. Most often cells are transferred directly into the skin of the recipient, then antigen is given either systemically or locally. The interval between the transfer of cells and the injection of antigen may also be varied. If both are administered at the same time, the reaction runs its course within the same time as in an actively sensitized animal. The antigen (tuberculin) is most often injected after the transfer of sensitized cells. In brief, all the manifestations of tuberculin allergy can be demonstrated on the recipient of cells from sensitized animals.

The mechanism of passive transfer. The successful passive transfer of delayed-type sensitivity by cells and, especially, the direct relation between the number of transferred cells and the degree of the resulting hypersensitivity, suggest that the transferred sensitized cells themselves react with the antigen in the course of the allergic reaction. This is also supported by the observation that in inbred animals the passive hypersensitivity persists longer than in random animals, in which the transferred cells remain viable for a shorter time. It is nevertheless possible that transferred cells participate in the reaction in an indirect way, i.e. by transmitting to the recipient information which induces a selection of immunologically competent cells, and, subsequently, their participation in the immunological process. Finally, as a third possibility, an immune complex might be formed as a consequence of primary interaction between the antigen and the sensitized cells or the antibodies produced by the latter; the immune complex attracts secondarily to the site of reaction the competent cells; thus cells both of the donor and the recipient animal participate in the reaction.

47

According to Metaxas and Metaxas-Bühler [97a, c] the transferred cells participate directly in the reaction. If sensitized cells were transferred intravenously, tuberculin allergy could be elicited in the recipient animal without latency, while in case of intraperitoneal transfer there was a latency of 12 to 20 h. According to these authors this time interval is necessary for the transferred cells to reach the circulation from the peritoneal cavity.

The direct role of the transferred cells is also supported by the observation that if several tuberculin tests are performed simultaneously, the individual reactions are less marked than the reaction induced with an identical amount of tuberculin applied at a single site. It is suggested that in case of simultaneous testing, there is a competition among the test sites for the limited number of transferred cells. The direct role is also supported by the fact that if cells are injected mixed with tuberculin, a local delayed-type reaction develops.

Studies in this field were considerably stimulated by the introduction of radioactive isotope techniques suitable for labelling cells. Tritiated cells from sensitized animals were transferred and Mantoux tests were performed with PPD on the ear of the recipient animal. Histological evidence pointed out that a part, though not all, of the cells participating in the reaction were labelled [102a, b, c]. Thus, it has been concluded that cells of the recipient animal also take part in the reaction. However, if cells of the recipient guinea pigs were labelled and allergy was transferred by unlabelled cells, almost all the cells of the infiltration were found to be labelled [94]. Similarly, the preponderance of cells of the recipient animals was observed following labelling of cells of the recipient animals in the course of lymphocyte transfer reaction [77].

The question arises whether allergy can be transferred with extracts of sensitized cells. Until now this has not been achieved in animal experiments either with cells enclosed in Millipore-chamber, or with extracts of sensitized cells. On the contrary, Lawrence made successful experiments in humans [82b, c]. He designated the substance which he held responsible for this phenomenon transfer factor. Table 72-I shows that the chemical characteristics of the transfer factor is not clear. It cannot be an antibody (protein), since trypsin digestion does not abolish its effect. It is not inactivated by DNase and RNase either. It has a molecular weight of 10,000 or less, and recent studies have raised the possibility that it might be a derepressor molecule of some sort [20a]. Though its nature remains one of the major enigmas of immunology, it is used for the therapy of various immune deficiency diseases in man more and more widely.

TABLE 72-I

Characteristics of Lawrence's transfer factor

Transfer factor is not influenced by:
      storage at 25 °C or 37 °C for 6 hours
      lysis in distilled water
      freezing and thawing 10 times
      deepfreezing for 5 months
      DNase
      RNase
      trypsin

Identification of the sensitized cells. The identification of the sensitized cells responsible for transferring tuberculin sensitivity would solve one of the basic questions in allergy. Theoretically, the problem seems simple: various cells of the sensitized animal should be separated and those transferring sensitivity should be determined. However, the situation is by far not so simple in practice. First of all, the exact morphological identification of the individual cells encounters difficulties because the ontogenesis of the cells potentially responsible for the transfer is not clear and the types of cells able to transform into other types have not been determined exactly. Furthermore, the production of pure suspensions of the individual cell types presents a serious methodological problem. In spite of these difficulties it can be stated that the sensitized cells responsible for passive transfer correspond to lymphocytes. This has been proved by the following: (*i*) All cell populations that have been used with success for passive transfer contained considerable amounts of lymphocytes. (*ii*) Allergy can easily be transferred with suspensions of cells from thoracic duct lymph; these are almost exclusively lymphocytes (80–90 per cent small lymphocytes, the rest large lymphocytes). (*iii*) Hypersensitivity can also be transferred with thymus cells, although these appear to be less competent in this respect. (*iv*) In homologous or secondary diseases (see Chapter 29 in Vol. 2) the immunological effect is proportional to the number of lymphocytes in the injected cell suspension. Similarly, runt disease could be induced in rats by small lymphocytes from the thoracic duct [15]. (*v*) With ablation experiments which markedly reduce the number of circulating lymphocytes (e.g. administration of anti-lymphocyte serum, cortisone, nitrogen mustard treatment, X-ray irradiation, etc.), the intensity of tuberculin allergy can be decreased to a great extent. (*vi*) The most convincing proof was yielded by experimental animals thymectomized early in life. In such animals the number of lymphocytes is low not only in the blood stream, but also in the lymph nodes and spleen. Delayed-type reactivity is very weak against all kinds of antigens and there is a convincing correlation between the decrease in the number of lymphocytes and the immunological unresponsiveness. However, the number of blood monocytes and large lymphocytes is normal [3] and in the lymph nodes and spleen the number of other cells is not decreased either [140]; even antibody formation may be normal. It should be noted that delayed-type allergy is not influenced by splenectomy performed in adult or newborn animals [66].

The above evidence, however, does not lead to the conclusion that the small lymphocyte is the only cell type which becomes sensitized by interaction with antigen; e.g. in peritoneal exudates macrophages may occur in greater number than lymphocytes, therefore, it is possible that these cells may also transfer sensitivity. Anti-macrophage serum, in contrast to the anti-lymphocyte serum, does not influence tuberculin reactivity, which is another fact pointing to the lymphocytes being responsible for the transfer. But it is beyond doubt that the reactivity of macrophages is also altered in sensitized animals (see below).

Even though there is no direct evidence for the sensitization of macrophages, they must play an outstanding role in the initiation of the immunological reaction for the antigen which has gained access to the organism is taken up first by the regional lymph nodes. It is possible that macrophages have a role not only in the primary uptake of antigen [40, 41]. From macrophages pre-incubated with bacteriophage, an RNA fraction was isolated which was able to induce antibody formation in lymphocyte culture. Thus, it is possible that the initial step of the immunological mechanism is the formation of an RNA-antigen complex in the macrophage.

In vitro techniques

Rich and Lewis described [116] that leukocytes of tuberculous individuals undergo cytolysis *in vitro* under the effect of tuberculin if complement is also present. Since, however, there is no correlation between the cytolytic effect and the intensity of the tuberculin skin test the cytolytic phenomenon seems to be of little interest.

By means of recent techniques delayed-type allergy can be reliably studied *in vitro*. It is a common feature of these techniques that the reaction given in response to the specific antigen by the cell population derived from sensitized animals shows a good correlation with the *in vivo* delayed-type reaction.

Macrophage migration inhibition. If a suspension of peritoneal exudate cells from tuberculin allergic guinea pigs is packed into a capillary tube and the end of the tube is led into a vessel (e.g. culture chamber) containing physiological saline, the cells will migrate into the vessel. If, however, the solution contains tuberculin, migration is inhibited. The phenomenon characterizes all delayed-type allergic reactions and shows a fairly good correlation with the allergic reaction *in vivo*. The reaction is specific for antigen that has sensitized the donor of the cells (Fig. 72-1). Two cell types participate in the reaction: lymphocytes and macrophages. For the development of the reaction the lymphocytes must be sensitized, while the macrophages need not. Sensitized lymphocytes while incubated with the specific antigen release into the medium a substance which also inhibits the migration of normal (non-sensitized) peritoneal exudate cells. This substance

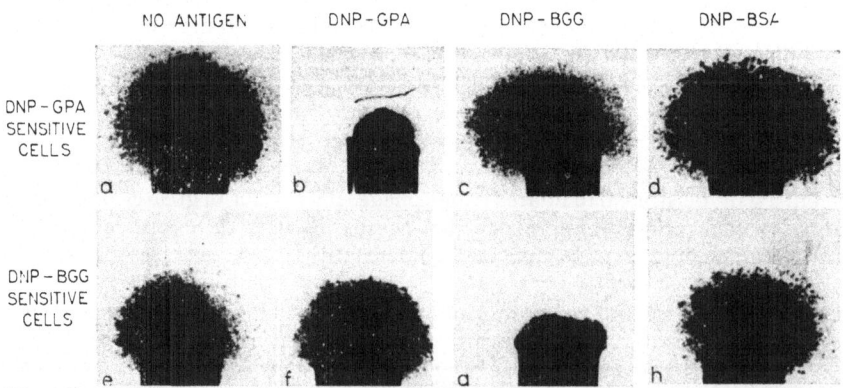

Fig. 72-1. Inhibition of macrophage migration. DNP = dinitrophenol; BGG = = bovine γ-globulin; BSA = bovine serum albumin; GPA = guinea pig albumin. The upper row indicates that the migration of cells of animals with a delayed-type allergy to DNP-GPA is only inhibited by DNP-GPA, while in the lower row inhibition of the migration of DNP-BGG sensitive cells is only evident to DNP-BGG (after David [34])

is called migration inhibition factor (MIF). Animals showing no delayed-type hypersensitivity do not produce MIF even if they have humoral antibodies.

The nature of MIF is not completely known, its synthesis is inhibited by puromycin and mitomycin C, it resists 56 °C for 30 min, it is non-dialysable, it is inactivated by trypsin but not by DNase or RNase [34]. From Sephadex G-200 column it is eluted in the peak which contains proteins of a similar mol. wt as albumin [34]. On the other hand, from sensitized cells an RNA fraction was extracted which was able to sensitize non-sensitized cells specifically against the antigen. The sensitization is demonstrable by the migration inhibition test. This RNA is of 8S–12S order of magnitude, its mol. wt. is more than 80,000 [134]. MIF is not identical with the transfer factor of Lawrence, which is resistant to both of trypsin and RNase.

Lymphocyte transformation. Small lymphocytes of animals exhibiting delayed-type allergy respond to the effect of specific antigen with blast transformation. The resulting lymphoblast cells are morphologically very similar to the pyroninophilic cells (immunoblasts which appear following *in vivo* antigen stimulus in lymph modes). Cytochemical techniques show in the transformed cells increased DNA, RNA and protein synthesis, which is finally followed by mitosis. The lymphocyte transformation ensuing on *in vitro* antigen stimulus is specific for the antigen responsible for sensitivity and is in good correlation with the delayed-type skin reaction demonstrable *in vivo*. The *in vitro* lymphocyte transformation can be demonstrated sooner than the positive allergic skin reaction, thus, it appears to provide a more sensitive technique for the demonstration of delayed-type allergy than the skin test [11, 28, 92, 100, 105, 115, 119].

Target cell destruction. This reaction serves first of all for the demonstration of transplantation immunity. Since tuberculin reaction and graft rejection are based on similar immunological mechanisms, the phenomenon of target cell

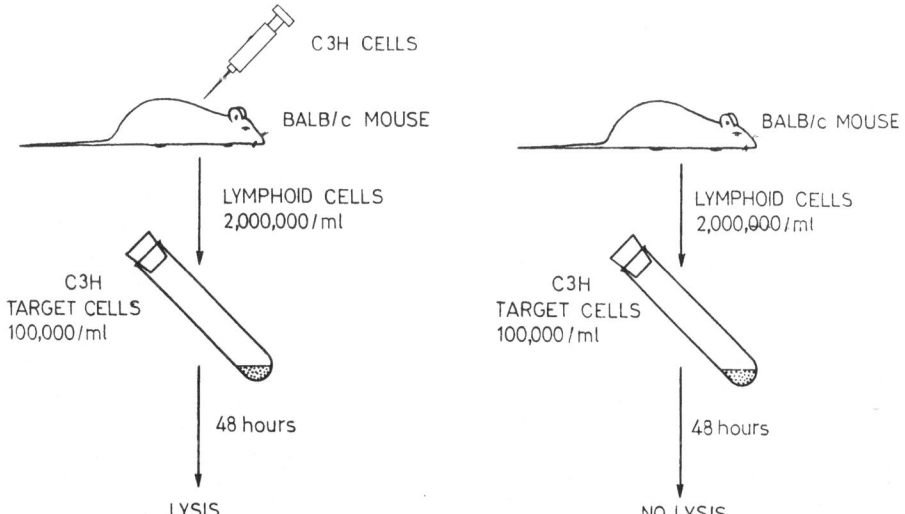

Fig. 72-2. Target cell destruction. Schematic drawing of the system by which lytic effect of the sensitized lymphocytes can be demonstrated (after Rosenau [118])

destruction is also discussed here. The essence of the reaction is as follows: if lymphoid cell suspension from animals immunized with immunologically non-identical cells of animals of the same species is added to the monolayer suspension of the target cells of the animal used for immunization, the target cells will be destroyed (Fig. 72-2). The reaction is specific, its mechanism has not been clarified. It is presumed that the reaction consists of two steps: (*i*) the lymphocytes of the specifically sensitized animals become attached to the target cells with antibodies or antibody-like structures bound on their surface and (*ii*) the lymphocytes produce substance(s) which cause lysis of the target cells [118].

Epidemiological significance

Since the positive tuberculin reaction reliably indicates that the organism has been exposed to the antigens of *M. tuberculosis*, it is suitable for screening large population groups. Such a screening, however, presents numerous problems. Firstly, in many countries, including Hungary, systematic BCG vaccinations are carried out, thus tuberculin positivity may be due either to vaccination or to natural infection. A reliable differentiation of tuberculin allergy caused by vaccination from that caused by natural infection has not been successful yet. Gel precipitation tests show no considerable difference between the antigenic structure of *M. tuberculosis* and BCG [85a, b]. Attempts have been made to overcome this difficulty by using in the skin test destroyed BCG bacteria (so-called BCG test) instead of tuberculin [45, 124, 129, 138]. Statistically significant differences could be demonstrated when only vaccinated and only naturally infected populations were comparatively tested with the two antigens but the origin of the allergy in a given individual cannot be decided on this basis alone.

Secondly, in the last decade it became known, primarily due to studies initiated and performed by the WHO, that the so-called atypical Mycobacteria (Runyon group I–IV) are in numerous, particularly tropical and subtropical areas widespread and in such areas a high percentage of the population may exhibit a slight tuberculin positivity. Since some antigen components of the atypical Mycobacteria are identical with those of *M. tuberculosis* or *M. bovis*, it is understandable that subjects previously exposed to atypical Mycobacteria may give a positive allergic response also to the tuberculins used in screening tests. However, the tuberculin reactions of such individuals are in general weak, and so-called minimal reactions are frequently noted. In such areas it is advisable to perform simultaneous skin tests with ordinary tuberculin on one arm and with sensitin prepared from atypical Mycobacteria on the other. A stronger reaction to sensitin indicates previous exposure to atypical Mycobacteria. In view of the minimal, so-called non-specific, skin reaction due to atypical Mycobacteria, the dose of tuberculin is of great importance. The minimal reaction does not develop in response to small doses of tuberculin and thus it does not disturb the screening. For comparative international screening tests therefore small doses, most often 1 TU, of the TWEEN-80-containing purified tuberculin (RT 23) are applied (1 U of RT 23 corresponds to 0.02 μg).

The tuberculin reaction is also suitable for checking the effectiveness of BCG vaccination. Although immunity against tuberculosis and the allergic reaction

are not necessarily parallel phenomena, it is beyond doubt that following successful BCG vaccination the vaccinated organism becomes sensitive to tuberculin.
This is the basis for estimating the success of BCG vaccination. Since, however,
according to widespread investigations, tuberculin allergy following vaccination
with an appropriate vaccine develops practically in 100 per cent of the vaccinees,
routine application of the tuberculin tests for this purpose can be omitted. It is
sufficient to control the allergy of the vaccinated population periodically.

Another field of application of the tuberculin reaction in epidemiology is the
selection of tuberculin-negative individuals to be vaccinated. Since, however,
BCG vaccination does not cause any harmful reactions in tuberculin-positive
individuals either, the view is widely accepted that BCG vaccination can safely
be applied even without any screening.

Finally, if tuberculin tests are systematically performed, the fresh conversion
(development of tuberculin positivity in previously negative individuals) reliably
indicates recent tuberculosis infection. Selection and, if necessary, adequate
therapy of such individuals may be a decisive factor in the effective fight against
tuberculosis.

IMMUNITY IN TUBERCULOSIS

It has been mentioned in the discussion of basic immunological phenomena
that resistance to both primary infection (or vaccination) and reinfection shows
a great variation. Even the well-known fact that only a small fraction of individuals infected with tuberculosis become manifestly sick indicates the decisive
importance of the immunological condition of the organism. In the following
the most important information concerning immunity in tuberculosis will be
summarized [21, 30, 57, 61, 62].

The concepts and characteristics of natural resistance (native immunity) and
acquired specific immunity have been defined in the foregoing. The question
arises whether it is justified to discuss the mechanism of these two categories
of immunity separately in relation to tuberculosis. On the basis of the arguments
listed below the answer is no.

1. The organism has no different defence mechanisms for the first, and for the
repeated exposures to *M. tuberculosis*. In both cases the same mechanisms are
active, i.e. phagocytosis, antibody formation, enzyme activity, etc. In agreement
with other investigators [49a, b, 147] we have found that the basic mechanism
of specific immunity is secondary, i.e. it is attained through factors which participate also in non-specific immunity of the organism. Acquired immunity signifies
an adaptation of the organism, in the course of which the defence mechanisms
responsible for natural resistance are greatly intensified [46a].

2. Due to well-known reasons, natural resistance (native immunity) to tuberculosis in man cannot be measured, while acquired immunity can be studied with
statistical-epidemiological methods.

3. Our knowledge concerning immunity in tuberculosis is mainly based on
examination of superinfection immunity in experimental animals. Measurement
of natural resistance is in general aimed at determining the resistance of a given
species, subspecies or strain.

HUMORAL ANTIBODIES AND THEIR SIGNIFICANCE

Antibodies in the blood of humans and experimental animals infected with tuberculosis have been known to be present since long. Various serological techniques have been applied for their demonstration [135].

Agglutination tests are carried out with suspended homogenized Mycobacteria as antigen. However, agglutination of *M. tuberculosis* encounters difficulties because the homogenization of Mycobacteria is almost impossible, first of all due to their high lipid content. Bacteria conglutinate even in the absence of antibodies, furthermore, the lipid-rich hydrophobic surface prevents interaction between antibodies, and bacterial cells. Therefore, agglutination could not gain general use.

For precipitation tests extract of tuberculous tissues or tuberculin were used as antigen. In practice, however, the precipitation tests also proved to be unsuitable.

C-fixing antibodies have also been demonstrated in the sera of tuberculous individuals [13, 23,a, b]. Old tuberculin was used as antigen. Many non-specific reactions were noticed, e.g. with the sera of individuals suffering from malaria, diphteria or syphilis. Since it was believed that the non-specific factor is bound to some lipid fraction, production of antigens prepared from lipid-free bacteria was initiated. In spite of numerous modifications, the C-fixation reaction did not meet the requirements either for the clinical diagnosis of tuberculosis or for judging the activity of the process or the immunobiological condition of the organism. The same is valid for the serological reactions involving large surface areas, e.g. the Middlebrook–Dubos reaction, in which antigen adsorbed on the surface of red blood cells reacts with the antibodies in the serum under testing [98, 99a, b]. Attempts to render this test suitable for clinical diagnosis and for following the course of the disease by pretreating the red blood cells with papain, tannin, trypsin and/or pepsin have failed. The same holds for the method of Takahashi [132, 133] who used kaolin as adsorbent.

Subsequently, gel precipitation and immunoelectrophoresis, i.e. serological reactions performed in a semisolid medium (agar gel, cellulose acetate, starch, acryl-imido-polymer, etc.), were introduced in tuberculosis research. In these reactions filtrates of the corresponding Mycobacterium are usually applied as antigen. These methods have brought remarkable development in the analysis of the antigenic structure of Mycobacteria and in the relatively gentle separation of different antigenic fractions (see below), however, for the clinical aspects of tuberculosis these reactions did not reveal any essential new correlations.

It may be concluded that humoral antibodies can be demonstrated by numerous methods in the serum of organisms which have undergone tuberculous infection. It is not proven, however, whether these antibodies would play an important role in shaping the immunological state of the organism and in the development of the clinical condition following tuberculous infection.

The idea has arisen that perhaps failure of serological reactions to fulfil expectations might be attributed to the fact that the tests did not differentiate between the classes of immunoglobulins. In recent years, the immunoglobulins of 81 infected and control individuals were studied by the Middlebrook–Dubos reaction. The haemagglutinating antibodies were identified as belonging to the

IgM class; in the haemagglutinating immunoglobulin IgG molecules were demonstrated only in one case [31a]. Studying the haemagglutinating antibodies of 80 tuberculous and control individuals with Boyden's method with respect to the immunoglobulin class, it was concluded that

1. neither the tuberculoprotein haemagglutination test nor the amount of antibody demonstrable with tuberculo-polysaccharides were in correlation with the condition of the patient;

2. in the haemagglutinating antibodies IgG, IgM and IgA molecules were demonstrated but no correlation was demonstrable between the amount of any of these and the condition of the patient [31b].

Thus for the time being, the study of the immunoglobulin types of serum antibodies demonstrated in tuberculosis has not enabled the serological reactions to be utilized in the clinical diagnosis of tuberculosis and in the estimation of the course of the already diagnosed illness.

The significance of the cytophilic antibodies [18] in the mechanism of tuberculin allergy and tuberculosis immunity cannot be regarded as verified either [10, 104].

On the basis of all these results only a subordinate role can be attributed to the mechanism of humoral immunity in tuberculosis.

In contrast to the poor results in the clinical utilization of immunological and serological techniques, the classification of Mycobacteria has been remarkably promoted by the procedures enabling the analysis of their antigenic structure. By means of gel precipitation and immunoelectrophoresis antigenic components

TABLE 72-II

Classification of Mycobacteria on the basis of group-specific antigens and serological identification according to Weissfeiler [142]

Group	Mycobacterium
A₁	M. tuberculosis
	M. bovis (BCG)
	M. microti
	M. avium
	M. xenopei
A₂	M. kansasii
	M. gastri
	M. marinum syn. balnei
	M. simiae No. 61
	M. aquae
A₃	M. simiae No. 29
B	M. smegmatis syn. butyricum
	M. phlei syn. moellers
C	M. fortuitum syn. minetti
D	M. abscessus syn. runyonii
	M. borstelense

can be separated from different Mycobacteria and thus mycobacterial species and strains can be characterized as regards their antigenic structure. For example, Lind [85a] succeeded in separating at least 17 antigenic components from *M. tuberculosis*. In the saprophytic Mycobacteria, in general, fewer components can be demonstrated. Different Mycobacteria often have common antigenic components [85a, b]. Up to now no antigenic difference has been demonstrated between human and bovine strains. This partly explains why the attempts to differentiate human and bovine infections by allergic tests have failed. According to the studies of Weissfeiler and his team [142], with gel precipitation methods even group-specific antigens, i.e. antigenic components common for several species of Mycobacteria, can be demonstrated. Classification on this basis is shown in Table 72-II.

CELL-MEDIATED IMMUNITY

This type of immunity in tuberculosis is not directly realized through the lymphocytes but through the activity of macrophages. On interaction with antigen macrophages become activated, proliferate and acquire an increased capacity to destroy mycobacterial cells. As a result of these processes, the digestive and bactericidal capacities of macrophages are enhanced, the macrophages increase in number and, consequently, the intracellular bacteria in the macrophages decrease in number [32]. This function of the macrophages is of decisive importance in the antituberculous defence mechanism of the organism.

Activation and proliferation of macrophages in cell-mediated immunity

The macrophage is the defensive cell the function of which influences the course of tuberculosis basically. Two phases can be differentiated in the activation of macrophages: an excitatory and an adaptive phase. The excitatory phase is characterized by an increase in oxygen uptake, glycolysis and lipid metabolism, thus, in general, by the acceleration of metabolic processes [33]. The adaptive phase is characterized by accumulation of lysosomes and mitochondria, furthermore, of lysosomal enzymes and by a rising protein content [32]. It has been proved experimentally that such an activated macrophage has an increased capacity for destroying intracellular bacteria. The mechanism of the latter process is not known. Nevertheless, from the observation that the increased bactericidal capacity and the activation phenomena can always be demonstrated together, it can be concluded that the destruction of bacterial cells will be realized by way of the activation phenomena described above. It has been supposed that the inhaled bacterial cells are taken up by macrophages of the pulmonary alveolus. In the case of primary infection a relatively long time (about 2 weeks) is needed until macrophage activation and, concomitantly, an increased bactericidal capacity develop. In case of superinfection the bacterial cells are taken up by macrophages already activated by the first infection (or vaccination), thus, their destruction ensues sooner. Accordingly, in the mechanism of both natural resistance and acquired immunity the function of the macrophages is of primary importance. The example of respiratory infection illustrates at the same time the accelerated, more effective, defence mechanism of acquired immunity. In the course of the process described the activated macrophage is transformed into a morphologically immature, then mature, epithelioid cell. The immature epithelioid cell is an activated macrophage rich in lysosomes, whereas the mature epithelioid cell is a macrophage in which at the site of digestive vacuoles and previous phagolysosomes much residual substance, i.e. undigested, mostly lipid, components are accumulated.

SYSTEMIC AND LOCAL IMMUNITY

As a consequence of sensitization the reactivity of the whole organism changes. In other words, tuberculin allergy is of systemic nature, the tuberculin reaction can be elicited in any organ and area of the sensitized organism. In contrast to this, the macrophagic, cell-mediated immunity manifests itself mainly locally, i.e. the degree of activation and bactericidal capacity of the macrophages are more marked at the site of the local lesion than elsewhere in the organism [32]. This is also indicated by the fact that at the sites of granulomatous lesions the enzyme activity of macrophages (β-galactosidase, acid phosphatase, β-glucuronidase, cytochrome oxydase, succinyl dehydrogenase, amino peptidase, phosphamidase, non-specific esterase and nicotinamide adenine dinucleotide diaphorase) is considerably more pronounced than in other parts of the organism [32, 52, 53, 58, 145]. The significance of local immunity is also indicated by the fact that tuberculosis superinfection in the area of the primary lesion generally shows slower progression. It is also known that the primary lesion may heal while in other parts of the organism the disease progresses.

This does not mean that following tuberculous infection (or vaccination) systemic immunity does not develop. In intravenously infected experimental animals or in human diseases of large extension *M. tuberculosis* invades the blood stream in great numbers and spreads in the whole organism. From experiments with bacteria labelled with radioactive isotope it is known that this process ensues not only after intravenous infection, but also in case of less extensive processes. Thus, following infection, also a systemic cell-mediated immunity develops, which is, however, in general less intensive than the local process.

SPECIFICITY OF ACQUIRED IMMUNITY

Tuberculin allergy is strictly specific, delayed-type allergy can only be elicited by the antigen responsible for sensitization. The so-called non-specific reactions (e.g. sensitization with saprophytic Mycobacteria followed by allergic reaction against tuberculin) can be explained by the existence of common antigenic components in the sensitizing and test antigens. In this sense the non-specific reactions are also specific. On the other hand, the macrophages of the organism sensitized with *M. tuberculosis* inhibit the multiplication not only of *M. tuberculosis* but also that of many other bacteria, and destroy them more intensely than the macrophages of non-sensitized organisms. For instance, alveolar macrophages of rabbits and peritoneal macrophages of mice both sensitized with BCG were found to inhibit listeriae and *Salmonella typhimurium*, respectively, more actively than macrophages obtained from a non-immune organism [37, 90]. Macrophages of the immunized organism take up also corpuscular materials of non-bacterial origin, such as carbon and collodion particles, to a greater extent. The cell-mediated immunity of the macrophage system cannot be regarded as strictly specific. Youmans [146b] has proposed the multiple response theory of immunity to tuberculosis because of the complex occurrence of specific and non-specific factors in acquired immunity. The components of the latter are: (*i*) non-specific activation of the RES, which is attributed to the thermostable endotoxin-like components to the bacteria; (*ii*) a more specific immunological mechanism attributable to the thermolabile components of living bacteria. In this mechanism also antibodies might participate; (*iii*) immunological response concomitant with granuloma formation which is connected with activation, accumulation and proliferation of macrophages. The latter is attributed to the direct or indirect effect of hypersensitivity to tuberculin and the adjuvant effect to the lipid components of Mycobacteria [146b].

Our present knowledge is insufficient to explain the mechanism of immunity against tuberculosis, but obviously non-specific factors have an important role in it.

MEASUREMENT OF ACQUIRED IMMUNITY

As mentioned above, the bulk of our knowledge concerning antituberculous immunity has been gained by experimental investigations of the so-called super-infection immunity in animals. The essence of these is that experimental animals are injected with some kind of vaccine, e.g. bacterial constituent, and, after an interval, the animals are challenged by a suspension of virulent bacteria. The reactions of the animals are in some way compared with the reactions of previously non-vaccinated and similarly challenged control animals.

As experimental animals mainly mice and guinea pigs, less commonly rabbits, red mice, Syrian hamsters and rats are used. As a rule, the vaccine to be examined is given intramuscularly, subcutaneously, intraperitoneally or intravenously while the challenging dose is administered intravenously, intraperitoneally, subcutaneously or by inhalation. In mice and rats almost exclusively the intravenous infection is used since this is the only way in which a progredient lethal disease can be produced.

To measure the response on the infective dose, numerous methods have been evolved. These can be grouped as follows [125]:

1. *Examination of survival*. Measurement of the average survival time is undoubtedly the simplest and most objective technique which includes the least methodological source of error. Another great advantage is that if sufficient numbers of animals are used the average survival times for the animal groups can be well analysed by biometrical methods. Its disadvantage is that if the inoculum is small (and as a rule this is so with natural infection of humans) the experiment can last for months and in this case the large standard deviation makes evaluation difficult. In order to eliminate this drawback, the method has been modified so that survival is only followed-up for a definite time, e.g. 30 days [146a], or mean half-life of the animals is compared.

2. *Macroscopic changes.* After a definite time following challenge the pretreated and the control animals are sacrificed and the macroscopically detectable tuberculous changes of the organs are scored according to the severity of changes and the mean values for each group are compared. For example, the so-called Feldman index is widely used [38]. The advantage of the procedure is that the duration of the experiment can be exactly predicted, the disadvantage is that judgement of the mascroscopic lesions may be very subjective, therefore, the comparison of the results of different laboratories encounters difficulties, furthermore, the results are strongly influenced by the time of killing of the animals.

3. *The method of bacterium counting.* The challenged animals are killed at a chosen time, then the number of colony-forming bacteria in the different organs (most often spleen and/or lungs) are compared among the different groups. The choice of time when to sacrifice the animals makes difficulties also here. This method is also technically more complicated and more expensive, and the results are subject to great individual variation.

4. The essence of the *index method* is that the animals are killed at a definite time following the injection of the challenge dose and organs are weighed; e.g. the spleen index = weight of the spleen/body weight. The mean values of indices for the different groups of animals are compared and statistically analysed. The method is very simple, the time of the experiment can be planned. However, the question remains open how far the index value really expresses the severity of the disease.

Other methods applied much less frequently include:

5. *Measurement of cutaneous ulcer.* Guinea pigs vaccinated intraperitoneally are superinfected with vole bacillus intradermally. The resulting cutaneous lesions are compared with those of non-vaccinated animals. The results thus obtained were found to be in good accordance with those of survival experiments [64].

6. *Lung density.* Specific gravity of the lungs of vaccinated and non-vaccinated animals are compared at a definite time after challenge [29a].

7. *Corneal lesion.* To intracutaneously or intracorneally vaccinated mice the challenge dose is given into the (contralateral) cornea. The developing pathological reactions can be well followed in the cornea and can be compared with the reactions of non-vaccinated animals [117].

Since literary data concerning the immunogenic properties of different vaccines and bacterial components are most contradictory, experiments with international co-operation were undertaken under the auspices of the WHO in 1967–1968 in order to establish the value of the methods used. In the experiments 9 laboratories from 8 countries participated.*

* Participating laboratories: Tuberculosis Research Institute, Prague (L. Sula, J. Galliova, J. Pruchova and J. Sulova); International Children's Center, Paris (F. Levy and G. Conge); Institute of Microbiology, Parasitology and Epidemiology, Bucharest (C. Oprescu); Korányi National Institute of Tuberculosis, Budapest (I. Földes and L. Lugosi); L. S. Tarasevich State Control Institute of Medical Biological Preparations, Moscow (T. Jablokova); Statens Seruminstitut, BCG Dept., Copenhagen (J. Guld, Miss Bunch-Christensen and Miss Ledefoged); Glaxo Laboratories Ltd., Greenford, Middlesex (P. Muggleton); National Institutes of Health, Rocky Mt. Laboratories, Hamilton, Montana, USA (E. Ribi and R. Anacker); University of Wisconsin, Madison, Wisconsin, USA (D. Smith, E. Wiegeshaus, D. McMurray and A. Grover).

The procedure was as follows. Five vaccines of supposedly different immunogenicity were produced by the Glaxo Laboratories. The vaccines were distributed among the participating laboratories. In the experiment the dose of vaccine and the interval between vaccination and challenge were standardized. The participating laboratories examined the vaccines by the method they generally used, the results were centrally evaluated by one of the participating laboratories on the basis of the collected protocols.*

Surprisingly there were no two laboratories obtaining consistent results about the immunogenic rank of any of the investigated vaccines. Furthermore, the results obtained in the same laboratory with different methods were also inconsistent (Table 72-III). Nevertheless, it could be unambiguously concluded that (i) the most severe tuberculous disease developed in the control (non-vaccinated) group and (ii) the live BCG vaccine proved to be the most effective.

BCG VACCINATION

In practice for vaccination against tuberculosis BCG vaccine is applied almost exclusively. BCG (Bacillus Calmette–Guérin) is an apathogenic variant of *M. bovis* developed by Calmette and Guérin by systematic passage performed for 13 years on a glycerol-bile-potato medium. It is a basic question whether there is any possibility for the strain to regain its original higher virulence. At the beginning wider application of BCG was strongly limited by this possibility. Experience of several decades has proved that this hazard can safely be excluded. The immunogenic capacity of BCG is quite a different question. Since the original strain was sent to numerous countries it has been sustained in numerous laboratories often under very different cultural conditions. Consequently, so-called BCG substrains have developed. The immunogenic and allergenic properties of these are very divergent. In spite of the fact that until now several hundred million people have been vaccinated with BCG the efficacy of vaccination in man has been debated for many decades. If, however, the results of well-controlled trials are taken into consideration (Table 72-IV), BCG vaccination must be accepted as effective. In half of the trials shown in Table 72-IV a protective effect of 78–82 per cent was achieved, in 4 trials the protection rate ranged between 31 and 59 per cent and there was only a single trial showing no significant protection.

The differences in protection rate may be attributed to (i) differences in the quality of the vaccines used; (ii) deviations between the vaccinated and control populations involved; (iii) the widespread occurrence of so-called atypical Mycobacteria and exposure of the population to them in some areas.

It is known from several investigations, in particular from the trials of the British Medical Research Council, that the morbidity hazards of tuberculin-positive and tuberculin-negative individuals are different, thus, the protection rate may be influenced by the ratio of tuberculin-positive and tuberculin-negative individuals in the population.

In spite of the inconsistent data BCG vaccination is the most efficient tool in the fight against tuberculosis. However, for its use a uniform scheme cannot be

* Evaluating laboratory: University of Wisconsin, Madison, Wisconsin, USA.

TABLE 72-III

Comparative determination of the protective value of 5 vaccines in various laboratories

| Examiner | Experimental animal | Method | Ranking of vaccines on the basis of protective value (1–6)* | | | | | |
			A Live BCG	B Live M. avium	C M. tuberculosis killed with formalin and suspended in physiological saline	D M. tuberculosis killed with formalin and suspended in oil-Arlacel	E 'Extraction residue' suspended in oil-Arlacel	Control
Bunch-Christensen	Red mouse	Survival	2.5	4	1	5	2.5	6
Földes, Lugosi	Mouse	Survival	2	3	1	4	6	5
Földes, Lugosi	Rat	Survival	1	6	4	2	3	5
Levy	Mouse	Bacterium count in lung	1	6	3	2	5	4
Oprescu	Mouse	Survival	3	1	2	4	6	5
Muggleton	Mouse	Macroscopic changes in lung	1	3	2	5	4	6
Muggleton	Mouse	Macroscopic changes in spleen	1	4	2.5	5	2.5	6
Ribi	Mouse	Survival	2	3	1	5	4	6
Ribi	Mouse	Bacterium count in lung	3	1	2	5	4	6
Smith	Guinea pig	Bacterium count in lung	2	4	5	1	3	6
Smith	Guinea pig	Bacterium count in spleen	1	4	5	3	2	6
Smith	Mouse	Bacterium count in lung	3	5	1	4	2	6
Smith	Mouse	Bacterium count in spleen	4	6	3	5	1	2
Smith	Guinea pig	Lung-index	1	6	3	2	4	5
Smith	Guinea pig	Spleen-index	1	5	4	3	2	6
Sula	Guinea pig	Lung-index	1	6	5	2	3	4
Sula	Guinea pig	Spleen-index	1	4	2	5	3	6
Sula	Guinea pig	Lung-index	6	3	5	1	2	4
Sula	Guinea pig	Spleen-index	1	4	2	5	3	6

* 1 = strongest protective effect.
6 = weakest protective effect.
2–5 = in-between values.

61

TABLE 72-IV

Results concerning the protective value of BCG vaccination

Author	Population studied	Vaccine applied	Criterion of vaccination	Basis of evaluation	Percentage value of vaccination
British Medical Research Council (1963)	15-year-old English students	Danish BCG intra-dermally, vole vaccine intradermally	Neg. 100 TU Neg. 100 TU	Tuberculosis morbidity	79 81
Aronson, Aronson and Taylor (1958)	0–20-year-old North-American Indians	Philadelphia BCG intradermally	2. Dose PPD	Tuberculosis morbidity	82
Rosenthal (1955, 1956)	Children from Chicago	Chicago BCG multiple puncture		Tuberculosis morbidity	78 79
Sergent, Catane, Ducros-Rougebief (1956)	Moslem children 0, 1, 3 and 7-year-old	Pasteur BCG orally		Total mortality	6 (0–2 years) 36 (3–7 years)
Frimodt-Moller, Thomas, Parthasarathy (1964)	All age groups South India	Madras BCG intradermally	Neg. 5 or 10 TU	Tuberculosis morbidity	59
U.S.P.H.S. Palmer, Shaw, Comstock (1958)	1–18-year-old Puerto-Ricans	New York BCG intradermally;	Neg. 10 TU	Incidence of tuberculosis revealed by routine examinations	31
	Southern part of USA >5 years	Chicago BCG multiple puncture	Neg. 5 TU		36

proposed for every country. The correct indications can only be stated after considering the epidemiological characteristics of a given area. In high-risk areas it is reasonable to vaccinate all newborn babies, then, since the immunity induced by BCG vaccination lasts only for a few years, it is wise to revaccinate those who prove to be tuberculin-negative when tested every third or fourth year. In those areas where, due to the more favourable epidemiological situation the risk of tuberculous infection is slight, vaccination of the high risk groups only is recommended.

In case of proper application, BCG vaccination is harmless, provided

1. The vaccine is good, i.e. adequately controlled and standardized (lyophilized if possible).
2. The vaccination technique is correct. On the basis of several decades' experience today only the intracutaneous vaccination technique can be recommended. Oral vaccination, originally suggested by Calmette, and the *"vaccinacao-concorrente"* of de Assis, applied especially in South America, (repeated oral introductions of 100 to 200 mg of BCG without previous tuberculin test) are only of historical interest.
3. Prevaccination tuberculin test, and the exclusive vaccination of tuberculin-negative individuals seems to be advisable, although recently indiscriminate vaccination, i.e. vaccination without a previously performed tuberculin test, has also been recommended (see p. 53).

In general a small infiltration and an exudating ulcer develop at the site of vaccination which then heal with a scar.

BCG vaccination is rarely followed by complication. These have been summarized by Mande as follows (cit. by [51]):

1. Infection in the local lesion
2. Perivaccinal pseudoeczematous reaction
3. Secondary auto-inoculation with BCG
4. Subcutaneous abscess
5. Cicatricial keloid
6. Lupus (skin tuberculosis)
7. Ostitis and osteomyelitis
8. Lymphadenitis

These complications heal in the majority of cases spontaneously in a few weeks, at most in a few months. From the data of the 12 lethal BCG vaccinations collected from the literature it is evident that in almost all the cases the affected children had hypo- or agammaglobulinaemia and death supervened in the majority of cases as a consequence of secondary infection [51]. On the basis of these data BCG vaccination cannot be regarded as more dangerous than any other immunizing procedure.

BCG vaccination seems to supply some protection also against leprosy since the pathogenic agent of leprosy is also a Mycobacterium, that bears antigenic components common with *M. tuberculosis*. In the practice of Fernandez a considerable part of lepromin-negative children became lepromin-positive following BCG vaccination [39]. In the field trial carried out in Uganda 26 and 44 months following vaccination the rate of leprous morbidity showed a decrease by 80 and 87 per cent, respectively, as compared to the non-vaccinated control group. In New Guinea the protective effect was found to be 50 per cent, whereas in Burma there was no appreciable difference in the rate of morbidity between the vaccinated and non-vaccinated group. More recently several authors have succeeded in infecting experimental animals with *Mycobacterium leprae* [114a, c, 123]; using this method, it was demonstrated that the multiplication of *Mycobacterium leprae* in mice was almost completely inhibited by BCG vaccination [114b].

Besides BCG vaccine antituberculous vaccine prepared from vole bacillus has been applied on relatively large population groups. Since, however, its protective effect did not prove to be stronger than that of BCG these experiments have been discontinued.

BCG vaccination has attracted renewed interest since toxic effects of the chemoprophylaxis against tuberculosis particularly liver damage became evident [43a]. In Hungary Weissfeiler and his co-workers prepared a vaccine of promising effect from the strain W 115 isolated by them. This vaccine has not yet been applied in man [143].

BACTERIAL COMPONENTS RESPONSIBLE
FOR ACQUIRED IMMUNITY

It is generally accepted that first of all bacterial proteins are responsible for the allergenic property of *M. tuberculosis*; only an adjuvant role is attributed to other constituents. Agreement is by far not so unanimous as to the factors responsible for immunity. The difficulties are due first of all to the fact that the immunity inducible by vaccination with either the killed whole bacterium or any of the isolated components is never equivalent to that achieved with live attenuated bacterium. Thus, it might be possible that the bacterium multiplying in the organism is necessary to induce immunogenic effect. This problem cannot be answered unequivocally, therefore, we have listed in Table 72-V the bacterial

TABLE 72-V

Immunogenic effect of different components of M. tuberculosis

Bacterial component studied		Immunogenic effect
lipids	Wax — A	—
	Wax — B	+ (weak)
	Wax — C	—
	(trehalose 6-6'dimycolate; cord factor)	
	Wax — D (PMK$_0$)	±
	Antigen methilique	
	(non-soluble phosphatide)	+
Extracts (chemically not defined)		±
Extraction residues (chemically not defined)		±
Polysaccharides		?
Proteins		+
Cytomembrane (Ribi, Larson)		+ (only in mice)
Protoplasm (Ribi)		—
Youmans' R-RNA		+ (only with adjuvant)

components studied so far indicating whether they have resulted in an immunogenic effect or not. However, even in case of an indisputable demonstration of the protective effect one cannot state that the component responsible for immunity has been found, since such a component ought to have a greater immunogenic capacity than the same quantity of the entire bacterium. Studies so far have not revealed such a component.

CORRELATION BETWEEN ALLERGY AND IMMUNITY

One of the most debated questions of the pathogenesis of tuberculosis is the correlation between allergy and protective functional immunity. Some authors emphasizing the differences between allergic and immune phenomena have suggested that the two processes are independent of each other. Calmette summarized [22] these differences as follows: (*i*) allergic reactions do not occur in organisms with high natural resistance; (*ii*) sensitized organisms that have become tuberculin-negative may remain immune against superinfection; (*iii*) certain factors (e.g. UV light) causing anergy (absence of reactions of cell-mediated immunity in a supposedly primed animal) may eliminate the allergy without affecting the immunity; (*iv*) with the administration of increasing doses of tuberculin the allergy can be eliminated without changing the immunity against superinfection; (*v*) many South-African Negroes show strong allergy without being immune [22].

Other authors emphasize the relation between allergy and immunity, pointing out that (*i*) both are brought about by the antigens of *M. tuberculosis*; (*ii*) the success of the vaccination is measured by allergic tests even by those workers who stress the independence of the two processes; (*iii*) desensitization never results in a complete elimination of allergy, since the development of the allergy induced by a repeated stimulus is accelerated (immunological memory) even in the maximally desensitized animal as compared to that induced by the primary stimulus.

Since the essence of the tuberculin-type allergy is that lymphocytes and (indirectly or directly) macrophages are sensitized to tuberculin with the consequence that macrophages, having a basic role in cell-mediated immunity, will become activated on contact with tuberculin, views emphasizing independence of allergy and immunity must be regarded as obsolete. These views originated at first from the correct observation that the intensity of allergic reactions does not in fact go parallel with measurable superinfection immunity. Much depends on the dose of the tuberculin applied. Appropriately low concentrations of tuberculin lead to the activation of macrophages while, under the same immunological conditions high concentrations cause a caseous necrosis involving the sensitized macrophages and the surrounding tissue. Thus, the long-debated question whether tuberculin allergy is harmful or useful can also be answered. It is by all means useful, since the sensitized lymphocytes and macrophages, i.e. the cells responsible for tuberculin allergy, play a basic role in the mechanism of cell-mediated immunity, but it can become harmful on account of the caseous necrosis developing if a large dose of tuberculin is introduced into the sensitized organism.

THERAPEUTICAL IMPORTANCE OF ALLERGY AND IMMUNITY

Since the discovery and clinical application of effective tuberculostatic drugs allergy and immunity in tuberculosis has obviously lost clinical interest. However, even in the face of optimal tuberculostatic therapy, cases resistant to therapy may occur. Therefore, besides other factors, the actual immunobiological state of the individuals must also be taken into consideration if an anti-tuberculous campaign is organized. The fact that, in spite of several decades' hard work, a reaction reliably reflecting the course, phases, direction and tendency of the disease could not be developed has led to a scepticism towards the value of clinico-immunological examinations. Serological reactions concerning tuberculosis can hardly be utilized in clinical practice, and this goes so far that in institutes for tuberculosis no efforts are made for the demonstration of antibodies. The situation is different with the allergic reaction. The positive tuberculin reaction reliably indicates that the organism has already been exposed to Mycobacterium. However, infection with *M. tuberculosis* induces a tuberculous process only in a small fraction of cases and, on the other hand, a positive allergic reaction can also be due to vaccination or exposure to atypical Mycobacteria. Nevertheless, by careful evaluation of individual cases the tuberculin reaction can still be utilized in many instances. Strong tuberculin reactions are suggestive of tuberculous infection, since vaccination, or atypical Mycobacteria do not elicit such reactions. Fresh conversion can also be of diagnostic value. Tuberculin reactions performed in series can particularly be valuable, since they reflect the changes in the reactivity of the organism relatively well. From the clinical point of view careful consideration of tuberculin sensitivity together with all the clinical symptoms is essential. The schemes developed earlier, e.g. the classification of Petruschky [110] and Ranke [113] used for decades, are not used any more. Reservation from the schemes cannot mean underestimation of clinical empiricism. At the bedside it should be seriously considered that strong tuberculin reactions are most frequently observed in acute tuberculous infection, in tuberculosis of lymph nodes, bones, joints and skin. In very strongly hyperreactive cases desensitization therapy may also be indicated.

On the other hand, the negative tuberculin test does not necessarily exclude the existence of a tuberculous disease. If, on the basis of other symptoms, tuberculosis may be supposed, areactivity due to poor general condition or toxic effects must be considered. Such conditions are commonly observed in severely progressed tuberculosis. Furthermore, simultaneous occurrence of tuberculosis and some other diseases, e.g. sarcoidosis or lymphogranulomatosis, which reduce tuberculin positivity should also be taken into account.

In summary, serological and allergic reactions in tuberculosis have no pathognomonic value, but with appropriate judgement they may be of help in clinical practice.

REFERENCES

1. Arima, J., Yamamoto, K., Morikawa, K. and Takahashi, Y.: *C. R. Soc. Biol.* **152**, 1292 (1958).
2. Arima, J., Yamamoto, K. and Takashashi, Y.: *C. R. Soc. Biol.* **153**, 1640 (1959).
3. Arnason, B. G., Janković, B. D., Waksman, B. H. and Wennersten, C.: *J. exp. Med.* **116**, 177 (1962).

4. Arnason, B. G. and Waksman, B. H.: *Fed. Proc.* **20**, 263 (1961).
5. Aronson, J. D.: *Amer. Rev. Tuberc.* **13**, 263 (1926).
6. Atkins, E.: Physiol. Rev. **40**, 580 (1960).
7. Baker, A. B.: *Amer. Rev. Tuberc.* **31**, 54 (1935).
8. Baldwin, E. R.: *J. med. Res.* **17**, 189 (1910).
9. Bauer, J.: *Beitr. Klin. Tuberk.* **13**, 383 (1909).
10. Benacerraf, B.: *Fed. Proc.* **27**, 46 (1968).
11. Benacerraf, B. and Bloon, B. R.: *Transplantation* **5**, 996 (1967).
12. Bentzon, J. W.: *Tubercle (Edinb.)* **34**, 34 (1953).
13. Besredka, A.: *Ann. Inst. Pasteur* **35**, 291 (1921).
14. Bessau, G.: *Klin. Wschr.* **4**, 337 (1925)
15. Billingham, R. E., Defendi, V., Silvers, W. K. and Steinmuller, D.: *J. nat. Cancer Inst.* **28**, 365 (1962).
16. Bloomfield, A. L. and Mateer, J. G.: *Amer. Rev. Tuberc.* **3**, 166 (1919).
17a. Boyden, S. V.: *Brit. J. exp. Path.* **38**, 611 (1957).
17b. id., *Progr. Allergy* **5**, 149 (1958).
18. Boyden, S. V. and Sorkin, F.: *Immunology* **3**, 272 (1960).
19. Branch, A. and Cuff, J. R.: *J. infect. Dis.* **47**, 151 (1930).
20. Brent, L., Brown, J. B. and Medawar, P. B.: In *Biological Problems of Grafting*. Ed. by Albert, F., Medawar, P. B., Blackwell, Oxford 1959.
20a. Burger, E. R., Vetto, R. M. and Malley, A.: *Science* **175**, 1473 (1972).
21. Burnet, F. M.: *Lancet* ii, 610 (1968).
22. Calmette, A.: *Ann. Inst. Pasteur* **49**, 279 (1932).
23a. Calmette, A. and Massol, L.: *C. R. Soc. Biol.* **71**, 341 (1911).
23b. id., *Ann. Inst. Pasteur* **28**, 338 (1914).
24. Canetti, G.: *L'allergie tuberculeuse chez l'homme.* Flammarion, Paris 1946, p. 40.
25. Canetti, G. and Lacaze, H.: *Ann. Inst. Pasteur* **65**, 435 (1940).
26. Chase, M. W.: *Proc. Soc. exp. Biol. Med. (N. Y.)* **59**, 134 (1945).
27. Corper, H. J., Cohn, M. L. and Damerow, A. P.: *Amer. J. clin. Path.* **10**, 361 (1940).
28. Cowling, D. C., Quaglino, D. and Davidson, E.: *Lancet* ii, 1091 (1963).
29a. Crowle, A. J.: *Amer. Rev. Tuberc.* **77**, 681 (1958).
29b. id., *Amer. Rev. resp. Dis.* **81**, 893 (1960).
30. Crowther, D., Hamilton Fairley, G. and Sewell, R. L.: *Nature* **215**, 1086 (1967).
31a. Daniel, T. M. and Baum G. L.: *Amer. Rev. resp. Dis.* **98**, 677 (1968).
31b. ibid., **99**, 249 (1969).
32. Dannenberg, A. M., jr.: *Bact. Rev.* **32**, 85 (1968).
33. Dannenberg, A. M., jr., Walter, P. C. and Kapral, F. A.: *J. Immunol.* **90**, 448 (1963).
34. David, J. R.: *Fed. Proc.* **27**, 6 (1968).
35a. Dienes, L. and Mallory, T. B.: *Amer. J. Path.* **8**, 689 (1932).
35b. id., *Proc. Soc. exp. Biol. Med. (N. Y.)* **34**, 59 (1936).
36. Enders, J. F.: *J. exp. Med.* **50**, 777 (1929).
37. Evans, D. G. and Myrvik, Q. N.: *J. Reticuloendothelial Soc.* **4**, 428 (1967).
38. Feldman, W. H.: *Amer. Rev. Tuberc.* **48**, 248 (1943).
39. Fernandez, J. M. M.: *Int. J. Lepr.* **23**, 243 (1955).
40. Fishman, M.: *J. exp. Med.* **114**, 837 (1961).
41. Fishman, M. and Adler, F. L.: *J. exp. Med.* **117**, 595 (1963).
42. Flax, M. H. and Waksman, B. H.: *J. Immunol.* **89**, 496 (1962).
43. Fleischner, E. C., Meyer, K. F. and Shaw, E. B.: *Amer. J. Dis. Child.* **18**, 577 (1919).
43a. Fogarty, J. E.: *Status of Immunization in Tuberculosis in 1971.* US Government Printing Office, Washington 1972.
44. Follis, R. H., jr.: *Bull. Johns Hopk. Hosp.* **63**, 283 (1938).
45. Fourestier, M. and Blacque-Belaire, A.: *Beitr. Klin. Tuberk.* **115**, 98 (1956).
46a. Földes, I.: In *A gümőkór.* (Tuberculosis.) Ed. by Telegdi, I. Medicina, Budapest 1959, p. 48.
46b. id., In *The Use of Radioactive Isotopes in Tuberculosis Research.* Ed. by Pasquier, J. F., Trnka, L. and Urbancik, R. Pergamon Press, London 1965, p. 93.
47. Földes, I. and Komlós, E.: *Tuberk. Kérd.* **9**, 97 (1956).
48. Földes, I. and Tomcsányi, A.: *Zbl. Bakt.* I. Abt. Ref. **194**, 213 (1964).

49a. Freerksen, E.: *Dtsch. med. Wschr.* **84**, 1533 (1959).
49b. ibid., **84**, 1617 (1959).
50. Freund, J., Laidlaw, E. H. and Mansfield, J. S.: *J. exp. Med.* **64**, 573 (1936).
51. Ganguin, H. G., Mydlak, G. and Zureck, A.: *Z. Erkr. Atmungsorg.* **130**, 101 (1969).
52. Gedigk, P. and Bontke, E.: *Arch. path. Anat.* **330**, 538 (1957).
53. Gedigk, P. and Fischer, R.: *Klin. Wschr.* **38**, 806 (1960).
54. Gell, P. G. H.: *Int. Arch. Allergy* **13**, 112 (1958).
55. Gell, P. G. H. and Hinde, I. T.: *Brit. J. exp. Path.* **32**, 516 (1951).
56. Good, R. A., Bridges, R. A. and Condie, R. M.: *Bact. Rev.* **24**, 115 (1960).
57. Gowans, J. L. and Knight, E. J.: *Proc. Soc. exp. Biol. Med.* (*N. Y.*) **87**, 249 (1964).
58. Grogg, E. and Pearse, A. G. E.: *Brit. J. exp. Path.* **33**, 567 (1952).
59. Guld, J., Bentzon, M. W., Bleiker, M. A., Griep, W. A., Magnusson, M. and Waaler, H.: *Bull. Wld. Hlth. Org.* **19**, 845 (1958).
60. Hall, C. H. and Atkins, E.: *J. exp. Med.* **109**, 339 (1959).
61. Hall, J. G.: *J. exp. Med.* **121**, 737 (1965).
62. Hall, J. G. and Morris, B.: *Lancet* **i**, 1077 (1964).
63a. Haxthausen, H.: *Acta derm.-venereol.* (*Stockh.*) **31**, 42 (1951).
63b. ibid., **31**, 659 (1951).
64. Iland, C. N. and Barker, R. M.: *Tubercle* (*Edinb.*) **40**, 235 (1959).
65. Inderbitzin, T.: *Int. Arch. Allergy* **8**, 150 (1956).
66. Jankovič, B. D., Waksman, B. H. and Arnason, B. G.: *J. exp. Med.* **116**, 159 (1962).
67. Johanovsky, J.: *Nature* **183**, 693 (1959).
68. Julianelle, L. A.: *J. exp. Med.* **51**, 625 (1930).
69. Kaliss, N.: *Cancer Res.* **18**, 992 (1958).
70. Kallós, P. and Kentzler, J.: *Beitr. Klin. Tuberk.* **79**, 584 (1932).
71. Kelly, W. D., Good, R. A. and Varco, R. L.: *Surg. Gynec. Obstet.* **107**, 565 (1958).
72. Kelly, W. D., Varco, R. L. and Good, R. A.: *J. clin. Invest.* **37**, 906 (1958).
73. Kertay, N. and Medveczky, E.: *Tuberkulózis* **12**, 222 (1959).
74. Kirchheimer, W. F. and Weiser, R. S.: *Proc. Soc. exp. Biol. Med.* (*N. Y.*) **66**, 166 (1947).
75. Klopstock, F.: *Dtsch. med. Wschr.* **49**, 1511 (1923).
76. Koch, R.: *Dtsch. med. Wschr.* **17**, 1189 (1891).
77. Kosunen, T. U.; cited by *Advanc. Tuberc. Res.* **13**, 1 (1964).
78. Kourilsky, R. and Decroix, G.: *C. R. Soc. Biol.* **146**, 235 (1952).
79. Landsteiner, K.: *The Specificity of Serological Reactions.* Harvard University Press, Cambridge 1947, p. 132.
80. Landsteiner, K. and Chase, M. W.: *Proc. Soc. exp. Biol. Med.* (*N. Y.*) **49**, 688 (1942).
81. Laporte, R.: *Ann. Inst. Pasteur* **53**, 598 (1934).
82a. Lawrence, H. S.: *Proc. Soc. exp. Biol. Med.* (*N. Y.*) **71**, 516 (1949).
82b. id., *J. clin. Invest.* **34**, 219 (1955).
82c. id., In *Cellular and Humoral Aspects of the Hypersensitive States.* Ed. by Lawrence, H. S. Hoeber, New York 1959, p. 279.
83. Levendel, L.: *Acta tuberc. scand.* **33**, 157 (1957).
84. Levendel, L. and Simon, T.: *Orv. Hetil.* **95**, 459 (1954).
85a. Lind, A.: *Serological Studies of Mycobacteria by Means of Diffusion-in-gel Technique.* Göteborg 1961, p. 311.
85b. id., *Amer. Rev. resp. Dis.* **92**, 54 (1965).
86. Long, E. R. and Seibert, F. B.: *Amer. Rev. Tuberc.* **13**, 448 (1926).
87. Long, J. B. and Favour, C. B.: *Bull. Johns Hopk. Hosp.* **87**, 186 (1950).
88. Lurie, M. B., Abramson, S., Heppleston, A. G. and Allison, J. M.: *Amer. Rev. Tuberc.* **59**, 198 (1949).
89. Lurie, M. B., Harris, T. N., Abramson, S. and Allison, J. M.: *Amer. Rev. Tuberc.* **59**, 186 (1949).
90. Mackaness, G. B. and Blanden, R. V.: *Progr. Allergy* **11**, 89 (1967).
91. Mantoux, C.: *Presse méd.* **18**, 10 (1910).
92. Marshall, W. H. and Roberts, K. B.: *Lancet* **i**, 773 (1963).
93. Massol, L., Breton, M. and Bruyant, L.: *C. R. Soc. Biol.* **74**, 185 (1913).

94. McCluskey, R. T. and Benacerraf, B.: cited by *Advanc. Tuberc. Res.* **13**, 1 (1964).
95a. Medawar, P. B.: *J. Anat. (Lond.)* **78**, 176 (1944).
95b. id., *Ann. N. Y. Acad. Sci.* **68**, 255 (1957).
96a. Meissner, J.: *Jber. Borstel* **5**, 841 (1961).
96b. id., *Rozhl. Tuberk.* **24**, 441 (1964).
96c. id., *Beitr. Klin. Tuberk.* **130**, 142 (1965).
97a. Metaxas, M. N. and Metaxas-Bühler, M.: *Proc. Soc. exp. Biol. Med. (N. Y.)* **69**, 163 (1948).
97b. id., *J. Immunol.* **75**, 333 (1955).
97c. id., In *Immunopathology.* 1st Int. Symp. Ed. by Graber, P. and Miescher, P. A. Schwabe, Basel 1958, p. 286.
98. Middlebrook, G.: *Amer. Rev. Tuberc.* **62**, 223 (1950).
99a. Middlebrook, G. and Dubos, R. J.: *J. exp. Med.* **88**, 521 (1948).
99b. id., *Amer. Rev. Tuberc.* **58**, 700 (1948).
100. Mills, J. A.: *J. Immunol.* **97**, 239 (1966).
101. Mitchell, A. G., Wherry, W. B., Eddy, B. and Stevenson, F. E.: *Amer. J. Dis. Child.* **36**, 720 (1928).
102a. Najarian, J. S. and Feldman, J. D.: *J. exp. Med.* **114**, 779 (1961).
102b. ibid., **115**, 1083 (1962).
102c. id., *Fed. Proc.* **21**, 41 (1962).
103. Nalbant, J. P.: *Amer. Rev. Tuberc.* **36**, 773 (1937).
104. Nelson, D. S. and Boyden, S. V.: *Brit. med. Bull.* **23**, 15 (1967).
105. Oppenheim, J. J.: *Fed. Proc.* **27**, 21 (1968).
106. Osgood, C. K. and Favour, C. B.: *J. exp. Med.* **94**, 415 (1951).
107. Patterson, P. Y.: In *Immunopathology.* 2nd Int. Symp. Ed. by Grabar, P. and Miescher, P. A. Schwabe, Basel 1962, p. 184.
108. Pepys, J.: *Amer. Rev. Tuberc.* **71**, 49 (1955).
109. Petroff, S. A.: *Amer. Rev. Tuberc.* **7**, 412 (1923).
110. Petruschky, J.: *Grundriss der spezifischen Diagnostik und Therapie der Tuberkulose.* Leineweber, Leipzig 1913, p. 38.
111. Pirquet, von C.: *Arch. intern. Med.* **7**, 259 (1911).
112. Platt, H.: *J. comp. Path. Ther.* **64**, 312 (1954).
113. Ranke, K. E.: *Beitr. Klin. Tuberk.* **52**, 212 (1922).
114a. Rees, R. J. W.: *Brit. J. exp. Path.* **45**, 207 (1964).
114b. id., *Int. J. Lepr.* **33**, 646 (1965).
114c. id., *Nature* **211**, 657 (1966).
115. Ribi, E.: Personal communication.
116. Rich, A. R. and Lewis, M. R.: *Bull. Johns Hopk. Hosp.* **50**, 115 (1932).
117. Robson, J. M., Sullivan, F. M. and Didcock, K. A.: *Brit. J. exp. Path.* **38**, 172 (1957).
118. Rosenau, W.: *Fed. Proc.* **27**, 34 (1968).
119. Schrek, R.: *Amer. Rev. resp. Dis.* **87**, 734 (1963).
120. Schwartz, P.: *Empfindlichkeit und Schwindsucht.* Barth, Leipzig 1935, p. 59.
121. Seeberg, G.: *Acta derm.-venereol. (Stockh.)* **27**, Suppl. 18 (1947).
122. Seibert, F. B.: *Chem. Rev.* **34**, 107 (1944).
123. Shepard, C. C.: *Amer. J. Hyg.* **71**, 147 (1960).
124. Sipos, K.: *Acta med. Acad. Sci. Hung.* **6**, Suppl. 1, 84 (1954).
125. Smith, D. W., Grover, A. A. and Wiegeshaus, E.: *Advanc. Tuberc. Res.* **16**, 191 (1968).
126. Spector, W. G.: *Brit. med Bull.* **23**, 35 (1967).
127. Stavitsky, A. B.: *Proc. Soc. exp. Biol. Med. (N. Y.)* **67**, 225 (1948).
128. Stetson, C. A.: In *Cellular and Humoral Aspects of the Hypersensitive States.* Ed. by Lawrence, H. S. Hoeber, New York 1959, p. 442.
129. Ström, L.: *Acta tuberc. scand.* **21**, 141 (1955).
130. Ström, L. and Widström, G.: *Acta paediat. (Uppsala)* **40**, 213 (1952).
131. Suter, E.: *Trans. N. Y. Acad. Sci.* Ser. 2. **24**, 281 (1962).
132. Takahashi, Y., Fujita, S. and Sasaki, A.: *J. exp. Med.* **113**, 1141 (1961).
133. Takahashi, Y., and Ono, K.: *Amer. Rev. resp. Dis.* **83**, 381 (1961).
134. Thor, D. E.: *Fed. Proc.* **27**, 16 (1968).
135. Tóth, F.: *Tuberkulózis és Tüdőbetegségek (Budapest)* **20**, 188 (1967).
136. Trudeau, E. L., Baldwin, E. R. and Kinghorn, H. M.: *J. med. Res.* **12**, 169 (1904).

137. Uhr, J. W. and Scharff, M.: *J. clin. Invest.* **38**, 1049 (1959).
138. Ustvedt, H. J. and Aanonsen, A.: *Acta tuberc. scand.* **23**, 1 (1949).
139. Vollmer, H.: *J. Pediat.* **39**, 22 (1951).
140. Waksman, B. H., Arnason, B. G. and Jankovič, B. D.: *J. exp. Med.* **116**, 187 (1962).
141. Waksman, B. H. and Matoltsy, M.: *J. Immunol.* **81**, 235 (1958).
142. Weiszfeiler, J. G.: *Die Biologie und Variabilität des Tuberkelbakteriums und die atypischen Mykobakterien.* Akadémiai Kiadó, Budapest 1969, p. 289.
143. Weiszfeiler, J. G. and Karasseva, V.: *Acta microbiol. Acad. Sci. hung.* **7**, 77 (1960).
144. Wijsmuller, G.: *Bull. Wld. Hlth. Org.* **35**, 459 (1966).
145. Yamori, T.: *Acta path. jap.* **14**, 1 (1964).
146a. Youmans, G. P. and Youmans, A. S.: *J. Immunol.* **78**, 318 (1957).
146b. id., *J. Bact.* **90**, 1675 (1965).
147. Zilber, L. A.: *Osznovü Immuniteta.* Medgiz, Moszkva 1948.
148. Zinsser, H.: *J. exp. Med.* **34**, 495 (1921).
149. Zinsser, H., and Grinnekk, F. B.: *J. Immunol.* **10**, 725 (1925).

CHAPTER 73

IMMUNOALLERGOLOGIC ASPECTS OF SYPHILIS

by

K. KIRÁLY

Abbreviations used in the text

BFP	biologically false positive
FTA	fluorescent treponemal antibody
FTA-ABS	absorbed fluorescent treponemal antibody

RPCF   Reiter protein complement fixation
RPR   rapid plasma reagin
STS   standard test(s) for syphilis
T   treponema
TPHA   *T. pallidum* haemagglutination
TPI   *T. pallidum* immobilization

INTRODUCTION

DEFINITION OF SYPHILIS AND OTHER TREPONEMATOSES. THEIR INTERRELATIONSHIP

Syphilis is a chronic infectious disease caused by *T.'pallidum,* systemic from the outset. Since virtually any organ or tissue may be affected, syphilis simulates many diseases. Short symptomatic phases alternate with long asymptomatic periods. A mother may transmit the disease to her offspring. If untreated, syphilis may give rise to vitally dangerous or disabling neurologic or vascular disorders. The variations of the clinical picture are the result of the changing relationship between the host and the pathogen, the degree of immunity, and the hyperergic inflammatory reaction. Many details of these relationships, and also the mechanism of the diverse clinical manifestations, are not yet clearly understood.

There are other treponematoses with an essentially benign course not causing involvement of internal organs or transplacental infection. Endemic syphilis is transmitted by direct or indirect, non-venereal contact in early childhood. It occurs in warm arid areas of the Middle East, Africa and Asia. Initially it is characterized by lesions on the mucous membrane of the mouth which is the most common site of infection. Skin and bone lesions resembling those of venereal syphilis appear later. Transplacental transmission to the foetus or destructive processes of the internal organs have not been observed. It conveys immunity against venereal syphilis. It is not known whether its benign course is inherent in the germ, due to ecological influences, or to specificity of the immune response of childhood.

Yaws is a treponematosis of humid tropical areas, beginning in early childhood. The causative organism, *T. pertenue,* is transmitted by direct contact. Its first sign is a primary papular skin lesion (mother yaw) followed by a generalized eruption of macular or typical raspberry lesions. A late stage is characterized by destructive incapacitating lesions of the the skin and bones, particularly of the superior maxilla (gundu), palatonasal structures (gangosa) and hyperkeratosis of the soles.

Another chronic benign disease, caused by *T. carateum* is pinta, often beginning between the ages of ten and fifteen years and occurring mainly in Central and South America, the Caribbean and, earlier, in Cuba. The clinical course is especially mild, characterized by an initial papular lesion on the hands or legs followed by a maculopapular scaling erythematous rash, lasting for years. In the late stage, permanent achromic or pigmented spots occur on the distal parts of the extremities.

Hudson [60] sees *T. pallidum* and *T. pertenue* as one, and ascribes the different clinical syndromes to environmental and social variables. The rather striking difference between yaws, endemic syphilis and venereal syphilis is the relative mildness and ubiquity of yaws and endemic syphilis in their favoured environment and the gravity of venereal syphilitic complications involving the central nervous system and the heart, and the possibility of congenital infections. The difference seems to be only in quantitative and locational degrees. Yaws is most commonly acquired under conditions of very close association and constantly moist skin. It has been noted in several tropical areas that the incidence of yaws decreases progressively with altitude. This effect becomes discernible at about 500 metres. Where the temperature falls more than about 2.5 °C below the mean characteristic of the equatorial lowlands, the occurrence of yaws is less frequent. Humidity is another variable to which yaws treponemes are very sensitive and areas of sub-humid climate or even those exposed to a high risk of drought should be regarded as precarious. The manifestation of the disease is complicated further by the microclimate of the human skin, variables such as the degree of skin exposure related to clothing habits and by levels of sanitation, use of soap, living densities and, possibly, soil types. Where yaws was prevalent but ecologically vulnerable as, for example, in Tahiti, the pattern of the disease may have been changed by human action so as to resemble gradually venereal syphilis.

A major effect of yaws, pinta and of endemic syphilis is that it confers a considerable immunity to venereal syphilis, so that the populations of most endemic tropical areas were protected to the extent to which they were ubiquitous. Until they were virtually eliminated by mass campaigns employing penicillin, venereal syphilis was practically unknown in rural populations inhabiting the more humid equatorial areas.

PATHOGENICITY OF TREPONEMES TO ANIMALS

T. pallidum does not affect animals in the natural state, but the rabbit and the higher apes are susceptible to experimental inoculation. Our present knowledge regarding the relationship between the pathogen and the host organism is based to a great extent on rabbit experiments. In addition, *T. pallidum* is capable of prolonged survival in the organism of certain animals (mouse, rat), in certain species (guinea pig, golden hamster) provoking any or slight clinical symptoms. Asymptomatic survival may be shown by transplantation of their organs into rabbits intratesticularly or subscrotally. All other animal species are resistant to *T. pallidum*. The cause and the mechanism of non-responsiveness are obscure.

Certain animals, however, may be affected by other pathogenic treponematoses. The rabbit treponematosis transmitted sexually is caused by *T. cuniculi*, a species not pathogenic to humans. A treponematosis, presumably caused by *T. pertenue*, is frequent among gorillas [49] and cynocephali [41] in certain parts of Africa. Kuhn and Brown [84] have found that about 15 per cent of chimpanzees tested were reactive in TPI test. The natural course of this monkey treponematosis has not been studied.

T. pallidum and the other pathogenic treponemes are not cultivable *in vitro*: they survive for 4 to 5 days in special media without multiplying. A large number of *T. pallidum* can be harvested, however, from intratesticularly infected rabbits. Several authors have claimed the cultivation of treponemes *in vitro* from syphilitic efflorescences. These so-called cultivable strains (Reiter, Kazan, Budapest, Noguchi, etc.) are non-pathogenic; they are presumably saprophytic treponemes invading the tissue together with *T. pallidum*. Several of them have the same antigenic structure as the treponemes isolated from the mouth [33]. Cultivable treponemes have the same requirements for growth as the pathogenic strains; their micromorphology and antigenic structure are also similar. Much of our knowledge regarding the biology of *T. pallidum* is based on the study of cultivable treponemes.

ANTIGENIC STRUCTURE OF TREPONEMES

ANTIGENICITY AND ELECTRON MICROSCOPIC ANATOMY

The ultrastructure of pathogenic and non-pathogenic treponemes is similar and quite complex. Different organelles are described; however, due to the lack of combined histochemical and electron-microscopic examinations, their function and chemical structure is rather conjectural. The pathogenic *T. pallidum* consists of the following main elements: a protoplasmic cylinder bounded by several semi-rigid limiting membranes somewhat analogous to the usual cell wall of bacteria; an outer envelope; a frail triple-layered membrane which encases the entire organism; between the cell membrane and the envelope a bundle of parallel series of round fibres traverse the length of the protoplasmic cylinder in a helical arrangement; an amorphous layer surrounding the organisms isolated from human syphilitic lesions. Within the protoplasmic cylinder the following main organelles are described: attached to the protoplasmic cell wall, and protruding both inward into the cylinder and outward into the intermediate space, multilaminated bodies, presumably analogous to the mesosomes of other bacteria; attached to the inside of the cell wall, and oriented in semi-longitudinal bundles, the deep fibres which contribute to the structural integrity and elasticity of the protoplasmic cylinder; osmiophilic bodies, thought to be ribosomes. At each extremity of the treponemes there are rather dense bodies resembling the heads of snakes. These serve as points of insertion or origin of the fibrils. The actual point of insertion of the fibril is slightly raised, disc-like, denser and larger than the fibril itself. This end piece, termed 'basal granule' or 'blepharoplast' lies within the cytoplasmic substance.

An unusual feature of the treponemes is the outer envelope membrane composed of protein, lipid and carbohydrate. The envelope is more pliable and is more easily ruptured than the protoplasmic cylinder wall. The latter structure corresponds to the bacterial cell walls of bacilli and cocci. The partial loss of the envelope 3 h after penicillin treatment [127b] suggests that it is built of mureinic acid, and the murein sacculus formation is inhibited by penicillin. The amorphous material surrounding the pathogenic treponemes may be a mucoid material: acid mucopolysaccharides which have been described in early orchitis of rabbits and in hard chancre, as well as in other lesions of secondary syphilis [170]. This material seems to protect the treponemes against the antibody response of the host and impede phagocytosis in a manner analogous to the hyaluronic capsule of streptococci. Its existence is in congruency with the fact that treponemes isolated freshly will not fluoresce in FTA test and are not affected by syphilitic sera in the TPI test [106]. The DNA-containing mesosomes are thought [180] to account for the beading fluorescence observed in FTA-ABS with lupus erythematosus sera [122].

74

As shown by absorption experiments, the lipids and the bulk of antigens shared with non-pathogenic treponemes are covered. .They may be present in the envelope and/or in the protoplasm. If the group-specific proteins are disguised either by ultrasonic treatment or digestion in macrophages during immunization, or by the destruction of heat labile membrane components, the lipid antigens and group-specific proteins or the corresponding antibodies may also be demonstrated immunologically.

IMMUNOCHEMISTRY

As may be predicted from their ultrastructure, the antigenic composition of treponemes is very complex. Extracts vary according to the method applied and contain different structural elements which are mosaics with different corpuscular size, chemical composition and antigenicity. As a rule they can be fractionated further by centrifugation, electrophoresis, gel filtration [153], ion exchange chromatography [3], precipitation by different chemical reagents, or simply by heat treatment. If a more harsh extraction method is applied, chemically characterizable, more or less homogeneous products result. The components of a crude extract or product are used either as antigens for syphilis serology, for the demonstration of antigens involved in treponemal tests, or for the study of the antigenic relationship between pathogenic and cultivable strains of T. pallidum or cultured strains of saprophytic treponemes.

Most of the work has been done on cultured treponemes, particularly on the Reiter strain, as sufficient quantities are available for analysis. Immunochemical study is hardly possible with pathogenic T. pallidum, since this organism has not so far been cultivated in the virulent state, if at all, and only relatively small quantities are procurable for investigation. The only practical source is cultivation in rabbit testes and as has been shown by immunological studies [102], the suspension, even after several centrifugations, cannot be freed from the testicular debris.

The disruption of treponemes for antigen analysis has been accomplished by cryolysis [20], ultrasonic disruption [80], chemical procedure [138b], trypsin digestion [47] and recently by Ribi cell fragmentation. This last technique, under highly controlled conditions of pressure, provides a method for obtaining protoplasmic antigens and facilitates the separation of cell wall and axial filaments [3].

Expressed in terms of coarse chemistry, desiccated treponemes contain about 67–70 per cent protein, 15–20 per cent lipids, 5 per cent carbohydrates and nucleic acids [58]. By freezing and thawing and consecutive precipitation with ammonium sulphate [20] or sonication and precipitation with trichloroacetic acid [131], a thermolabile antigen specifically reactive with human sera of patients with venereal syphilis and endemic treponematoses can be obtained from T. reiteri and other cultured treponemes [53]. The extract is widely used in the serodiagnosis of treponematoses. Its bulk consists of protein(s) shared with pathogenic treponemes [23], and it is referred to as group-specific protein antigen. The antigen contains two components when separated by electrophoresis [20] and three in gel diffusion with specific immune serum; one is reactive with syphilitic serum [134].

In ultrasonically disrupted pathogenic *T. pallidum* suspension two proteins may be detected: the group-specific protein shared with non-pathogenic treponemes and a protein present only in pathogenic ones [70d]. The latter can only be obtained in pure form, after ether-acetone and deoxycholate treatment. The extract reacts with syphilitic serum but fails to do so with rabbit anti-*T. reiteri* serum [138a]. Judging from its failure to inhibit the TPI test, this protein does not seem to be involved in the immobilization of treponemes [70e]. The antigen may, however, be used for diagnostic tests.

Polysaccharides may be extracted from cultivable [29, 118a] and pathogenic [13a] treponemes. The fraction isolated by Nell and Hardy [118a] from the Reiter treponeme appears to be among those which are purer chemically with only traces of proteins. This antigen seems to be species-specific [134]. The antigen was active in the usual *in vitro* test with specific antisera to the Reiter treponeme and also with sera from animals immunized with other strains of cultivable treponemes – non-reactive, however, with syphilitic rabbit serum. Polysaccharide extracts from pathogenic treponemes obtained from rabbit testes are shown to be immunologically active, but essentially similar fractions have been obtained from normal rabbit testicular extracts [13b]. With due reservation concerning impurity caused by tissue debris, there seems also to be a difference between polysaccharides of pathogenic treponemes: an ultracentrifugally homogeneous polysaccharide isolated from the Nichols strain reacts with homologous rabbit but not with human syphilitic sera [112]. Heat stable polysaccharide antigens may be involved in the TPI test [22].

A lipopolysaccharide antigen has been isolated from *T. reiteri* [21] and from the rabbit-adapted Nichols strain [113]. This antigen reacts only occasionally with human serum.

Lipids account for about 15–20 per cent of dry weight of treponemes. Beside triglycerids, cardiolipin, lecithin and other phospholipids could also be detected. Biochemical analysis did not reveal much difference in the cellular fatty acid composition of pathogenic and cultivable treponemes. The antigen responsible for seroreactivity is cardiolipin. Cardiolipin is widespread in nature. It has been prepared from many mammalian tissues, some bacteria and even budding plants (sitolipin). Cardiolipins isolated from different sources vary regarding the number of free OH groups, length of fatty acids and the number of double bonds in the molecule. Though homogeneous fractions may be obtained chromatographically, due to the variety of antibodies produced during the infection, these homogeneous fractions have no advantage over the original crude mixture obtained by chemical extraction. Due to their inexpensive preparation, lipid antigens containing cardiolipin, lecithin and cholesterol are used routinely in screening tests for treponematoses. Glucolipids may also be isolated from Reiter treponemes. Antibodies, cross-reacting with them are present in patients suffering from demyelinating processes of the central nervous system [31].

Cardiolipin is a hapten which becomes antigenic if combined with proteins, as it is present originally in treponemes. Wassermann antibody can be produced in rabbits with a precipitate consisting of the lipid antigen used for syphilis serodiagnosis and syphilitic human or rabbit serum.

Only cultivable and pathogenic treponemes may be differentiated by immuno-chemical and immunological methods as described above; no differences can be demonstrated between different pathogenic strains, or even species of treponemes. Antibodies produced in endemic treponematoses and venereal syphilis are the same. All attempts to show the existence of yaws-specific antibodies have failed. Superinfections, and the different clinical course of infection in humans and animals indicate difference in the pathogenicity (and presumably antigenicity) of the different strains and species of treponemes. Some strains have shown the following preference for skin symptoms according to animal host [174]:

Strain	Skin symptom		
	rabbit	guinea pig	golden hamster
Nichols strain of veneral syphilis	+	±	—
Bosnia strain of endemic syphilis	+	+	+
Brazzaville strain of yaws	+	—	+

ANTIBODIES FORMED IN THE COURSE OF SYPHILITIC INFECTION

WASSERMANN ANTIBODY (REAGIN)

This antibody reacts with the cardiolipin component of treponemes. It is produced in large quantities in all treponemal infections, and appears 3–6 weeks after infection. The amount of antibody tends to correlate directly and quite immediately with the number of treponemes: it waxes as the number and tissue reaction increases and wanes as they decline. Its detection remains the chief procedure used for the laboratory diagnosis of syphilis. The Wassermann anti-body is characteristic but not absolutely specific for syphilis: sometimes it is present in sera of healthy individuals, or patients without any clinical evidence of syphilis (biologically false positive reactors — BFP). With refined methods [66, 94] it can be shown in minute amounts in almost all human sera. In the presence of certain non-treponemal conditions the amount of Wassermann anti-body may increase to the point of giving positive results with the standard tests for syphilis (STS).

There is no indication that the Wassermann antibody plays any role in the immune process. The antibody is not treponemicidal nor does it give protection against infection. Sera of rabbits immunized with Kahn precipitate or BFP human sera do not immobilize treponemes; rabbits immunized with Kahn pre-cipitate, remain susceptible to syphilis [32]. It is a well-known clinical finding too, that early syphilitic patients, though Wassermann positive, may be reinfected after treatment. The quantity of Wassermann antibody bears no direct relation-ship to immunity. The titre of the antibody is often high at a time when resistance to infection is poorly developed, and the titre is often low when resistance is high.

As was shown by separation with gel filtration [4], ultracentrifugation [24], preparative electrophoresis [88, 89, 90] and mercaptoethanol treatment [166], Wassermann antibody could be found in the IgG (7S or slow) and IgM (19S, fast or mercaptoethanol sensitive) classes of immunoglobulins, both in syphilitic and BFP sera. IgM antibodies are the first to appear after infection in humans [166], as well as in rabbits [125]. The majority of BFP sera contain only IgM class Wassermann antibodies [167]. These observations have not found an interpretation in clinical terms. Despite the higher C fixing capacity of IgM type antibodies, no difference between C fixing and precipitating antibodies has been shown: both are absorbed with a lipid antigen emulsion. There is evidence [147, 152] of the existence of univalent antibodies.

The origin of Wassermann antibody has been extensively discussed. Its presence in sera of patients without clinical and other laboratory evidence of treponematoses (BFP reactors) suggests that it is an autoantibody developed in response to tissue cardiolipins liberated during the infection. This hypothesis does not explain why Wassermann antibodies are produced almost uniquely and certainly spectacularly in treponemal infections, even if the course is asymptomatic. Bacterial or other diseases causing serious tissue damage elicit a positive STS only rarely. On the other hand, rabbits immunized with killed *T. pallidum* produce Wassermann antibodies without any destructive tissue reaction.

As has been shown by experimental disease in rabbits, and several decades of clinical experience, the level of Wassermann antibodies reflects in a general way the activity of syphilis. Its quantitative determination is a routine follow-up of patients to establish the end result of treatment.

IMMOBILIZIN

Nelson [119a, 120] while conducting experiments on the survival of *T. pallidum*, discovered, that its motility is arrested in the presence of syphilitic serum and C. The antibody responsible for this phenomenon is called immobilizin. It is not identical with the Wassermann antibody, since it cannot be absorbed from syphilitic serum by lipid antigens; on the other hand, sera containing Wassermann antibody do not immobilize treponemes [120], neither do immune sera prepared with non-pathogenic *(T. microdentium)* or cultivable (Reiter and Kazan) treponemes [46, 69]. Only pathogenic strains *(T. pallidum, T. pertenue, T. carateum, T. cuniculi)* induce the production of immobilizin. Several antiviral and antibacterial immune sera have been examined for their effect on *T. pallidum* and none of them caused immobilization [123]. Immobilizin seems to be specific for pathogenic treponemes.

Immobilizin belongs to the IgG class of immunoglobulins: its sedimentation constant is 7S [175a, b], in continuous flow electrophoresis it appears in the slow γ-globulin fraction [137], and in Sephadex gel filtrate in the IgG peak [73]. It is resistant to heating at 70–72 °C for 10 minutes [120] and to storage in the sterile state at 37 °C for 5 weeks [55]. Its titre remains unchanged in lyophilized sera and in sera stored at − 20 °C.

The antigen which induces immobilizin production has not so far been identified. It survives the death of *T. pallidum*, as immobilizin can be absorbed from syphilitic sera by means of killed treponemes [141], and is produced also in animals so immunized [53a]. As shown by immunization experiments in rabbits and by absorption of syphilitic sera with heat-treated treponemes, the antigens reacting with immobilizin are both thermolabile and thermostable [22], which is why heated treponemes are less efficient antigens than those unheated.

The immobilization of treponemes is a slow process, lasting for 16 to 18 hours: some 12 to 14 hours are necessary for the binding of the immobilizin, and the major part of this time is required for the dissolution of the slimy envelope. The latter may be speeded up by lysozyme [106], trypsin or papain [77] which shorten the incubation time necessary for specific immobilization aggravating the damage inflicted immunologically [115a]. Immobilized treponemes are non-viable: rabbits [120] and mice [91a] cannot be infected with such treponemes. Even motile treponemes incubated with syphilitic serum for a certain time become non-pathogenic [163].

The ultrastructure of specifically immobilized treponemes indicates that lysis is occurring: the outlines of the cells become blurred, the convolutions are less marked, the cell wall is discontinuous and protoplasm extrudes through the gaps [50].

FLUORESCENT TREPONEMAL ANTIBODY (FTA)

Antibodies present in syphilitic serum are bound to the surface of treponemes fixed on a slide and become visible when examined by dark ground microscopy with an ultraviolet light source if stained with fluorescein-labelled anti-human globulin. There is no fluorescence unless there is antibody in the serum [25].

During syphilis, two types of antibody detectable by indirect immunofluorescence tests with treponemes are produced. One is specific for *T. pallidum* and for other pathogenic treponemes; the other is a group-reactive antibody which reacts with *T. pallidum* and with a wide variety of cultivable [27] and commensal treponemes [68, 74] and with *Borrelia hispanica* [42] because of shared antigens. After absorption with Reiter treponemes, the titre of syphilitic sera is reduced to 20–25 per cent of the original level [70c]. The group-reactive antibody is found in most normal non-syphilitic sera at a low titre, probably produced in response to the normal flora of commensal treponemes. Higher titres of group-reactive antibodies are found in the sera of elderly persons [57] and in some diseases (balanitis, stomatitis) accompanied by a heavy growth of saprophytic treponemes [70c]. The fluorescent antibody is distinct from the reagin: the latter can be absorbed from the serum without a reduction of the FTA titre [133, 181]. Differences in the kinetics of the tests and of their behaviour in the course of syphilis suggest that the antibodies involved in the TPI test are different from those involved in the FTA test.

The antibody is resistant to physical influences. Dried blood absorbed on blotting paper rondelles and eluted in saline can be used for the test [176]. Heating is also tolerated; the antibody is inactivated above 62 °C [160].

As was shown by monospecific conjugates reacting with a single immunoglobulin class, antibodies are present in IgA, IgM and IgG classes of immunoglobulins [71, 103]. They are present in the peaks containing IgM and IgG globulins after Sephadex gel filtration [64, 73] as well as in the fast and slow fractions of electrophoretically separated sera [137].

The antigen reacting with FTA has not so far been identified. Both the group- and the T. pallidum-specific antigens consist of a thermolabile and a thermostable component [70e].

Foetal antibodies produced in response to intrauterine infections occur in the IgM fraction of foetal blood, whereas passively transferred maternal antibodies are found in the IgG fractions. The total serum IgM levels are also commonly elevated in infants with neonatal infections. Serological tests designated to diagnose or exclude congenital syphilis after birth have been developed. Their basis is the FTA or FTA-ABS technique, demonstrating IgM class antitreponemal antibody. The presence of IgM antitreponemal antibody in the newborn infant's serum suggests that congenital infection has occurred. Transplacental leakage is con- trolled by the presence of ABO isoagglutinins. Lack of IgM antibodies in the sera of newborns does not exclude the possibility of syphilitic infection. If the mother was infected in the last months of pregnancy, IgM antibodies may appear only from 3 to 5 weeks after birth [63]. In this case it may be presumed that the deficiency of antibody production in the newborn is a reflection of the presence of high levels of transmitted maternal antibodies. After birth the newborn is released from this inhibitory 'blanketing' effect.

IgM class antibodies disappear from sera earlier after adequate treatment. Primary syphilis cases with non-reactive STS remain IgM positive for 1 to 6 months after treatment (average 3 months), treated seropositive primary syphilis for an average of 6 months (range 3–16 months), treated secondary and early latent cases for an average of 8 months. IgM type antibodies disappear, even from sera of patients with congenital syphilis, 2.5 years after treatment. IgM positivity seems to be a better indicator of therapeutic success than classical STS: only in 28 per cent of patients treated was IgM class antibody positive. Persistence of IgM for years seems to indicate relapse or reinfection. An indirect proof of this is the higher prevalence of IgM antibodies in promiscuous male homosexuals frequently exposed to reinfection and the negativation of resistant cases after retreatment [126].

AGGLUTININ

Agglutinin was one of the first antibodies described in syphilitic patients [186] but it has scarcely been studied.

Freshly prepared suspension of T. pallidum is but weakly agglutinated by syphilitic serum. Agglutinability may be increased by heating to 65 °C or prolonged storage at 4 °C [53a] as also by lysozyme, papain or trypsin digestion [108a], after dissolution of the slimy layer covering the treponemes [108b]. The agglutina- tion may be enhanced by conglutinin of bovine serum [96c], or by binding Ca ions with EDTA inhibiting the agglutination.

Two antigens are involved: a thermostable and a thermolabile [53b], presumably proteins, as they may be destroyed by treatment with trypsin [108c]. A tissue antigen must be present on the surface of T. pallidum, as treponemes are aggluti- nated also by the serum of chickens or goats immunized by rabbit testis [65]. The antigen responsible for the agglutination depends, therefore, on the method of the treatment of treponemes. Both reagin and treponemal antibodies are involved in the agglutination of heat-treated treponemes: the suspension is agglutinated by the serum of rabbits immunized with the lipid hapten [53a]; the agglutinin titre of most syphilitic sera decreases [53a] or sometimes disappears completely [70a] after absorption with lipid antigens. The *T. pallidum* agglutination test is not used for diagnostic purposes: BFP sera agglutinate treponemes in 14.5 to 29.0 per cent of cases [35, 53a]. However, cross-agglutination is used for the comparison of different treponemal species and strains. On the other hand, agglutination using *T. reiteri* suspension as antigen is a sensitive diagnostic test for examination of the cerebrospinal fluid [145].

IMMUNE ADHERENCE ANTIBODY

T. pallidum, if incubated with syphilitic serum and C at 37 °C for one hour, adheres to human erythrocytes and disappears from the supernatant after the centrifugation of the red blood cells. The treponemes reappear if the red cells are haemolysed. The phenomenon is called the immune adherence of treponemes [119b]. *T. pallidum* adheres also to bacteria, e.g. to *E. coli*, *Str. pyogenes*, *S. lactis*, etc., to the platelets of man, rabbit and guinea pig, and further, to collodion particles [87]. The adherence of treponemes to corpuscle elements promotes their phagocytosis: if the reaction mixture contains leukocytes, hardly one-third of the treponemes added may be recovered from the sediment [119b]. The phenomenon occurs with treponemal suspensions exposing different antigenic receptors (intact living, killed either by storage or by heat, enzymatically digested, etc.) i.e. with different antibodies having the common feature of fixing C [79]. Beside the reagin [87], adherence is observed in the presence of syphilitic sera absorbed with lipid antigen [19, 119b]. The antibodies involved are distinct from immobilizin: they appear in experimental syphilis earlier than immobilizin. The reaction, though simple to carry out, is not used for the laboratory diagnosis of syphilis.

When treponemal suspension and syphilitic serum were mixed and injected into the peritoneal cavity of normal guinea pigs, a similar disappearance of treponemes from the punctate was observed [158]. This procedure has been shown to work also as a verification test for problem sera [1, 116, 175c].

COMPLEMENT FIXING ANTIBODIES

Syphilitic sera contain at least four antibodies which fix C: immobilizin, immune adherence antibodies reacting with the surface antigens of the treponemes, reagin, and antibodies reacting with protoplasmatic components of treponemal cells. The last of these are partly group-specific antibodies reacting also with non-pathogenic treponemes, and species-specific antibodies, reacting with pathogenic treponemes. The immunological role of the latter antibody class has not been studied. The demonstration of group-reactive antibodies as used in the Reiter protein C fixation test is one of the serological procedures used in syphilis diagnosis. Several attempts have been made to use *T. pallidum* extracts as diagnostic antigens [70b, 138b, 139]. Though a specificity and sensitivity almost equivalent to the TPI test was claimed [6, 54, 98], C fixation using *T. pallidum* extract has not received general acceptance. It has not been shown that the extract is really free from tissue impurities and it is doubtful if it has any advantage over the inexpensive Reiter protein antigen, which can be produced on a large scale.

C fixing group-reactive antibodies could be detected in the slow gamma fraction after separation by continuous flow electrophoresis at the onset of infection, and only later in the secondary stage in the fast fraction [137].

DELAYED HYPERSENSITIVITY

T. pallidum suspension, or extract of syphilitic rabbit testicle (Luetin), given intracutaneously induces, in late syphilis, a hyperaemic area of 10 mm diameter with a papule of about 5 mm in its centre. The reaction reaches its peak after 48 hours, a slight induration is palpable even after one week. Histologically, an infiltrate consisting of lymphocytes and histiocytes around the vessels and the appendages of the skin may be seen. In tertiary syphilis, histiocytes and fibro-blasts predominate, with a few giant cells [110].

Intracutaneous injection of treponemal suspension may also cause an imme-diate reaction; it has been shown by the method used for the demonstration of passive cutaneous anaphylaxis: after i.v. Evans blue injection the site of the i.c. test stained blue [15].

For a positive reaction, an injection of about 200 million treponemes is required. The antigen involved is thermostable [82] and is shared by *Borrelia hispancia* [142] and cultivable treponemes. It cannot be replaced by cardiolipin or lipid extract of treponemes [82].

The reaction becomes positive only 2–4 years after infection unless large doses of antigen are injected. It is positive in a third of patients with late latent syphilis or neurosyphilis [81] and invariably so in patients with aortitis and gummata [17, 81, 101, 151, 162]. In tertiary syphilis the reaction is strongly positive and it is not influenced by treatment [38]. The presence of delayed hypersensitivity modifies the clinical picture at reinfection: patients develop gummata [99].

The intracutaneous test is positive in 1–2 per cent of non-syphilitic individuals. It may be explained by the group-specific antigens present in non-pathogenic and pathogenic treponemes and by sensitization with saprophytic treponemes of mucous membranes.

Why delayed hypersensitivity develops only after 2 years of infection is not known. Weak antigenicity of the treponemes may be one of the reasons. It is possible, too, that the antigen is blocked by circulating antibodies in early syphilis. There is, indeed, a lack of correlation between the outcome of STS and the Luetin reaction. On the other hand, a positive reaction is observed even in early syphilis if the antigen was injected repeatedly after a short time in the same area [9].

The Luetin test has no diagnostic value: it gives a high rate of non-specific reaction in healthy individuals and sometimes it does not react in late syphilis. Its positivity indicates, however, that the unexpected serological positivity is due to late syphilis.

SEROLOGICAL TESTS FOR SYPHILIS

There are two types of serological tests: (*i*) non-specific, screening, lipoidal or standard tests (STS) which detect Wassermann antibody, and (*ii*) specific tests using treponemal antigens.

STANDARD TESTS FOR SYPHILIS (STS)

These tests are universally used, are well known and described in all relevant manuals. The antigen employed is an extract of tissue lipids, having cardiolipin, a phospholipid: found in mammalian heart muscle as the active principle [128]. If this is mixed with lecithin and cholesterol in suitable proportions, it forms a stable suspension for the detection of reagin. The antigenic ingredients are chemically well characterized, reproducible and suitable for standardization. Two types of STS based on different methods of detection have been developed: flocculation and C fixation tests. The earlier precipitation tests using antigens not chemically characterized (Kahn, Kline, Meinicke etc.) have now generally been abandoned and replaced by a simple slide test, the VDRL, using cardiolipin antigen or its modified variant applicable for the examination of unheated serum (rapid plasma reagin test — RPR) [136]. RPR antigen sensitized with charcoal is used in an automated device for serial screening [95].

False positive reactions, in the absence of Wassermann antibody, may occur because of undue handling of specimens, insufficient laboratory technique and faulty reagents. Wassermann antibody may be present, however, in healthy individuals and in diseases other than syphilis (BFP), when the specific tests are non-reactive. BFP may be acute or chronic. In acute, transitory forms the STS becomes negative spontaneously within 6 months. It is usually observed during acute febrile infectious diseases (particularly with rickettsial pneumonia, infectious mononucleosis) or provoked by strong immunological stimuli such as vaccination and pregnancy. The duration of chronic BFP is longer than 6 months. It may be caused by chronic infectious diseases (tuberculosis, leprosy, tropical parasitic diseases), systemic lupus erythematosus, other autoimmune diseases (rheumatoid arthritis [8*a*, 115], chronic persistent hepatitis [67], autoimmune thyroiditis [148]). As BFP may precede the clinical manifestations of systemic lupus erythematosus or other autoimmune diseases, patients presenting chronic BFP need constant supervision. Chronic BFP is frequently seen in the elderly [168] as a symptom of tissue wear and tear.

The results of C fixation and precipitation tests in BFP are generally equivocal; the reagin titre is low. Sera of chronic BFP patients may show a variety of other pathological laboratory findings: increased erythrocyte sedimentation rate, hyperglobulinaemia, positive McLagan and Hanger tests [114], rheumatoid and antinuclear factors [83], lack of β_1C line in the immunoelectrophoretogram, increased IgM and IgG levels [75], mitochondrial antibodies [8*b*]. A positive Kveim test is an unexplained finding [83].

The mechanism of BFP is varied and has to be elucidated for each case. It may be the result of: (*i*) infection with microorganisms containing cardiolipin; (*ii*) tissue destruction and liberation of cardiolipin from mitochondria; (*iii*) serum protein disturbance. Wassermann antibody is also present in minute quantities in the sera of healthy individuals, as may be shown by hypersensitivity reactions [66, 94]. Normally it is inhibited by a globulin, known as the inhibitor [121]. If the level of the inhibitor is reduced, as has been shown in acute hepatitis [177], the minute amount of Wassermann antibody present renders the STS positive.

The frequency of BFP depends upon the type of test used; it is more frequent with traditional than with cardiolipin antigens. On the other hand, the lower the prevalence of treponematoses in the population, the higher is the relative percentage of BFP among the seroreactors.

REITER PROTEIN COMPLEMENT FIXATION (RPCF) TEST

The group-specific protein antigen shared by pathogenic and non-pathogenic treponemes is the active principle of the following commercially available diagnostic antigens prepared from *T. reiteri*: (*i*) *T. reiteri* saline suspension (Pallingnost, Tréponine); (*ii*) sonicate (Pallida, [44]; (*iii*) 'protein' extracts: supernatant of centrifuged sonicate [80, 134] or protein precipitated from the supernatant with ammonium sulphate [20] or trichloroacetic acid [131]. Group-specific proteins may be absorbed to polystyrene-latex particles which agglutinate in the presence of syphilitic serum [37]. The antibodies detected by the RPCF test are distinct from those detected by STS in treponematoses and differs from those causing false positive reaction with reagin. The likelihood of their coexistence in the same patient is small. Because all treponemal tests depend upon the presence of different specific antibodies there may not be complete correlation between their results. TPI and RPCF tests are in agreement, however, in some 90 per cent of cases. Due to its high sensitivity the RPCF test can detect syphilitic infection at an early stage but when the disease is of many years' duration, especially in a treated case, the RPCF is not as sensitive as the other treponemal tests. False positive reactions, due to a group antigen shared with a variety of saprophytic treponemes, and cross-reaction between Wassermann antibody and the lipopolysaccharide impurity present in commercial antigen preparations, may be observed in about 0.5–2.0 per cent of non-syphilitic individuals [72]. Though the frequency of false positive reactions varies with different antigens, the diagnostic value of the RPCF test is limited by such reactions. From a practical standpoint this antigen appears to have little advantage over the common cardiolipin antigens. RPCF may also be carried out with the cerebrospinal fluid. Being more sensitive than STS, it is nevertheless of high diagnostic value.

T. PALLIDUM IMMOBILIZATION (TPI) TEST

Of the many tests described for the serologic diagnosis of syphilis, the TPI test seems to be theoretically the most specific and the most reliable for the verification of syphilis and other treponematoses. The TPI test is basically a bactericidal reaction in which *T. pallidum* are killed by the action of antibody (patient's serum) and C (fresh guinea pig serum) when they are incubated together at 35 °C for 18 hours. The death of treponemes is shown by the loss of their characteristic motility, ascertained by microscopic examination. If 50 per cent or more trepo-nemes are immobilized the test is reported as positive, if 20 per cent or less, as negative, and results in between are regarded as weakly reactive. For the test, sterile serum is required and it is important that the patient should not have had recent treatment with treponemicidal drugs, particularly penicillin, which may interfere with the validity of the test.

Despite its specificity, technical difficulties have greatly limited the use of the TPI test. One major problem has been the acquisition of suitable treponeme suspensions. The virulent treponemes required for the test must be obtained from rabbits infected intratesticularly, the supply of organisms being perpetuated by serial passage of infected material intratesticularly from one rabbit to another. A delicate balance of host-parasite relationship must be achieved in order to acquire and adequate number of organisms relatively free of tissue component and devoid of host-induced antibody. In general, this requires a 6–8 day infection and thus TPI testing must be scheduled at least a week in advance. A newer development of tremendous advantage is the preservation of treponemal sus-pension with 10 per cent DMSO in liquid nitrogen [118b]: frozen treponemes used in this fashion yielded TPI test results comparable to those of fresh suspen-sion. Antigen of known quality can be prepared beforehand and kept available for use whenever required.

The TPI is the most reliable test, but it can only be carried out in specifically equipped laboratories and the costs are very high. Its particular value is in distin-guishing between syphilitic and non-syphilitic reactions to STS and in the diag-nosis of certain cases of late syphilis, particularly those of the cardiovascular system, in which the STS may have become negative in the course of time.

Since immobilizin may be present in the cerebrospinal fluid, its demonstration may be the only laboratory sign of neurosyphilis [34].

FLUORESCENT TREPONEMAL ANTIBODY (FTA) TEST

This test, as originally described, gives false positive results in 2 to 5 per cent of cases. To get above the normal threshold of group antibody, sera were tested at a dilution of 1 : 200 (FTA-200) [26]. This test had a good specificity but was relatively insensitive and was replaced by the absorbed fluorescent treponemal antibody (FTA-ABS) test described by Hunter et al. [62]. In this, sera are tested in a dilution of 1 : 5 after absorption with ultrasonically disrupted Reiter trepo-nemes. An evaluation of the test in parallel with the TPI test has shown it to be more sensitive than, and as specific as, the TPI test [28]. The Reiter sonicate was later replaced by a heated and concentrated culture filtrate of Reiter trepo-nemes [154] and this reagent (sorbent) was recommended and is now generally used. Its activity was ascribed to the presence of antigenic material. The FTA-ABS test is more sensitive than the TPI and all the other serologic tests in every stage of syphilis. It is usually the first to become positive in untreated primary syphilis and like the TPI test it reverts to negative if treatment is given early in the disease, but not very often if it is delayed until the later stages. The FTA test can be carried out with dried blood eluate, a great advantage in tropical countries where laboratory facilities are scarce.

The FTA test is a sensitive method for the detection of specific antibodies in the cerebrospinal fluid, giving four times higher titres than the TPI test, though group-reactive antibodies are also demonstrable [70e]. The absorption of material is not necessary.

Due to the simplicity of the technique, especially of the semi-automated variant [154], the FTA-ABS test has replaced the TPI test in certain laboratories. The specificity of the test, however, has not been proved unequivocally. The reaction taking place between the sorbent and serum to be examined is not a purely immunological one. The uninoculated autoclaved medium used for the cultivation of Reiter treponemes might also block the reaction of group antibody and *T. palli-dum* [7, 182]. High osmolarity [184] and acid pH of the sorbent [53c] are thought to play an important part in the decrease of original reactivity. A sonicate of Reiter treponemes is a more reliable and a more effective reagent than the sorbent. Difficulties in production of sonicate in sufficient quantities unfortunately limit its use in practice.

Other factors, the frequency of which has not been assessed, limit the specificity of the test. Testicle tissue antigens adhering to the surface of treponemes may react with certain sera [161], as may treponemal antibodies, produced by the rabbit, with rheumatoid factor [183]. The antinuclear factor present in the sera of patients with systemic lupus erythematosus gives a characteristic bead-like staining pattern [122] with certain antigen suspensions.

Modifications of the test were described which have proved [76] less reliable than the FTA-ABS test. Such procedures, which represent a certain theoretical interest, are: blocking of the group-specific antigens on the surface of treponemes with anti-*T. reiteri* immune serum produced in rabbits [61]; the blocking test, using conjugated syphilitic serum for staining of smears. In this test, if the antigenic receptors on the surface of treponemes are covered by antibodies of the serum tested, they cannot bind the conjugate and the treponemes remain invisible. If antibodies are not present in the serum the treponemes are stained [146]. Labelled anti-guinea pig C was also suggested [135]. The sandwich consisting of treponemes and antibodies bind C which may be made visible by labelled anti-C. This method is handicapped by the presence of group antibodies in guinea pig sera [70e].

As a further development, peroxidase-labelled conjugates have been used for the reaction. The advantage is that smears may be examined by the conventional light microscope. A very good correlation was described between the tests performed with peroxidase and isothiocyanate conjugates [132, 150].

T. PALLIDUM HAEMAGGLUTINATION (TPHA) TEST

As the TPI and FTA tests — the present major treponemal tests — require highly trained personnel, a procedure such as the TPHA test seems to be of great interest because of the simplicity of its performance. In this test, sheep erythrocytes sensitized with cell components of virulent *T. pallidum* obtained from syphilitic rabbit testicles are used as antigen. Reiter treponemes and rabbit testis are used for the absorption of sera to be examined [165]. The specificity and sensitivity of the test favourably compares with the TPI and FTA tests [143, 164]. Its sensitivity in cases of primary untreated syphilis is slightly less than that of the FTA-ABS procedure [63]. Data obtained in testing sera of rabbits and chimpanzees infected with pathogenic treponemes, as well as sera of normal rabbits immunized with cultivable treponemes or bacteria, have shown the high specificity and sensitivity of the TPHA procedure [16]. The only drawback observed is an agglutination of unsensitized sheep red cells in approximately 0.5 per cent of sera [45]. The reagent for TPHA is now commercially available. More recently the manual macrovolume procedure was modified in a microvolume technique by the use of•an automatic serial dilution instrument [93]. The simplicity and good reproducibility of the test, the low cost and availability of the reagent, with the possibility of their standardization, are arguments in favour of its use as a verification test.

SEROLOGICAL TESTS IN THE COURSE OF SYPHILIS
THEIR INTERPRETATION

While the amount of the individual antibodies varies from person to person, there is some consistency in the time of appearance of Wassermann antibodies and of the antibodies detected by the specific tests.

In untreated early syphilis the FTA and RPCF tests may be found positive as early as 3 weeks after infection, TPHA and tests performed with lipid antigens in the following two weeks, while the TPI test becomes positive somewhat later, sometimes only when secondary symptoms have been established. The antibody titre reaches its peak in secondary syphilis, the titres of TPHA and FTA being the highest and C fixation and precipitation tests the lowest. There is no set of pattern in the order of disappearance of antibodies after specific treatment. Certain general tendencies may be discerned, however, after the clinical stage. Commencement of treatment does not immediately stop antibody production in primary syphilis. After an initial rise, serological tests revert to negative usually between 3 and 6 months after treatment. In secondary syphilis their reversion to non-reactive takes a longer time; TPI and FTA tests may even remain positive for many years after successful treatment.

The level of antibodies can be followed by titration of sera and it is usually determined to check the therapeutic success. A steady decrease of antibody titre is predictive for successful treatment, while a rise after an initial drop suggests a serological relapse or reinfection, which may be followed by a clinical relapse. Due to their simplicity, availability and early reversal, quantitative STS are used generally for the control of the treatment.

Owing to the widespread use of the broad-spectrum antitreponemal antibiotics for conditions other than syphilis, some patients with asymptomatic syphilis may have received inadequate treatment before their infection is discovered. This can make serological diagnosis quite difficult. Late latent syphilis is usually discovered by a positive VDRL screening test. C fixation tests give usually equivocal results. In this case, the specificity of VDRL positivity has to be confirmed by specific (TPI, FTA-ABS and TPHA) test. When clinical signs indicating late symptomatic syphilis (aortic incompetence, aneurysm, stenosis of the opening of coronary arteries, oligosymptomatic tabes dorsalis, etc.) are present,

STS may be non-reactive. In these cases the specific tests confirm the clinical suspicion. The reversal of STS tests after treatment takes a long time, with a slow and fluctuating drop of titre. The treponemal tests usually remain positive still longer, sometimes for life. Such patients, if treated adequately, do not show, however, any clinical progress or deterioration of the existing symptoms, nor will prolonged treatment improve the serological pattern. At present there is no test to predict the elimination of *T. pallidum* from the organism.

Patients suffering from tropical treponematoses (bejel, pinta, yaws) produce the same antibodies as patients with syphilis. Therefore, by serological methods, it is impossible to differentiate between venereal syphilis and other treponematoses.

THE RATIONAL ORGANIZATION OF SEROLOGICAL TESTING

Because of their economy and relative ease of performance, the STS are invaluable as screening tests and follow-up tests after treatment. When correlated with history and clinical evidence of syphilis, a reactive STS is confirmatory. When used in conjunction with epidemiological investigations, a reactive STS in a contact, suspect, or associate is highly significant. Treponemal tests (TPI, FTA-ABS or TPHA, according to laboratory facilities) are reserved for problem cases, where routine serological findings, history and physical examination are not diagnostically decisive. They do not substitute for clinical judgement and should not be performed on a routine basis. In some tropical areas, however, where the rate of serological positivity is between 10–50 per cent with a varying high percentage of false positivity, the qualitative cardiolipin test does not have any value for the clinician. It is necessary to make a quantitative cardiolipin test and, if feasible, a treponemal test as well.

IMMUNOALLERGOLOGIC PHENOMENA IN SYPHILIS

THE NATURAL COURSE OF SYPHILIS

The natural course of syphilis is similar in many respects to other infectious diseases except that the time course is stretched out over a much longer span. Such a chronic infectious process may be related to the low rate of multiplication of the treponemes or to the particular immune response of the host.

T. pallidum invades the body via a mucous membrane, usually genital, or by a minuscule break in the skin. From the earliest minutes after implantation some treponemes make their way beyond the immediate site of entry, quickly reaching the regional lymph nodes and the blood, and establish what is in effect a generalized infection. In congenital syphilis there is a blood-borne infection of the foetus via the placenta. The time interval elapsing between implantation of the organism and appearance of a lesion at that site usually takes about 15–24 days and is known as primary incubation. The primary lesion or chancre, as it is traditionally called, is an inflammatory tissue reaction to the presence and multiplication of treponemes. Defective blood supply results in erosion or deeper necrosis of the lesion. A similar tissue response results in characteristic enlargement of the regional lymph nodes although no necrosis of the glands takes place. The primary lesion heals slowly and spontaneously frequently leaving a scar. Concomitantly treponemes, which have found their way through the blood stream and have been disseminated to all tissues of the body, multiply. There may be transient signs of involvement of internal organs. Most characteristic, however, are the muco-cutaneous lesions, e.g. a maculo-papular generalized skin rash. This is the secondary stage, manifesting itself 6–8 weeks after the beginning of the primary sore. The lesions disappear slowly and spontaneously. They are likely to relapse, with diminishing frequency, until the patient reaches a stage of latency with no symptoms and signs of the disease, yet the infection is present and active treponemes may be demonstrated in the blood and in some other body fluids. During this stage of early latency, lesions may reappear occasionally, but usually not after the second year of infection. All early lesions are potentially contagious but those on moist skin sites are invariably and dangerously so, with *T. pallidum* abounding in the exudates. Tissue reactions in early syphilis may be so slight that they escape notice.

The early latent stage may continue into late latency, the latter lasting for many years with treponemes producing no evident tissue reaction. Or the balance between organism and host may suddenly be altered, and a gumma, the characteristic reaction of the tertiary stage, ensues: between 3 and more than 30 years after infection. A gumma is a nodule of considerable size, with necrosis of the central or surface tissue which is apt to be severe and very destructive. It may not be possible to demonstrate treponemes in the tissues involved except by animal inoculation. Late lesions are therefore practically not contagious. The gumma may affect any organ, usually the skin and the bones. The original lesion on the skin heals slowly, with scar formation, but new lesions may appear peripherally and these tertiary lesions may continue to extend over a period of many years showing an arciform and circinate pattern. After varying intervals of latency they may appear at several sites. Treponemes that reach the cardiovascular and nervous systems early in the disease produce a similar chronic cellular reaction but gross tissue necrosis is rare and progression is apt to be so slow that destruction of tissue and degenerative changes may take many years to produce clinical symptoms (aortitis, tabes, general paresis of the insane). In about two-thirds of the cases the latent stage continues for the rest of the patient's life without the development of any clinical lesions.

PATHOGENESIS OF CLINICAL SYMPTOMS

Early lesions are probably induced by the accumulation of treponemes and their metabolites beyond a critical threshold in the tissues. No evidence of the production of exotoxin by *T. pallidum* has ever been produced. The general symptoms (malaise, low grade fever) of the early secondary stage may be ascribed to tissue destruction. The assumption of a critical number of treponemes necessary to evoke lesions in the rabbit is supported by the fact that the primary incubation period is shortened proportionately with the increasing number of treponemes inoculated. *T. pallidum* divides in rabbits in an average of about 33 h. It was calculated that the incubation period could be shortened by about 4 days for each tenfold increase of treponemes inoculated within a fairly narrow limit [170]. The slow multiplication and the critical number of treponemes to elicit tissue symptoms may also explain the length of primary latency in man. Factors causing the generalized rash of the secondary stage are not known. In general, single secondary lesions tend to be smaller than the primary sore, a phenomenon that can be ascribed to the progressive development of immunity. Once immunity is well established, treponemes, while present in many tissues, are less abundant and the lesions tend to decrease in size. Finally the disease may be clinically asymptomatic. Latency indicates the absence of readily detectable signs and symptoms of the disease and not a 'dormant' state of treponemes in microscopic foci: e.g. in rabbits many months after infection, during the course of latent syphilis treponemes may be shed into the blood at intervals [39]. The immunological background of relapsing secondary lesions is not clear: the antigenic structure of treponemes may be changed by the influence of antibodies—as is shown in *Borrelia duttoni* isolated from rats or mice after hyperpyretic attacks, or a waning of immunity may occur, or the treponemes may be protected by 'enhancing' antibody against cellular antibodies.

A unique symptom of late syphilis in man, which cannot be reproduced in rabbits, is the gumma. It is characterized by massive infiltration of lymphocytes and epitheloid cells with necrosis due to tissue destruction and by a paucity of treponemes. The fact that the size of the hypertrophic lesion is disproportionate to the number of treponemes suggests that allergy is operative in the process. The same is also suggested by studies showing that reinoculation of patients having late syphilis with *T. pallidum* resulted in similar proliferative and destructive skin lesions devoid of treponemes [99]. Parenchymatous keratitis, as has been shown to develop in rabbits injected intracorneally with killed treponemes 3 to 10 months after a syphilitic infection, seems to be a similar delayed-type allergic reaction [105].

Congenital syphilis manifests itself sometimes, after an asymptomatic period of several decades, with interstitial keratitis. This stable and long-lasting equilibrium between treponemes and the human organism is reminiscent of the phenomenon of immunological tolerance. Its experimental reproduction in rabbits, however, failed. Since rabbits do not transmit syphilis to their offspring through the placenta, newborn animals non-receptive immunologically were infected and treated [36, 130] or injected with killed treponemal suspension [179] and reinfected again. The clinical course of syphilis was, however, either the same as in the controls infected after immunological maturation with the production of the same antibodies, or it took a more serious course as in older rabbits.

As a cellular immune phenomenon, phagocytosis of treponemes may play a role in the spontaneous healing of syphilitic lesions. This may be the first step in the induction of cell-mediated immunity as antigen-processing by macrophages. The first indirect proof of phagocytosis was the disappearance of treponemes injected into the peritoneal cavity of syphilitic rabbits or healthy guinea pigs, if the treponemes were mixed with syphilitic serum [158]. The phagocytosis of treponemes was shown only recently by means of electron microscopy.

T. pallidum may exist in a rabbit chancre both inside and outside the cells, as may be seen by electron microscopy. The phagocytosis of treponemes by cells is clearly visible: they sink into a hollow in the cell membrane, which then closes over them. This process is commonly observed in lymphocytes, neutrophils, plasma cells and endothelial cells. Macrophages usually grasp the treponemes with their numerous pseudopods. These intracellular treponemes, especially in plasma cells, are frequently covered with a kind of membraneous sheath and provided with dense envelopes. In this way, treponemes in plasma cells are well protected, evade destruction and may survive for a long time. Treponemes in macrophages may be later greatly altered and may become digested. An active role in this process is played by lysosomes or phagosomes [127b]. Digestion is enhanced after an injection of penicillin.

Humoral and cell-mediated immunity can be separated only for purposes of analysis. They act in concert to protect the host against extra- and intracellular pathogens. The interplay between humoral and cellular immunity is important in creating the great variability of clinical symptoms in syphilis and may even contribute to the recurrence of the disease.

SPIRAL ORGANISMS IN LATE SYPHILIS AFTER TREATMENT

Serological reactions, especially the specific tests in late syphilis, remain positive after treatment for several years, sometimes for life. It was long supposed that their persistence was caused by treponemes surviving treatment. The frequent occurrence of neurosyphilis in persistently seropositive patients treated with neoarsphenamine-bismuth before the Second World War supported this assumption.

Collart et al. [14] found corkscrew-shaped structures resembling *T. pallidum* in silver-stained smears taken from lymph nodes of rabbits a year after infection and treatment with adequate amounts of penicillin. Attempts to infect rabbits with lymph nodes harbouring this spiral organism were, however, unsuccessful even after immunosuppression. Since then these experiments were repeated by several workers [30, 187] using other methods (darkfield examination, direct immunofluorescent staining) for the detection of spiral organisms, and showing their pathogenicity by rabbit transfer. Though the finding of 'persistent treponemes' was frequent, only in a few instances was the material infectious.

This phenomenon was recently studied by the same methods in humans. A few patients with late syphilis, remaining seropositive after adequate penicillin treatment, harboured spiral organisms in the aqueous humour, lymph nodes, aorta and cerebrospinal fluid. Syphilis could only exceptionally be transferred to rabbits. The possibility of reinfection could not, however, be excluded, with certainty. The only recovery of *T. pallidum* after treated early syphilis was described by Hardy et al. [52]: a baby with congenital syphilis died in spite of continuous penicillin treatment for 17 days. Non-motile treponemes were found by darkfield in the spinal fluid and aqueous humour. The latter, and also tissue from the eye, produced orchitis by inoculation into rabbits. The *T. pallidum* strain isolated was, however, penicillin sensitive. No correlation has been found between the presence of spiral organisms, and the stage and activity of late syphilis. It was even difficult to find them for a second time in the same patient. Sometimes they could be found even in controls without any evidence of syphilis [30].

To explain the finding several hypotheses were proposed. Due to the immune response of the host slowly dividing treponemes were selected which could not be killed by penicillin, which acts only on dividing specimens. Benzyl or benzathine penicillin penetrates unsatisfactorily in the aqueous humour. Based on electron micrographs showing treponemes in plasma cells [2] and endothelial cells of capillaries [127a] their survival has been explained by the low level of penicillin within the cells of the host. It was found eventually [140] that certain human syphilitic sera contain a substance reducing the sensitivity of treponemes to penicillin and bismuth. In such cases, huge penicillin doses (6.0 M.U. daily) were required for serological reversal.

It is not known for sure whether these spiral organisms were really treponemes with altered biological properties or whether they were artefacts or tissue filaments; anyway, they seemed to be of low virulence and harmless. The world-wide experience of penicillin treatment for more than 25 years has shown that symptomatic disabling late syphilis can be prevented by adequate treatment, even in long-standing cases.

IMMUNITY IN SYPHILIS

NATURAL IMMUNITY

It is not clear whether man and rabbit possess some natural immunity to syphilis. Both are highly receptive to infection with $T.$ $pallidum$. Earlier studies [97] indicated that infection in rabbits could be established with a very small number of treponemes, or even with one treponeme. The smallest number of organism required to infect 50 per cent of rabbits (the ID_{50} dose) was 23, the ID_{50} of the same inoculum for man being 57 [99]. One can only speculate about the relative infectivity of treponemes for man. Assuming that a critical number of treponemes is required to induce a clinically recognizable lesion, it can be postulated that, starting with a single treponeme, the longest incubation period should be of the order of 60 days. It is known that approximately 20 to 50 per cent of contacts of primary and secondary syphilis become infected. This fact gives no clue to natural resistance, since the degree and duration of contact, the number and viability of the organisms at the contact site, and physical influences are unknown.

Despite the high susceptibility of humans to infection, an immobilizing, heat sensitive natural antibody has been found in sera of healthy humans in varying but low levels [40, 55] and has been studied in detail [56b, c]. The lag period of immobilization is shorter than that seen in the TPI test. However, both lag periods could be shortened by adding lysozyme to the reaction mixture. The shortening depends on the quantity of lysozyme added. Immune immobilizin has an enhancing effect: if it is added to serum with high normal anti-treponemal antibody content, the lag period of specific immobilization could be shortened. Based on the different kinetics, it may be assumed that the two antibodies attack different antigenic receptors.

Normal human serum loses its lytic activity against sheep red cells and its immobilizing activity against $T.$ $pallidum$ upon heating at 56 °C for thirty minutes. The immobilizing activity is, however, more sensitive to heat treatment and the two actions can be separated either by storage, or different heat treatment regimes. There is no correlation between immobilization and haemolytic activity of sera. C is involved in normal immobilization. However, more C is needed to immobilize treponemes than to lyse erythrocytes. All the C factors are necessary for the immobilization reaction to occur. If C reagents each lacking one of the C factors are used, prepared from a serum with a high immobilizing capacity, immobilization ceases.

The immobilizing factor may be absorbed with treponemes from sera at 0 °C, without a significant decrease of C activity. The responsible antibody belongs to the IgM class of antibodies: it is present in the first (19S) peak of sera separated by Sephadex filtration, is sensitive to mercaptoethanol treatment and does not pass the placental barrier. It is, however, different from the natural group-specific antibodies detected in the FTA reaction. It is not identical with lysozyme or properdin. No correlation was found between the lysozyme content of sera and their immobilizing titres; after absorption with zymosan, properdin activity disappeared, the treponemicidal effect was somewhat reduced. The relationship of natural antibody to receptiveness to infection is obscure.

ACQUIRED IMMUNITY

Infectious versus true immunity

From clinical observations of reinfections observed in humans after treatment and chancre immunity in untreated late syphilis came the notions that immunity in syphilis is a unique phenomenon differing qualitatively from immunity in many other infectious diseases and that resistance appears to be closely linked to the presence of the infecting agent. The term 'infectious immunity' promulgated by Neisser [117] carried the implication that cure of the disease leads to the disappearance of resistance.

Chesney [10], in experiments with treated rabbits, showed that syphilis immunity, as could be anticipated from the persistence of antibody production after long-standing infection, follows the same pattern as immunity in other infectious diseases. Rabbits, at least, may acquire during the course of syphilis an immunity which will persist after the infection has been treated. This refractory state—as has been shown by reinfections in man—is, however, not absolute, i.e. largely dependent on the size of the infectious dose. The validity of Chesney's ideas regarding the persistence of immunity after treatment have been confirmed by recent experiments.

Experiments on rabbits with immunizing infection

Immunity develops in rabbits during the course of experimental syphilis. They begin to show some degree of immunity within 3 weeks after infection. As the untreated disease progresses, resistance to challenge increases, reaching a maximum about 12 weeks after the initial infection and remaining high for the rest or the animal's life. If this so-called 'immunizing infection' is terminated with penicillin in less than 12 weeks, at a time when resistance has not fully developed, animals can be consistently re-infected. However, if treatment is delayed for 12 weeks or longer, at a time when the immune response appears to be maximal, a high degree of resistance or even complete immunity to challenge persists for at least one year following therapy.

Establishment of immunity in rabbits happens with intradermal challenge: 10^2–10^5 treponemes are injected into the shaved skin of the back. The level of immunity is measured with the reaction in response to the different challenge doses: lack of chancre, asymptomatic infection, prolonged incubation period or decrease of the size of the chancre in comparison with the controls. Asymptomatic infection in the symptom-free rabbits is detected by removal and transfer of a popliteal lymph node to a recipient animal intratesticularly or subscrotally, followed by testicular palpitation, darkfield examination in the case of infiltration, and serological testing of the recipient animals over a 6-month period, or by the rise of antibody titre following the challenge.

Besides the duration of infection, the level of immunity conveyed by infection is also influenced by the size of the infecting inoculum, i.e. by the degree of antigenic stimulus stemming from the multiplication of treponemes in the host [173]. If subclinical infection is maintained by subcurative penicillin injections over a period of months, no immunity ensues, and the evolution of the syphilitic process after the cessation of therapy will be the same, as might have been expected after fresh infection [100].

Resistance is highest to challenge with the homologous 'immunizing' strains. Rabbits infected with the Nichols strain exhibited a lesser degree of immunity to reinfection with some heterologous rabbit-adapted strains than with the homologous strain [170]. Rabbit-adapted strains ensured immunity against non-adapted strains, whereas the immunity conveyed by the latter was insufficient to protect rabbits against superinfection with stronger rabbit-adapted strains. Beside adaptation, antigenic differences between *T. pallidum* strains may also be involved. The Nichols strain, highly pathogenic to rabbits, failed to confer immunity against challenge with three freshly isolated strains, not adapted to rabbits. On the other hand, rabbits infected with two of these strains were not resistant to infection with the Nichols strain. If a mixture of different strains is used for immunization, reinfection by a 'wild' strain produces no symptoms [185].

Some degree of cross-immunity may exist between different treponemal species. *T. pertenue* infection protected approximately 75 per cent of rabbits against a challenge with *T. pallidum* [96d], while *T. cuniculi* protected only 33 per cent of the animals [172]. However, rabbits given an immunizing infection with *T. pallidum* developed lesions on challenge with *T. pertenue* Haiti B strains.

The multiplication of treponemes in immunized rabbits is inhibited. If the immunity is incomplete, the inoculation-time of the chancre is prolonged [18], or syphilis cannot be transferred as regularly by the popliteal lymph nodes to healthy animals as it may be with non-immunized rabbits infected simultaneously [178]. If the immunity is complete, treponemes may be demonstrated around a piece of chancre graft containing treponemes for 8–24 days, afterwards disappearing completely [156]. They do not enter into the draining lymph nodes and the infectivity of the graft ceases after about four days [144].

Immunization of rabbits with killed or attenuated T. pallidum

Despite the ability of virulent *T. pallidum* to stimulate host resistance during experimental disease, early attempts to induce immunity with massive doses of *T. pallidum* inactivated by heat, merthiolate, lyophilization, mapharsen, and protein antigens or ultrasonic lysates prepared from *T. pallidum* or cultivable treponemes remained uniformly unsuccessful. Suspensions of killed treponemes are, however, complete antigens, inducing reagin and immobilizin production and booster effect in infected animals. Recently, Metzger et al. [107] succeeded in protecting rabbits against symptomatic infection by inoculating them with suspensions of *T. pallidum* killed by storage at 4 °C for 7–10 days. As shown by lymph node transfer, the animals challenged with living treponemes developed asymptomatic infection. Penicillin inactivated *T. pallidum* antigen gave a lesser degree of immunity, as may be seen from the development of chancres in 25 per cent of rabbits immunized after challenge [109]. These studies suggest that the antigens responsible for inducing resistance are extremely labile. The possibility that irradiation might render freshly isolated *T. pallidum* non-infectious without appreciably affecting their highly sensitive immunogenic antigen was shown by Miller [111a]: freshly isolated *T. pallidum* when exposed to γ-irradiation from a ^{60}Co source lost their ability to infect rabbits with no appreciable effect upon motility. Animals immunized over a 24-week period showed evidence of partial immunity to challenge based upon the delay and growth of chancres as compared to the non-immunized control animals. Recently rabbits immunized intravenously over a 37-week period with a total of 3.71×10^9 γ-irradiated treponemes exhibited complete resistance to massive homologous challenge (10^5 treponemes) which persisted for at least one year after the last immunizing dose of organisms [111d]. Cross-protection against *T. pertenue*, Haiti B strain was, however, minimal.

The complete protection achieved with freshly isolated irradiated treponemes in contrast to the significant but lesser degree of immunity obtained with treponemes inactivated by storage in a refrigerator, strongly suggests that an antigen may be present in the mucopolysaccharide-containing superficial layer surrounding freshly isolated treponemes which is coincidentally lost during cold storage.

The inability to separate adequately *T. pallidum* from rabbit host testicular tissue during preparation of vaccine precludes the use of such suspensions in humans. Their administration in rabbits gives rise to enhanced homograft rejection and testicular antibodies [102]. The ability, however, to confer complete protection in rabbits for at least one year with γ-irradiated treponemes lends encouragement to the feasibility of a human vaccine.

IMMUNITY IN MAN

The natural course of syphilis indicates that mportant immune mechanisms are involved in the host-treponeme relationship. A great part of present knowledge on the natural course of infection comes from the patient material of Boeck, Bruusgaard and Gjestland in Norway where about 1,000 untreated patients were observed 30–50 years after the infection [5, 48]. About 25 per cent of the patients developed secondary relapses, the majority during the first year; about 13 per cent developed benign late syphilis, about 10 per cent cardiovascular syphilis, and 6 per cent neurosyphilis. About 60–70 per cent of untreated patients go through life without, or with minor, physical or mental consequences of infection.

About a hundred years ago, reinoculation and autoinoculation experiments in humans, carried out largely to differentiate primary sclerosis and chancroid, provided clear evidence that syphilitic infection gives rise to partial immunity, and the degree of resistance, at least in the early stages of the disease, in general bears direct relationship to the duration of infection. Though these studies are far from exact from the point of view of the methods used, a few facts can be gleaned from them. Healthy individuals are susceptible to infection with *T. pallidum* if the infectious material is introduced into the skin. In patients with syphilis, superinfection takes a different course. As the duration of untreated disease increases, lesions following challenge with homologous or heterologous strains occur less frequently. The lesion tends to conform to the stage of the disease reached by the original infection, i.e. chancre in primary, a papule or nodule in secondary syphilis; nodes or gumma follow challenge in individuals who had late syphilis (Finger-Landsteiner's rule). Except for the chancre, treponemes can be demonstrated only rarely in lesions of superinfection. Skin lesions remain restricted to the place of inoculation or its immediate neighbourhood. Patients with general paresis react rarely to challenge.

The only study under well controlled quantitative conditions was performed by Magnusson et al. [99]. It confirmed the information already obtained from experiments performed in rabbits and in humans. Sixty human volunteers were inoculated with the Nichols strain of *T. pallidum*. The diagnostic categories and the results of challenge of the volunteers are shown in Table 73-I. The Nichols strain, though passed through rabbits for many years, is still infectious to man and produced a skin lesion quite similar to chancre in all controls and receptive patients with syphilis treated earlier. Five patients with untreated latent syphilis showed no clinical or serological response to challenge and were assumed to be

TABLE 73-I

Results of inoculation of human volunteers with Nichols strain of T. pallidum [99]

Diagnosis	No. of patients	Lesions at the inoculation site			Increase of STS titre
		Darkfield		Gumma	
		+	−		
Controls	8	8			
Latent syphilis, treated	5				
Early syphilis, treated	11	9	2		11
Reinfection, treated	3	1	1		2
Late latent syphilis, treated	26	1	11*	1	9
Congenital syphilis, treated	5	1	2	1	4
Asymptomatic neurosyphilis, treated	2				

* No increase of STS titre in 3 volunteers.

resistant to superinfection. Of the eleven patients previously treated for early syphilis, all were reinfected and all responded with increased STS and TPI titres. Of 26 patients treated for late syphilis 13 could not be infected at all and those who had darkfield negative lesions had considerable residual immunity to challenge. In a general way, the patients who had previously had syphilis differed from non-syphilitic controls in their reaction to infection. Despite the individual differences the immunity was influenced by the duration of the original infection. After the treatment of syphilis there remains immunity against superinfection both in man and in rabbit, but due presumably to their respective life spans there is a significant difference between the duration of infection necessary to elicit a conspicuous immunity. While rabbits are immune to reinfection after three months of immunizing infection, man remains susceptible. On the other hand, rabbits can be reinfected two years after treatment, whereas humans remain immune for some 10 to14 years.

As was stated above, there are theories that syphilis, yaws, pinta and bejel are the same disease influenced only by ecological factors. In areas where yaws is prevalent there is no venereal syphilis, i.e. adults are protected as a result of yaws contracted during childhood. By superinfection, Medina [104] studied the cross-immunity between yaws, syphilis and pinta in 515 patients. Some of the treated pinta patients were susceptible to challenge and all untreated pinta patients were resistant. Yaws patients, whether treated or untreated were resistant, as were untreated syphilis patients. In contrast, about 30 per cent of treated syphilitics were susceptible to challenge with *T. pertenue*. One treponemal disease thus provides a sufficient degree of protection against the others.

ARTIFICIAL IMMUNIZATION TO TREPONEMATOSES IN HUMANS

The basic problem of artificial immunization is that an insufficient antigenic mass can be obtained from rabbit testicles. Another difficulty, however, arises in selecting methods of inactivation and preservation for conserving the protective antigenic capacity which at best can be present only to a limited degree. Magnusson et al. [99] injected three healthy persons with 50 million killed *T. pallidum*. They responded to inoculation of living treponemes as did the unimmunized controls. The component conveying resistance was, however, present in the antigen used. Only 26 per cent of their patients treated previously because of syphilis reacted to reinfection with lesions, against 70 per cent of the non-immunized group, i.e. resistance to reinfection could be reinforced by anamnestic reaction.

Nature has achieved, however, an attenuated treponeme species in the disease of pinta, which gives a conspicuous resistance against syphilis. Until recently it had not been possible to pass pinta to animals for study purposes. A considerable advance was the passage of the disease to the chimpanzee [85, 86]. The course of the disease in the chimpanzee is, however, rather torpid, with long-lasting erythematous plaques showing an insignificant tendency to spontaneous healing and sluggish and insignificant immune response as far as the reversal of serological tests is concerned. The animals can be reinfected from the plaques to the healthy skin within the first year.

It is probable, too, that the potential of *T. cuniculi* as an immunizing agent has not been fully explored. Rabbits infected experimentally with this species of treponemes develop resistance to syphilis and yaws. Fragmentary information in the old literature suggests that this treponeme does not produce a local lesion in man on artificial inoculation but these observations cannot be regarded as definitive.

There is another difficulty inherent in the use of effective vaccines based on virulent treponemes. They would make all recipients — as has been shown by experiments in animals — STS and TPI positive and therefore make diagnosis by blood tests impossible.

IMPORTANCE OF IMMUNE MECHANISMS IN THE COURSE AND IMMUNITY IN SYPHILIS

There is direct and indirect evidence regarding the role of immune mechanisms involved in the clinical course and spontaneous healing of syphilis and syphilitic lesions. If the immune system of the organism is impaired, the disease takes a more serious course. Newborn, immunologically immature rabbits may succumb after syphilitic infection; if they survive, the disease may manifest itself in generalized skin eruptions [123]. Treatment of rabbits at the time of infection with immuno-suppressive agents (X-rays, cortisone, nitrogen mustard) results in a very high yield of treponemes in the orchitis.

The protection is associated with the circulation. Syphilitic lesions of rabbits connected parabiotically with animals infected 100–450 days earlier disappeared much sooner than did those connected with non-infected animals [157]. It is a well-known fact that the cornea of syphilitic rabbits is susceptible to reinfection. If it is vascularized by means of killed *M. tuberculosis*, reinfection becomes impossible [11].

The protection is due partly to circulating antibodies. Suspensions of *T. pallidum* incubated with sera of patients with tertiary syphilis or of rabbits infected more than 6 months earlier failed to infect rabbits [34, 159]. Sera of patients with early syphilis have shown hardly more protective effect than normal human sera [171]. Since the protective effect could be demonstrated with sera negative in lipoidal tests, it can hardly be ascribed to the Wassermann antibody. On the other hand, based on the similar kinetics (long incubation requested for neutralization, need for C [169a], lack of protective action in early syphilis) it can be assumed that immobilizin may be one of these protective antibodies. It is, however, not the chief antibody responsible for protection. Rabbits immunized with killed *T. pallidum* suspension [96b] or infected with *T. pertenue* [96a] could be infected with syphilis despite the reactive TPI test. On the other hand, rabbits treated after long-standing syphilis were resistant to reinfection despite a negative TPI test [91b]. The correlation between the level of immobilizin and the number of treponemes in humans is quite poor. Skin efflorescences of patients with secondary syphilis and the brains of patients with general paresis harbour huge numbers of treponemes despite high titres in the TPI test, both in serum and cerebrospinal fluid.

Rabbits injected several times with large quantities (20 ml) of syphilitic rabbit serum did not develop chancre to a simultaneous heavy (8×10^5 germs) intracutaneous, treponemal challenge [149]. As indicated, however, by the rise of FTA titre following the disappearance of passively injected antibodies, the infection was taken, i.e. the immunity transferred passively by the serum was only relative.

The importance of cell-mediated immunity is shown by the positivity of delayed i.c. tests to treponemal extracts in the late, non-infective stages of the disease, whereas such tests are usually negative or weak in the early infectious stage. It was shown recently [92] that delayed hypersensitivity is impaired-in-this-stage of the disease. Lymph nodes removed from patients with early syphilis and spleens of babies who died of congenital syphilis showed depletion of lymphocytes in the paracortial areas similar to that found in lymph nodes of patients and experimental animals deficient in cell-mediated immunity. The response of peripheral blood lymphocytes to phytohaemagglutinin *in vitro* was reduced in comparison with that of the normal population. This impairment of cell-mediated immunity in congenital and secondary syphilis is related to the generalized spread of *T. pallidum* in the host early in the disease.

Despite the availability of *in vitro* models to analyse cell-mediated immunity little work was done regarding syphilis. Lymphocyte transformation test has been found to be increased by stimulation with cardiolipin and Reiter protein antigen in patients at all stages of syphilis [12, 91]. These results could be related as much to antibody production as to cell-mediated immunity. Experiments to show the toxic effect of immune lymphocytes on the motility or infectivity of treponemes, however, failed [111c]. Leukocyte migration using Reiter protein antigen was examined recently [43]. Stimulation of migration was observed in primary syphilis and inhibition in active late syphilis. In secondary syphilis neither stimulation nor inhibition of migration was seen (presumably as a sign of the suppression of cell-mediated immunity). The wide range of results observed in latent syphilis raises the possibility of distinguishing between early and late latent syphilis. The *in vitro* data at present are, however, insufficient to explain the role of histiocytic infiltration in late syphilitic lesions.

Local factors of immunity as well as general ones are also operative. Rabbits cannot be re- (super-) infected with syphilis in the testis after a syphilitic orchitis has taken place. It is a well-known clinical fact that the gumma strictly spares the scars left by previous gummata. Pasini [129] failed to superinfect humans in gummatous scars. The mechanism of this localized non-responsiveness is unknown.

The autoantibodies which are formed during the infection are also of great interest. A classical autoantibody as discussed earlier, is the Wassermann antibody which reacts with mitochondria. The Donath–Landsteiner cold–warm haemolysin antibody is seen occasionally in syphilitic patients. At low temperatures it combines with specific antigen found on erythrocytes, platelets and perhaps other body cells to produce their agglutination. On subsequent warming, the cells are lysed in the presence of C. The relationship between these antibodies and the clinical manifestations of syphilis is unknown.

EPIDEMIOLOGICAL CONSIDERATIONS

On a community level the incidence of syphilis and treponematoses results as a balance between ecological forces influencing the host-agent relationship. At least two ecological factors are operating simultaneously to create changing environments to the decrease and changing aspects of treponematoses: the improvement of living conditions on a world-wide level, especially in the developing countries, and mass examinations and effective penicillin treatment. Yaws, under the impact of control programmes, has been reduced in terms of both seriousness and incidence. It seems that there is less syphilis than there used to be, again in terms of both seriousness and attack rate. Due to the increased incidence of early syphilis since the mid-fifties, however, the haunting thought arises that maybe in some instances the infection has only been driven underground, ready to return. The causes of this recrudescence are, indeed, deeply rooted in contemporary human society: a tolerant attitude to homosexuals and prostitutes, both highly promiscuous groups; permissive male and female patterns in sexual life; urbanization and industrialization, migrant labour and tourism; unconcern in regard to syphilis among the public, health administrations and doctors. There are, however, also medical and biological factors operating in favour of the spread of venereal syphilis. Penicillin is now prescribed by doctors for treatment of different ailments less frequently, and coincidental syphilis treatment does not occur so often as when penicillin was the only antibiotic available. Unfortunately, it is an antibiotic too good for the treatment of syphilis: it acts promptly after short administration schedules. While promiscuous patients in the past received lengthy treatment with bismuth and neoarsphenamine, assuring an effective chemoprophylaxis against new infection, immunity developed, too, during the long and less effective treatment. Reinfections in the past were observed occasionally, while nowadays they are quite common. In yaws endemic areas the population attained immunity against venereal syphilis in childhood. The mass campaigns against treponematoses have rendered the population unprotected against venereal syphilis. Continuous medical and epidemiological surveillance of the patients and of the population as a whole is probably the only available weapon to prevent the gradual return of syphilis.

REFERENCES

1. Allegra, F., Marchessetti, W., Santini R. and Csermely, B.: *Riv. 1st Sieroter. ital.* **37**, 12 (1962).
2. Azar, H. A., Pham, T. D. and Kurban, A. K.: WHO/VDT/RES/72.255, unpublished working document.
3. Berg, R. N., Duncan W. P. and Thornton, C. G.: *Brit. J. vener. Dis.* **481**, 489 (1972).
4. Bonomo, L., Pinto, L., Marano R. and Damacco, F.: *Boll. Soc. ital. Biol. sper.* **39**, 1369 (1963).
5. Bruusgaard, E.: *Arch. Derm. Syph. (Berl.)* **157**, 309 (1929).
6. Cannefax, G. R. and Garson W.: *Publ. Hlth. Rep. (Wash.)* **72**, 335 (1957).
7. Cannefax, G. R., Hanson, A. W. and Skaggs, R.: *Publ. Hlth. Rep. (Wash.)* **83**, 411 (1968).
8a. Catterall, R. D.: *Quart. J. Med.* **30**, 41 (1961).
8b. id., *Mitochondrial and Other Antibodies in Chronic BFP Reactors. Overseas Meeting of the Medical Society for the Study of Venereal Diseases, Budapest, June 16, 1969.*

9. Charpy, J., Ranque, J. and Tramier, G.: *Bull. Soc. franç. Derm. Syph.* **64,** 18 (1957).
10. Chesney, A. M.: *Medicine (Baltimore)* **5,** 463 (1926).[1]
11. Chesney, A. M. and Woods, A. C.: *J. exp. Med.* **80,** 369 (1944).
12. Chieregato, G. and Faldarini, G.: *Minerva derm.* **43,** 264 (1968).
13a. Christiansen, A. H.: *Acta path. microbiol. scand.* **50,** 106 (1960).
13b. ibid., **61,** 141 (1964).
14. Collart, P., Borel, L. J. and Durel, P.: *Brit. J. vener. Dis.* **40,** 81 (1964).
15. Cottini, C. B., Lazzaro, C., Randazzo, S. D. and Giardina, A.: *Minerva derm.* **39,** 205 (1964).
16. Cox, P. M., Logan, L. C. and Norins, L. C.: WHO/VDT/RES/69.174, unpublished working document.
17. Csonka, G.: WHO/VDT/136, unpublished working document.
18. Cumberland, M. C. and Turner, T. B.: *Amer. J. Syph.* **33,** 201 (1949).
19. Daguet, G.: *Bull. WHO* **14,** 303 (1956).
20. D'Alessandro, G. and Dardanoni, L.: *Amer. J. Syph.* **37,** 137 (1954).
21. D'Alessandro, G. and Del Carpio, C.: *Nature* **181,** 991 (1958).
22. D'Allesandro, G., Zaffiro, P. and Dardanoni, L.: *Minerva med.* **53,** 2933 (1962).
23. Dardanoni, L. and Censuales, S.: *Riv. 1st. Sieroter. ital.* **32,** 489 (1957).
24. Davis, B. D., Moore, D. H., Kabat, E. A. and Harris, A. D.: *J. Immunol.* **50,** 1 (1945).
25. Deacon, W. W., Falcone, V. H. and Harris, A.: *Proc. Soc. exp. Biol. (N. Y.)* **96,** 477 (1957).
26. Deacon, W. E., Freeman, E. M. and Harris, A.: *Proc. Soc. exp. Biol. (N. Y.)* **163,** 827 (1960).
27. Deacon, W. E. and Hunter, E. F.: *Proc. Soc. exp. Biol. (N. Y.)* **110,** 352 (1962).
28. Deacon, W. E., Lucas, J. B. and Price, E. V.: *J. Amer. med. Ass.* **198,** 624 (1966).
29. de Bruijn, J. H.: *Antonie v. Leeuwenhoek* **27,** 98 (1961).
30. Dunlop, M. M.: *Brit. med. J.* ii, 577 (1972).
31. Dupouey, P.: Mise en evidence et étude d'haptens lipidiques nouveaux dans certaines espèces de tréponèmes. Etude des anticorps correspondants. Thèse. Paris, 1972.
32. Eagle, H.: *J. exp. Med.* **55,** 667 (1932).
33. Eagle, H. and Germuth, F. G.: *J. Immunol.* **60,** 223 (1948).
34. Eberson, F.: *Arch. Derm. Syph. (Chic.)* **4,** 490 (1921).
35. Ehrmann, G. and Nielsen, H. A.: *Brit. J. vener. Dis.* **31,** 249 (1955).
36. Festenstein, H. and Bokkenhauser, V.: *Brit. J. exp. Path.* **42,** 158 (1961).
37. Fischman, A.: *Brit. J. vener. Dis.* **40,** 225 (1964).
38. Földvári, F., Károlyi, S., Király, C. and Lazarovits, L.: *Arch. klin. exp. Derm.* **219,** 249 (1964).
39. Frazier, C. M., Bensel, A. and Keuper, C. S.: *Amer. J. Syph.* **36,** 167 (1952).
40. Fribourg-Blanc, A.: *Presse méd.* **64,** 1396 (1956).
41. Fribourgh-Blanc, A., Mollaret, H. H. and Niel, G.: *Bull. Soc. path. exot.* **59,** 54 (1966).
42. Fribourg-Blanc, A. and Niel, G.: WHO/VDT/RES/67.115, unpublished working document.
43. Fulford, K. W. M. and Brostoff, J.: *Brit. J. vener. Dis.* **48,** 483 (1972).
44. Fühner, F. and Gaethgens, W.: *Z. Hyg. Infekt.-Kr.* **138,** 573 (1954).
45. Garner, M. F., Backhouse, J. L., Daskalopoulos, G. and Walsh, J. L.: *Brit. J. vener. Dis.* **48,** 411 (1972).
46. Gastinel, P., Vaisman, A. and Hamelin, A.: *Ann. Inst. Pasteur* **90,** 249 (1956).
47. Gelperin, A.: *Amer. J. Syph.* **35,** 1 (1951).
48. Gjestland, T.: *Acta derm.-venereol. (Stockh.)* **35,** Suppl. 34 (1955).
49. Gregory, W. K.: Cit. by Guthe *The Henry Cushier Raven Memorial Volume*, Columbia University Press, (1950).
50. Greifelt, A.: *Derm. Wschr.* **129,** 181 (1954).
51. Guthe, T.: *Acta derm. venereol. (Stockh.)* **49,** 343 (1969).
52. Hardy, T. P., Hardy, P. H., Oppenheimer, E. H., Ryan, S. J. and Sheff, R. N.: *J. Amer. med. Ass.* **212,** 1315 (1970).
53a. Hardy, P. H. and Nell, E. E.: *J. exp. Med.* **101,** 367 (1955).

53b. id., *Amer. J. Hyg.* **66**, 160 (1957).
53c. id., *Amer. J. Epidem.* **96**, 141 (1972).
54. Harris, A., Falcone, V. H., Price, L. S. and Brown, W. J.: *Publ. Hlth. Rep.* (*Wash.*) **73**, 210 (1958).
55. Harris, A., Portnoy, J., Falcone, V. H. and Olansky, S.: *Amer. J. Syph.* **37**, 101 (1953).
56a. Hederstedt, B.: *Acta path. microbiol. scand.* **54**, 126 (1962).
56b. id., WHO/VDT/RES/72.275, unpublished working document.
56c. id., WHO/VDT/RES/72.277 & Corr. 1, unpublished working document.
57. Henschler-Greifelt, H.: *Ärztl. Wsch.* **14**, 987 (1959).
58. Heymann, G. and Siefert, G.: *Z. Immun.-Forsch.* **116**, 257 (1958).
59. Horváth, I.: Unpublished data (1970).
60. Hudson, E. H.: *Non-venereal Syphilis.* Livingstone, Edinburgh 1958.
61. Hunter, E. F.: *Proc. World Forum on Syphilis and Other Treponematoses.* U. S. Government Printing Office, Washington 1964, p. 269.
62. Hunter, E. F., Deacon, W. E. and Meyer, P. E.: *Publ. Hlth. Rep.* (*Wash.*) **79**, 410 (1964).
63. Johnston, N. A.: *Brit. J. vener. Dis.* **48**, 474 (1972).
64. Julian, A. J., Logan, L. C. and Norins, L. C.: WHO/VDT/RES/69.166, unpublished working document.
65. Julian, A. J., Portnoy, J. and Bossak, H. N.: *Brit. J. vener. Dis.* **39**, 30 (1963).
66. Kahn, R. L.: *An introduction to Universal Serologic Reactions in Health and Disease.* Commonwealth Fnd., New York 1951.
67. Károlyi, I. and Király, K.: *Orv. Hetil.* **97**, 36 (1956).
68. Kent, J. F., Covert, S. V., Reilly, H. W., Kinch, W. H. and Lawson, W. B.: *Proc. Soc. exp. Biol.* (*N. Y.*) **109**, 584 (1962).
69. Kahn, A. S., Nelson, R. A. and Turner, T. B.: *Amer. J. Hyg.* **53**, 296 (1951).
70a. Király, K.: *Z. Immun.-Forsch.* **117**, 317 (1959).
70b. id., *Bőrgyógy. Vener. Szle.* (*Budap.*) **13**, 261 (1959).
70c. id., *Path. et Microbiol.* (*Basel*) **29**, 75 (1966).
70d. id., *Hautarzt* **19**, 36 (1968).
70e. id., unpublished data (1970).
71. Király, K., Backhausz, R., Jobbágy, A., Lajos, J. and Kováts, L.: *Acta derm.-venereol.* (*Stockh.*) **48**, 362 (1968).
72. Király, K. and Csomay, T.: *Bőrgyógy. vener. Szle.* (*Budap.*) **44**, 1 (1968).
73. Király, K. and Jobbágy, A.: *Bőrgyógy. vener. Szle.* (*Budap.*) **45**, 1 (1969).
74. Király, K., Jobbágy, A. and Kováts, L.: *J. invest. Derm.* **48**, 98 (1967).
75. Király, K., Káldor, I., Jobbágy, A. and Karsay, K.: *Acta derm.-venereol.* (*Stockh.*) **46**, 506 (1966).
76. Király, K. and Kováts, L.: *Dermatologia* (*Basel*) **135**, 443 (1967).
77. Király, K., Laurenszky, J. and Tihanyi, E.: WHO/VDT/RES/72.268, unpublished working document.
78. Király, K., Orbán, T. and Károlyi, I.: *Psychiat. Neurol. med. Psychol.* **11**, 378 (1958).
79. Király, K. and Porgányi, M.: *Z. Immun.-Forsch.* **119**, 183 (1960).
80. Király, K. and Prerau, H.: *Z. Immun.-Forsch.* **134**, 32 (1967).
81. Király, K. and Rácz, I.: *Arch. klin. exp. Derm.* **209**, 583 (1960).
82. Király, K., Rácz, I. and Jobbágy, A.: *Bőrgyógy. vener. Szle.* (*Budap.*) **46**, 235 (1970).
83. Király, K., Rácz, I., Vereczkei, I. and Tokodi, I.: *Arch. klin. exp. Derm.* **255**, 353 (1966).
84. Kuhn, U. S. G. III. and Brown, W. J.: cited in Cannefax, G. R., Norins, L. C. and Gillespie, E. J.: Immunology of Syphilis. *Ann. Rev. Med.* **18**, 471 (1967).
85. Kuhn, U. S. G. III. Medina, R., Cohen, P. G. and Vegas, M.: *Brit. J. vener. Dis.* **46**, 311 (1970).
86. Kuhn, U. S. G. III. Varela, G., Chandler, F. W. and Osuna: *J. Amer. med. Ass.* **206**, 829 (1968).
87. Lamanna, C. and Hollander, D.: *Science* **123**, 989 (1956).
88. Laurell, A. B.: *Acta path. microbiol. scand.* Suppl. 103, (1955).
89. Laurell, A. B. and Lindau, A.: *Acta path. microbiol. scand.* **42**, 67 (1958).

90. Laurell, A. B. and Malmquist, J.: *Acta path. microbiol. scand.* **51**, 187 (1961).
91. Lazzaro, C. and Lanza, C.: *Bull. Soc. med.-chir. Catania* **33**, 287 (1965).
91a. Levaditi, C., Vaisman, A. and Hamelin, A.: *Ann. Inst. Pasteur* **82**, 635 (1952).
91b. id., *Bull. Acad. nat. Méd. (Paris)* **136**, 367 (1952).
92. Leven, G. M., Wright, D. J. M. and Turk, J. L.: *Proc. roy. Soc. Med.* **64**, 426 (1971).
93. Logan, L. C. and Cox, P. M.: WHO/VDT/RES/69.175, unpublished working document.
94. Lund, R.: *Amer. J. Syph.* **26**, 1 (1942).
95. McGrew, B. E., DuCross, M. J., Stout, G. and Falcone, V.: *Amer. J. clin. Path.* **50**, 52 (1968).
96a. MacLeod, C. P. and Magnusson, H. J.: *J. Vener. Dis. Inform.* **32**, 305 (1951).
96b. id., *Amer. J. Syph.* **37**, 9 (1953).
96c. id., *Publ. Hlth. Rep. (Wash.)* **68**, 747 (1953).
96d. id., WHO/VDT/140, unpublished working document.
97. Magnusson, H. J., Eagle, H. and Fleischman, R.: *Amer. J. Syph.* **32**, 1 (1948).
98. Magnusson, H. J. and Portnoy, J.: *Amer. J. publ. Hlth.* **46**, 190 (1956).
99. Magnusson, H. J., Thomas, E. W., Olansky, S., Kaplan, B. I., de Mello, K. and Cutler, J. C.: *Medicine (Baltimore)* **35**, 33 (1956).
100. Magnusson, H. J., Thompson, F. A. and Rosenau, B. J.: *Amer. J. Syph.* **34**, 219 (1950).
101. Marshak, L. C. and Rothman, S.: *Amer. J. Syph.* **35**, 35 (1951).
102. Matej, H., Metzger, M. and Smogor, W.: WHO/VDT/RES/72.276, unpublished working document.
103. Matuhasi, T., Mizuoka, K. and Usui, M.: *Bull. Wld. Hlth. Org.* **34**, 566 (1966).
104. Medina, R.: WHO/VDT/RES/63.64, unpublished working document.
105. Merté, H. J.: *Bericht über die 62. Zusammenkunft der Deutschen Ophthalmologischen Gesellschaft in Heidelberg.* 1959, p. 282.
106. Metzger, M., Hardy, P. H. and Nell, E. E.: *Amer. J. Hyg.* **73**, 236 (1961).
107. Metzger, M., Michalska, E., Podwinska J. and Smogor, W.: *Brit. J. vener. Dis.* **45**, 299 (1969).
108a. Metzger, M. and Podwinska, J.: *Arch. Immunol. Ther. exp. (Warsaw)* **13**, 16 (1965).
108b. id., WHO/VDT/RES/66.95, unpublished working document.
108c. ibid., WHO/VDT/RES/66.99, unpublished working document.
109. Metzger, M. and Smogor, W.: *Brit. J. vener. Dis.* **54**, 308 (1969).
110. Mezzadra, C.: *Minerva derm.* **35**, 119 (1960).
111a. Miller, J. N.: *J. Bact.* **90**, 297 (1965).
111b. id., *J. Immunol.* **99**, 1012 (1967).
111c. id., *Progress report to WHO*, 1973.
111d. id., *J. Immunol.* **110**, 1206 (1973).
112. Miller, J. N., Bekker, J. H., De Bruijn, J. H. and Onvlee, P. C.: *J. Bact.* **99**, 132 (1969).
113. Miller, J. N., De Bruijn, J. H., Bekker, J. H. and Onvlee, P. C.: *J. Immunol.* **96**, 450 (1965).
114. Miller, L. J., Brodey, M., Hill, J. H.: *Arch. Derm.* **79**, 206 (1959).
115. Moore, J. E. and Mohr, C. F.: *J. Amer. med. Ass.* **150**, 467 (1952).
115a. Müller, F., Feddersen, H. and Segerling, N.: *Immunology* **24**, 711 (1973).
116. Neblett, T. R., Merriam, L. R., Burnham, T. K. and Pine, G.: *J. invest. Derm.* **43**, 439 (1964).
117. Neisser, A.: *Arbeiten an dem kaiserlichen Gesundheitsamte* **37**, 1 (1911).
118a. Nell. E. E. and Hardy, P.: *Immunochemistry* **3**, 233 (1966).
118b. id., *Cryobiology* **9**, 404 (1972).
119a. Nelson, R. A.: *Amer. J. Hyg.* **75**, 339 (1948).
119b. id., *Science* **118**, 733 (1953).
120. Nelson, R. A. and Mayer, M. M.: *J. exp. Med.* **89**, 368 (1949).
121. Neurath, N., Volkin, E., Ericson, O., Craig, M. W., Putnam, M. W. and Cooper, C. R.: *Amer. J. Syph.* **31**, 397 (1947).
122. Nicolau, S. C., Bădănoiu, A. and Nicolau, G.: Communication à la 6ème semaine médicale balcanique. Bucarest, Mai 1962.

123. Nielsen, H. A.: WHO/VDT/RES/7, unpublished working document.
124. Nielsen, H. A. and Metzger, M.: *Brit. J. vener. Dis.* **35**, 241 (1959).
125. Norins, L. C., Logan, L. C. and Julian, A. J.: cited in Cannefax G. R. Norins, L. C. and Gillespie, E. J.: Immunology of Syphilis. *Ann. Rev. Med.* **18**, 471 (1967).
126. O'Neill, P. and Nicol, C. S.: *Brit. J. vener. Dis.* **48**, 460 (1972).
127a. Ovcinnikov, N. M. and Delektrosky, V. V.: *Brit. J. vener. Dis.* **48**, 227 (1972).
127b. ibid., 327 (1972).
128. Pangborn, M., Maltaner, F., Tompkins, V. N., Beacher, T. and Thompson, W. R.: *Bull. Wld. Hlth. Org.* **4**, 151 (1951).
129. Pasini, A.: *Urol. Cutan. Review* **32**, 249 (1928).
130. Pautrizel, R., Szersnovicz, G. and Marcenach, J.: *C. R. Soc. Biol. (Paris)* **150**, 632 (1962).
131. Pautrizel, R., Szersnovicz, F. and Rollet, M.: *Bull. Soc. Pharm. (Bordeaux)* **92**, 141 (1954).
132. Petts, V. and Roitt, I. M.: *Clin. exp. Immunol.* **9**, 407 (1971).
133. Pillot, J. and Borel, L. J.: *C. R. Acad. Sci. (Paris)* **252**, 954 (1961).
134. Pillot, J. and Faure, M.: *Ann. Inst. Pasteur* **96**, 196 (1959).
135. Pillot, J. and Wattré, P.: *C. R. Acad. Sci. (Paris)* **265**, 1769 (1967).
136. Portnoy, J. and Garson, W.: *Pub. Hlth. Rep. (Wash.)* **75**, 985 (1960).
137. Portnoy, J., Julian, A. J., Smith, J. F. and Harris, A.: *Brit. J. vener. Dis.* **39**, 33 (1963).
138a. Portnoy, J. and Magnusson, H. J.: *Amer. J. clin. Path.* **26**, 313 (1956).
138b. id., *J. Immunol.* **75**, 748 (1955).
139. Price, I. N. O.: *Brit. J. vener. Dis.* **34**, 91 (1958).
140. Rabito, C. and Marson, G. B.: *Boll. Soc. ital. Biol. sper.* **36**, 633 (1960).
141. Ranque, J. and Moignoux, J. B.: *C. R. Soc. Biol.* **146**, 1762 (1952).
142. Ranque, J. and Quilie, M.: *Méd. trop.* **27**, 519 (1967).
143. Rathlev, T.: WHO/VDT/RES/77.65, unpublished working document.
144. Reynolds, F. W.: *Bull. Johns Hopk. Hosp.* **69**, 53 (1941).
145. Roemer, G. B. and Schlipköter, H.: *Dtsch. med. Wschr.* **78**, 345 (1953).
146. Ruczkowska, J.: WHO/VDT/RES/73.65, unpublished working document.
147. Ruge, H.: *Dtsch. med. Wschr.* **76**, 991 (1951).
148. Selenkov, H. A., Cline, M. J., Fudenberg, H. and Brooke, M. S.: *Amer. J. Med.* **31**, 144 (1961).
149. Sepetjian, M., Salussola, D. and Thivolet, J.: WHO/VDT/RES/72.279, unpublished working document.
150. Sepetjian, M., Thivolet, J., Leung-Tack, J. and Monier, J. C.: WHO/VDT/RES/73.300, unpublished working document.
151. Simeray, A.: *Bull. Soc. franç. Derm. Syph.* **60**, 186 (1953).
152. Sinecker, H.: *Z. Immun.-Forsch.* **11**, 191 (1959).
153. Stevens, R. W.: *N. Y. State Health Department: Annual Report of the Division of Laboratory Research.* 1963, p. 79.
154. Stout, C. W., Kellogg, D. S., Falcone, V. H., McGrew, B. E. and Lewis, J. S.: *Hlth. Lab. Sci.* **4**, 5 (1967).
155. Stout, G. W., McGrew, R. E. and Falcone, V. H.: *J. Publ. Hlth. Lab. Div.*, **26**, 7 (1968).
156. Strempel, R. and Armuzzi, J.: *Derm. Z.* **50**, 423 (1927).
157. Tani, T. and Aikawa, A.: *Jap. J. exp. med.* **14**, 465 (1936); ref. *Zbl. Haut-Geschl. Kr.* **46**, 209 (1937).
158. Tani, T., Matsubara, M. and Hayasi, T.: *Jap. J. med. Sci. Biol.* **81**, 303 (1955).
159. Tani, T. and Ogiuti, K.: *Jap. J. exp. Med.* **14**, 457 (1936); ref. *Zbl. Haut-Geschl. Kr.* **56**, 210 (1937).
160. Thatcher, R. W.: *Brit. J. vener. Dis.* **45**, 10 (1969).
161. Thivolet, J. and Cherby-Grospiron, D.: *Ann. Inst. Pasteur* **101**, 869 (1961).
162. Thivolet, J., Simeray, A., Rolland, M. and Challut, F.: *Ann. Inst. Pasteur* **85**, 23 (1953).
163. Thompson, F. A., Greenberg, B. G. and Magnusson, H. J.: *J. Bact.* **609**, 473 (1950).
164. Tomizawa, T.: *Jap. J. clin. Med.* **26**, 304 (1968).
165. Tomizawa, T. and Kasamatsu, S.: *Jap. J. med. Sci. Biol.* **19**, 305 (1966).

166. Tringali, G., Del Carpio, C. and Giammanco, N.: *Riv. 1st. Sieroter. Ital.* **41**, 291 (1966).
167. Tringali, G., Julian, A. J. and Halbert, W. M.: *Brit. J. vener. Dis.* **45**, 202 (1969).
168. Tuffanelli, D. L.: *Brit. J. vener. Dis.* **42**, 40 (1966).
169a. Turner; T. B.: *J. exp. Med.* **69**, 867 (1939).
169b. id., In *Infectious Agents and Host Reactions.* Saunders, Philadelphia, 1970, p. 346.
170. Turner, T. B. and Hollander, D. H.: *Biology of Treponematoses.* WHO monograph series No. 35 Geneva 1957.
171. Turner, T. B., Kluth, F. C., McLeod, C. and Winsor, C. P.: *Amer. J. Hyg.* **48**, 173 (1948).
172. Turner, T. B., McLeod, C. and Updyke, E. L.: *Amer. J. Hyg.,* **46**, 287 (1947).
173. Turner, T. B. and Nelson, R. A.: *Trans. Ass. Amer. Physicians* **63**, 112 (1950).
174. Vaisman, A.: *Proph. Sanit. Morale* **45**, 41 (1973).
175a. Vaisman, A. and Hamelin, A.: *C. R. Soc. Biol. (Paris)* **146**, 52 (1952).
175b. id., *C. R. Acad. Sci. (Paris),* **234**, 156 (1952).
175c. id., *Presse méd.* **68**, 1297 (1960).
176. Vaisman, A., Hamelin, A. and Guthe, Th.: *Bull. Wld. Hlth. Org.* **29**, 1 (1968).
177. Volkin, E., Neurath, H., Erickson, J. O. and Craig, H.: *Amer. J. Syph.* **31**, 397 (1947).
178. Waring, G. W. and Fleming, W. L.: *Amer. J. Syph.* **36**, 368 (1952).
179. Wicher, K. and Rogalows, D.: *Polish Med. Sci. Hist. Bull.* **3**, 62 (1960).
180. Wiegland, S. E., Strobel, P. L. and Glassman, L. H.:*J. invest. Derm.* **58**, 186 (1972).
181. Wilkinson, A. E.: *Brit. J. vener. Dis.* **37**, 59 (1961).
182. Wilkinson, A. E. and Ferguson, H. C.: *Brit. J. vener. Dis.* **44**, 291 (1968).
183. Wilkinson, A. E. and Rayner, C. F. A.: *Brit. J. vener. Dis.* **42**, 8 (1966).
184. Wilkinson, A. E. and Wiseman, C. C.: *Proc. roy. Soc. Med.* **64**, 422 (1971).
185. Worms, W.: *Brit. J. vener. Dis.,* **18**, 18 (1942).
186. Zabodotny, D. and Maszlakowetz, N. N.: *Zbl. Bakter. I. Orig.* **44**, 532 (1907).
187. Yobs, A. R., Rockwell, D. H. and Clard, J. W.: *Brit. J. vener. Dis.* **49**, 248 (1964).

CHAPTER 74

ALLERGY AND IMMUNITY IN LEPROSY

by

K. SIPOS and I. RÁCZ

Leprosy (recently also called hanseniasis) is a chronic disease caused by *Mycobacterium leprae*, infectious in some cases, primarily affecting peripheral nerves and secondarily affecting skin and certain other tissues. Progress in the study of human leprosy has brought into prominence the importance of allergo-immunological processes in the development and course of the disease.

M. leprae is an obligate intracellular parasite composed of protein, polysaccharide, phospholipid fractions, glycerides and waxes [1, 55, 62, 67, 89, 102]; no satisfactory method for its cultivation has so far been found [19, 30, 32c, 36, 49b, 70, 110, 147], although recently evidence has been produced of a limited multiplication within macrophages derived from human peripheral blood; the applicability of this method is, however, restricted by the limited survival of the host cells. In certain forms of the disease (the foci of lepromatous leprosy) the affected tissues are invaded by an enormous number of bacteria. There are two methods (Fernandez and Castro [46], and Dharmendra, [39a, b]) for separating bacteria from such tissues [89, 134, 144], yet the bacterial suspensions obtained in this way are not yet quite suitable for appropriate biological, allergic, serological, etc. tests [35, 133b, 134, 143, 144].

Animal inoculations (mice, rats, golden hamster) with *M. leprae* are increasingly successful [17a, 18, 19, 38, 62, 82, 86, 106, 120, 137, 155, 161]; not only local infections could be obtained by inoculation into the foot pads of mice, but also generalized infection could be induced in thymectomized and whole-body X-ray irradiated mice by intravenous injection of leproma homogenates. The dissemination can be rendered even more effective by pretreatment with antilymphocyte globulin [19, 49a, b, 103, 118a, b, c, d]. More recently successful infection of the armadillo has been reported. About one-third of the animals inoculated developed a disseminated infection [73]. So far no inoculated armadillo has developed leprosy of tuberculoid or of borderline type. This is where the mouse provides a useful counterpart in the study of the immunological complexities of leprosy, as the mouse (if not immunologically suppressed) is capable of producing cell-mediated immunity to *M. leprae*, whereas the armadillo is not. Another important aspect of lepromatous leprosy in the armadillo is that it provides a rich source of supply of leprosy bacilli for research centres all over the world.

CLINICAL PICTURE

The cutaneous infection escapes notice, and even its conditions have not yet been clarified [112]. The infection proceeds along the superficial branches of cutaneous nerves, most frequently along the radial, ulnar, peroneal and post-auricular nerves to the Schwann cells and from there into the cells of the RES [32c, 157]. As regards the pathogenesis of nervous damage it has been supposed that in tuberculoid leprosy, the cell-mediated immune response against *M. leprae* destroys both the bacilli and the Schwann cells that contain them, whereas in the lepromatous type bacilli multiply freely in the Schwann cells and in perineurial cells. Their presence in perineurial cells impairs the functional efficiency of these cells, allows leakage of extracellular fluid into the endoneurium, thus causing impairment of nerve function, which is probably reversible. In an attempt to repair the perineurium, Schwann cells take on the form and function of peri-neurial cells and form multiple layers of pseudoperineurium. This slow loss of Schwann cells is the major cause of irreversible nerve damage in lepromatous leprosy.

The incubation takes a long time, 7 to 20 years [32d, 35, 83]. During the invasive stage only non-specific symptoms are observed (e.g. gastro-intestinal, psychic, neuralgic and other nervous symptoms, pruritus, formication, etc.), and the early erythematous lesions only appear after a number of years. The great majority of the latter consist of various forms of erythemas, less frequently small papulae or nodules and ulcers, varying considerably in both number and size, may be seen. At this stage the organism is incapable of any resistance and it cannot be predicted which form of leprosy will develop. Subsequently, depending on the immune response, the progress of the disease shows a dichotomy, resulting in the two main forms of leprosy different in both symptoms and course.

LEPROMATOUS LEPROSY OR NODULAR LEPROSY
(LEPRA TUBEROSA)

In this form of leprosy, which is strongly contagious [44], numerous bilaterally and symmetrically distributed macules, papules and nodules (nodular form) develop in the place of earlier exanthems. Sensation and hairgrowth in these areas are normal. Subsequently, oedema and lacerations, scars and mutilations occur owing to the destruction of mainly the nasal, mandibular and digital bones; further lesions of the peripheral, often cranial, nerves ensue. If the patient remains untreated, the lines of the forehead become deeper as the skin becomes thickened (leonine facies), the eyebrows become thinned or lost, the nose becomes broadened and deformed, the ear lobes are thickened, the voice becomes hoarse, the upper incisor teeth loosen or fall out, and a slow fibrosis takes place in the peripheral nerves resulting in nerve thickening and glove and stocking anaesthesia. The two commonest causes of death are pulmonary tuberculosis and renal failure due to chronic glomerulonephritis, chronic interstitial nephritis, or renal amyloidosis [68].

There are no signs of immunity of any kind and the lesions are crowded with an enormous number of bacteria [7, 32b, 83, 140]. The bacteraemia is constant even in the first four months of antibacterial therapy. A high incidence and persistence of Australia antigen, probably related to the depression of cell-mediated immunity, was shown in lepromatous leprosy as opposed to the tuberculoid form which is found to be negative for Australia antigen [41a].

The *histological picture* of lepromatous leprosy is characterized by diffuse infiltration, well separated from the epidermis by normal connective tissue. The infiltration consists of various cells from histiocytes in different stages to large vacuolated cells with clear cytoplasm, transforming into the typical lepra cells of Virchow [8]. Apart from the presence of mast cells and giant cells, a marked decrease in the number of lymphocytes [151a] and an accumulation of plasmacytes [6, 149, 151a] are characteristic findings. Almost all the tissue elements and nasal mucosa are invaded by a large number of bacterial cells, arranged frequently in typical cigar-bunches or clusters [81b, 84a, 91, 108, 150] which nearly fill up the macrophages [6] (Fig. 74-1).

Early during treatment the histiocytes and the lepra cells in lepromatous leprosy show an increased acid phosphatase activity, indicating an enhanced phagocytotic activity of macrophages. Subsequently, in the regressive phase, the

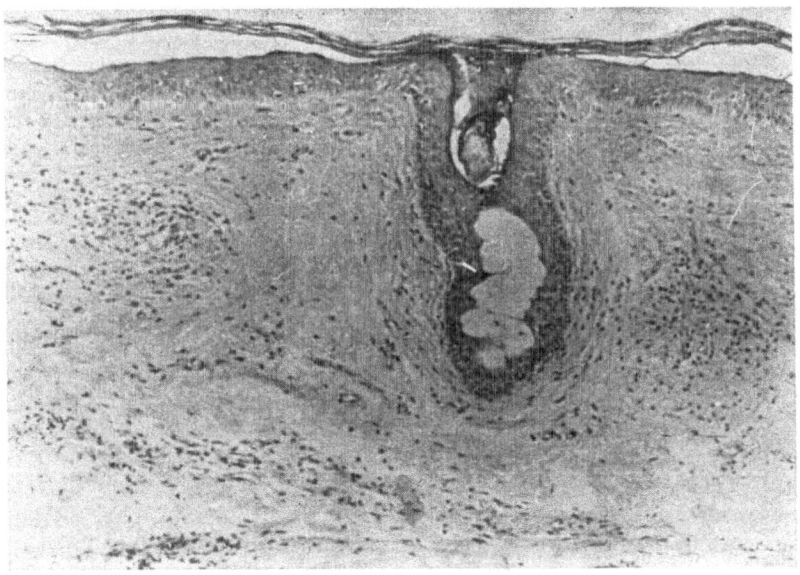

Fig. 74-1a. Histology of lepromatous leprosy

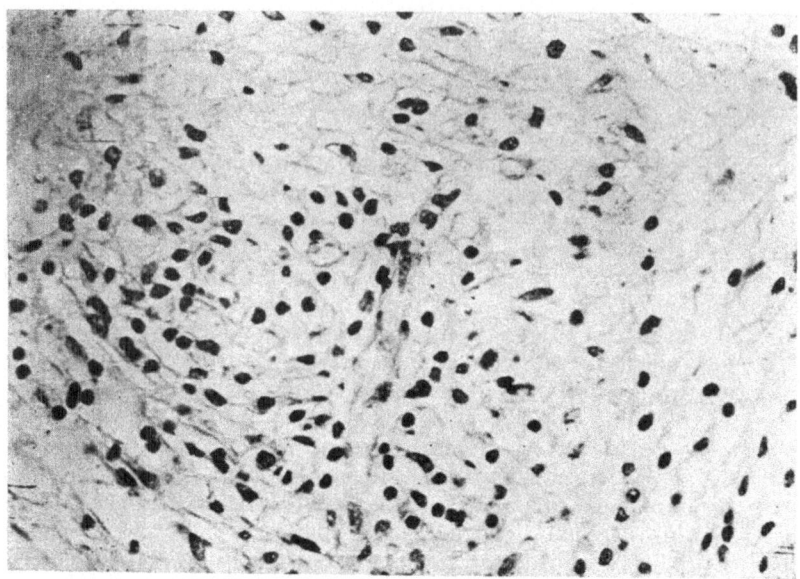

Fig. 74-1b. Histology of lepromatous leprosy

degenerating lepra cells are replaced by lymphoid elements also showing increased acid phosphatase activity. The lymphoid infiltration indicates the development of delayed hypersensitivity [78]. The difference between the two forms of leprosy is clearly seen in the histological picture of the lymph nodes [151c]. Lepromatous leprosy is characterized by cells of the histiocytic-macrophage type in the paracortical areas; these cells are unable to eliminate mycobacteria. The more intensive the resistance against the infection, the more differentiated are the histiocytes and the more they are resembling epitheloid cells.

TUBERCULOID LEPROSY
(BENIGN OR NEURAL TYPE)

This type of leprosy, which is not contagious [44], is characterized by a tuberculoid granulomatous structure containing very few bacteria. The granulomas are of variable numbers (mostly two or three) and usually of a moderate size. Only the skin and the nerves are involved. The lesions consist of erythematous or hypopigmented macular or papular foci with dry surface and well defined edges. There is a central flattening and hair loss resembling tuberculosis verrucosa. If the local resistance is weak, haematogenous dissemination occurs. The nervous symptoms (early nerve thickening) may precede those of the skin such as anaesthesia and trophic ulcerations. The clinical condition is not severe since the bacilli invading the skin give rise to tuberculoid granuloma formation, but subsequently no acid-fast bacteria can be found [32b, 34, 82, 97, 101]. No bacteria are detected in the skin excised 4 h after lepromin injection. Similarly, bacteria are found to be absent from nasal mucus cultures. In this way tuberculoid leprosy differs from the lepromatous type lesions which invariably contain the pathogen [132].

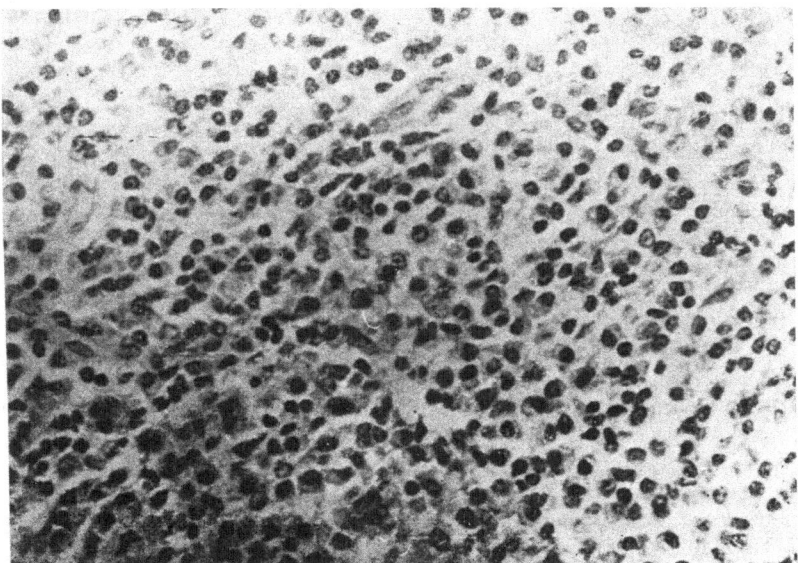

Fig. 74-2. Histology of tuberculoid leprosy

The histological picture of tuberculoid leprosy is characterized by the absence of the connective tissue zone between the infiltration and the dermis. The inflammatory exudate invades the epidermis as well as the deep layers of the subcutis. At the beginning, macrophages containing phagocytosed bacteria may be seen [107], but soon thereafter tubercles consisting of epitheloid cells predominate. Giant cells surrounded by numerous lymphocytes and few plasmocytes may be seen mainly in active progressive cases. Necrobiosis and caseation may also occur. At this time mycobacteria are absent or rather scarce; they can be detected mostly on the progressive borderline of the active lesion [72, 91, 101, 107, 150]. The histological picture of the lymph nodes in tuberculoid leprosy is similar to that in sarcoidosis and the paracortical area is populated by lymphocytes and immunoblasts [151c] (Fig. 74-2).

OTHER CLINICAL FORMS

The above-described two major forms of leprosy are distinct conditions without transition from one into the other [32d, 65, 83]. In addition to the differences in clinical picture and histology, there are very important distinguishing characteristics in the pathogenesis especially from the immunological point of view.

There are, besides the two basic types, a number of borderline or intermediate clinical forms. Some of these are still disputed owing mainly to the great variability of leprosy in geographically remote countries (e.g. India, South America). Briefly the following forms may be mentioned [10, 19, 32a, 35, 74, 82, 101, 114, 123a, b, 150]:

Borderline (dimorphous) leprosy. This type of leprosy, characterized by weak contagiousness [44], is immunologically unstable and usually evolves into one of the polar types in the course of time. Two groups are usually distinguished: one on the tuberculoid side of the borderline spectrum and one on the lepromatous side [72, 149, 155]. Since almost all types of the cellular elements of the organism are mobilized (tissue panic), the clinical and histological pictures are highly variable. Typically macules, plaques, annular lesions and punched-out lesions appear. Macules have well-defined edges; plaques have edges which are not consistently well defined and have little central flattening. All show some degree of sensory loss; they are too numerous and not dry enough for tuberculoid; they are too few and not shiny enough for lepromatous. Early nerve thickening occurs. Acid-fast bacilli are numerous or moderate in the borderline-lepromatous form, moderate in the mid-borderline form and few or absent in the borderline-tuberculoid form.

Indeterminate leprosy. This type of leprosy, which is not contagious [44], and the immunological aspects of which have not yet been determined, is a transitory phase in the disease process. It may last for months or years before disappearing or giving way to one of the major types of the disease depending on the influence of the immunological factors in the host. At this stage the histology alters accordingly. Lesions consist only of macules which are nondescript in character and asymmetrical in distribution. Cellular reaction is of simple inflammatory type and acid-fast bacilli are absent (rarely present in cutaneous nerves).

Early stage (silent phase) of leprosy may persist for years. In this almost no specific defence is shown and later on it progresses into one of the polar forms.

Lazarine leprosy resembles tuberculoid leprosy, its prognosis as well as its healing tendency being benign.

Diffuse lepromatous leprosy (Lucio and Alvarado Mexican type, spotted leprosy) is characterized by gangrenous ulcers. In this form the highest degree of anergy of the host is found.

Not only may peripheral nerve damage be the first sign of leprosy, but in some cases the disease may remain *purely neural* [68], the patient possessing a high degree of cell-mediated immunity. Presenting symptoms are either sensory or motor, or both, depending on the type of nerve involved, and nerve thickening will be found on palpation. It should be noted that three cranial nerves can be damaged in leprosy—the first, fifth, and seventh—the reason being that they have courses outside the skull, and leprosy bacilli prefer the cooler portions of nerves [66].

IMMUNOLOGICAL ASPECTS

LEPROSY REACTIONS (REACTIONAL STATES)

These are the bugbear of treatment and call for patience and skill in their management [66]. They are not drug reactions and may occur in patients not under treatment, but are more likely to complicate chemotherapy. One type of reactions, so-called *type I reaction*, represents an extremely rapid change in cell-mediated immunity, for better or worse, and is particularly liable to complicate borderline leprosy; the concept of upgrading and downgrading reactions has been proposed by Ridley [122], reflecting an increase or decrease in cell-mediated immunity. The reaction is characterized by swelling and redness of skin lesions, oedema of face, hands and feet and pain and swelling in one or more nerves [66].

Another type of reaction, commonly known as *erythema nodosum leprosum* or *type II reaction*, is an immune complex syndrome and occurs only in lepromatous leprosy [44, 49c, 66]. It is characterized by transient erythematous nodules and patches occurring in crops on any part of the skin but particularly on the face, arms, and thighs, usually fading in a few days and being replaced by fresh lesions but sometimes becoming necrotic [122, 135, 159, 161]. Oedema of face and limbs are a usual symptom. When it develops during sulphone therapy, analogy to the Jarish–Herxheimer reaction has been suggested [32a, 156a]. Owing to the extensive destruction, the number of bacterial cells is very small. Histologically it corresponds to allergic vasculitis. The clinical picture may suggest intermediary forms between classic erythema nodosum and polyarteritis nodosa [7, 12]. Its incidence is low (approximately 2.3 per cent of the cases), but recurrences are frequent [101]. It may be prevented by calcium and antihistamine drugs [17a]. The sera from patients with active erythema nodosum leprosum tested with the precipitin assay technique react more frequently with the C1q component of C [49c]. This is further, although circumstantial, evidence for the immune complex aetiology of this condition [124]. Electron microscopic study of erythema nodosum leprosum by means of the ferritin conjugated antibody method revealed that the antigenicity of leprosy bacilli is localized in the cytoplasm of leprosy bacilli [107a]. As antibodies to the cytoplasm of leprosy bacilli are present in the serum, the outflow of cytoplasmic substance of leprosy bacilli results in an antigen–antibody reaction which leads to erythema nodosum. Other manifestations, which may correspond to symptoms of the immune complex syndrome, include fever, neuritis, swollen joints, swollen fingers, painful tibiae, swelling and tenderness of lymph nodes, epistaxis, epididymoorchitis, iridocyclitis, and laboratory findings of proteinuria, anaemia, raised erythrocyte sedimentation rate and serum globulin, and a polymorphonuclear leukocytosis [66].

In all these forms the cellular reactions differ according to the immunological status. The immunological status is all-important in deciding the clinical picture, course and prognosis. It can be accepted as a rule: the more pronounced the tuberculoid character in the histological picture, the more intensive is the development of immunity and *vice versa*. The absence of a tuberculoid histological picture indicates the failure of the defense mechanism. In tuberculoid leprosy the considerable immune resistance is based, like in tuberculosis, on cellular function [25, 81b, 133a, 150].

IMMUNOLOGICAL DIFFERENCES BETWEEN THE TWO MAJOR TYPES OF LEPROSY

The differences between the two polar forms of leprosy cannot be attributed to the pathogen itself, but to the affected organism. Leprosy is contagious even through the skin. The significance of the circumstances and route of infection are well known in the development of the different types of tuberculosis; in this respect there are no reliable data available in leprosy [32c, 147]. The difference between the two types may be the function of processes exerting their influence upon the disease from the very beginning of the infection and through its entire course. Obviously, the pathogen is well tolerated by the tissues, and owing to this tolerance, the cellular immune reaction requires several years to develop in tuberculoid leprosy. Such a reaction never develops in the lepromatous form, in which the insufficient native resistance is not supported by any other defensive function. The essence of the tolerance is not clear. In the majority of the cases of lepromatous leprosy only an atypical variant of the pseudocholinesterase is present, in contrast to healthy persons and patients suffering from tuberculoid leprosy. As specific HLA antigens were not associated with tuberculoid or lepromatous leprosy [120a], it has been rejected that genetic factors play an important role in developing the lepromatous form of leprosy [145]. A primary deficiency of cell-mediated immunity might come into consideration [25]. This deficiency may result, probably secondarily rather than primarily, in the absence of lymphocytes in the paracortical areas and in their functional insufficiency, characterizing the lepromatous form [24b, 37, 151a]. The reaction to intracutaneous and subcutaneous transfer of lymphocyte concentrates is weaker than that to normal lymphocytes [94], i.e. the leprous lymphocytes are weak in inducing graft-versus-host reaction [57, 81a]. Lepromatous leprosy patients with lymph node cells from a lepromin positive tuberculoid donor converted lepromin negativity to positivity in skin test and in vitro lymphocyte transformation test [7a]. Replacement of paracortical area by a massive infiltration of histiocytes [40] and a repopulation of this area with lymphocytes had been described as the result of successful treatment of lepromatous leprosy with intravenous lymphocyte infusions [87]. A deficiency of immunity in the lepromatous form is also shown by the marked depression or total absence of the delayed-type intracutaneous hypersensitivity reactions [24a, 25, 71, 81b, 84a, 94, 107, 156] against lepromin, bacterial and fungal antigens as well as against haptens and transplantation antigens [25, 71, 131, 156]. It may occur that the lepromin reaction is negative [64b], but a positive PPD test can be obtained [142]. The failure of, or highly reduced ability for, lymphocyte transformation seems to be proved, despite the somewhat divergent results [6, 81a, 104, 153]; both the PHA and the streptolysin O reactions are depressed [40, 109, 136, 142]. Moreover, it has been shown that blastic transformation of lymphocytes from patients with tuberculoid leprosy cannot be induced with minced rat lepromas or with M. leprae obtained from such nodules by ultracentrifugation, using lymphocytes from active lepromatous cases and even by the non-specific stimulus of PHA [96]. It is suggested that C reactive protein in autologous serum may, in part, be responsible for the depression of 3H thymidine incorporation into DNA of leukocytes of leprosy patients [61a]. This depression was reversed by the subsequent addition of choline phosphate. In lepromatous leprosy patients the deficit in lymphoblastic transformation was accompanied by a high percentage of failure to sensitize with DNCB [10a]. The divergent results of lymphocyte transformation tests may have been due to the circumstance that the response varied with the status of the patient [93]. Leukocytes from untreated cases of lepromatous leprosy showed a depressed response to PHA, whereas the leukocytes from patients treated with sulphones gave an enhanced response. T lymphocytes of lepromatous leprosy patients do not form rosettes with sheep erythrocytes spontaneously [87a]. Lymphocytes from lepromatous leprosy patients do not produce lymphotoxin demonstrable by lepromin in HeLa cell culture [56]. There is also inability to produce the migration inhibition factor under lepromin action [71]; antigen effect induces the appearence of a DNA synthesis inhibiting factor [25]. The macrophages in lepromatous leprosy have completely lost their ability to digest bacteria [34, 50, 51]. In the absolute majority of the cases there was lack of production of the macrophage aggregating factor, whereas in tuberculoid leprosy this factor was present in most cases [142]. Response to irritants (benzalkonium chloride and potash soap) is also depressed in the majority of patients with lepromatous leprosy [94a]. A reduction in number of a subpopulation of T lymphocytes was noted in lepromatous leprosy cases with high bacillary load [103a]. Tuberculoid and treated lepromatous patients, who were bacillary negative, had normal levels of these cells. In patients with active lepromatous leprosy the percentage of B lymphocytes assessed by means of an immunofluorescent technique was very high (60 to 85 per cent) [48] irrespective of bacillary load [103a] and rose still higher from time to time as a result of effective sulphone therapy [48]. The excess of B lymphocytes may represent on overcompensation by B cells when the T cell population is numerically and functionally deficient [48]. The increase in the absolute number of B lymphocytes and the decrease in that of T lymphocytes suggest that the anergy of the cell-mediated immune systems in patients with lepromatous leprosy may be secondary to the destruction of T lymphocytes or some disturbance in their recirculation [42]. The residual T cell function together with a very vigorous humoral response may adequately protect patients against other bacterial, fungal and viral infections. Indeed, it has been shown that leprosy patients who failed to be sensitized to DNCB [19, 71, 81b, 116] were able to develop delayed-type hypersensitivity to keyhole limpet haemocyanin [151b]. Recent evidence has suggested that the anergy in leprosy can be reversed with the transfer factor [26] or allogeneic cell infusions [87b].

A disturbed equilibrium between cell-mediated and humoral immunity may be found [44]. The Mitsuda reaction is positive in tuberculoid leprosy, while the patients' serum does not contain anti-Hansen-bacillus antibodies. On the other hand, the Mitsuda reaction is negative and humoral antibodies can be demonstrated in lepromatous leprosy. In the sera of patients with lepromatous leprosy precipitable immune complexes were found in 70 per cent. On the other hand, the sera of only 2 out of 9 patients with tuberculoid leprosy were found to contain precipitable complexes [124]. Thus it seems that while in lepromatous leprosy the patient is incapable of cell-mediated immune reactions, he produces a special protein in the serum. This immunoglobulin is known as humoral antibody, but is incapable of eliminating M. leprae from the tissues, and the bacilli multiply unhindered. Hence lepromatous leprosy is a progressive disease involving many tissues [66]. The anergy, however, is incomplete, and is not directed toward other Mycobacteria [81b, 151a, b]. In the clinically involved skin of patients with lepromatous leprosy fine granular deposits of IgM have been found at the dermoepidermal junction [24c]. Electron microscopically within the glomeruli dense, amorphous deposits in subendothelial and intramembranous position were also demonstrated [24d]. These suggest that lepromatous leprosy may be associated with immunologic disturbances of both skin and glomerular basement membranes. Others [116a] have found by direct immunofluorescence technique deposition of IgM at the dermoepidermal junction only in 50 per cent of the cases, and in the other 50 per cent along the dermal collagen and elastic fibers in the skin. By indirect immunofluorescence circulating IgG antibodies to intercellular substance of epithelial cells were found in 25 per cent of patients with lepromatous leprosy. These antibodies appeared to be different from the skin-bound immunoglobulin deposits. Although there were bacilli present in biopsy specimens, the immunoglobulin deposits did not correspond to the deposits of bacilli [116a]. However, it is also possible that antimycobacterial antibodies may cross-react with basement membrane antigens [24c]. It is possible that the occurrence of anti-intercellular-substance antibody may be related to the tissue damage brought about by the lepromatous process [116a].

The cellular defence in the tuberculoid form resembles that found in tuberculosis of the skin, but is much more effective [32c, d]. The lymphocytes of the tuberculoid leprosy patients are not defective in their response to PHA and lepromin (blast transformation) [64b], and respond to lepromin with an increased production of the migration inhibition factor [11, 15, 71]. The patients can readily be sensitized by dinitrochlorobenzene and respond to various common allergens with a satisfactory delayed-type reaction. Also, the existence of a yet unknown humoral protective mechanism, independent of cellular defence, or rather cooperating with the latter, cannot be excluded [25, 108]. Summarizing it may be stated that in tuberculoid leprosy the patient is able to produce lymphocytes that are capable of reacting specifically with *M. leprae*. The presence of these specially sensitized lymphocytes makes it possible for macrophages to destroy *M. leprae* and thereby contain the infection [66].

In borderline leprosy antigenic heterogeneity has been established by lymphocyte transformation test [11a].

LEPROSY COMPARED WITH TUBERCULOSIS

Despite the identical mechanism, there are prominent differences between tuberculosis and leprosy, concerning both the quality and the degree of immunity [84a, 105, 123b].

Tuberculosis of the skin is highly variable in clinical appearance, but each type invariably retains its character. Contrarily, in leprosy only the two polar types maintain constantly their peculiar features [101].

In tuberculosis the initial non-specific histological picture turns, inevitably and within a short time (in 2 to 3 weeks), into the typical specific picture (tuberculous structure), always accompanied by acquired immunity. In leprosy this picture will only develop after years and even then only in the tuberculoid form, whereas in the lepromatous form this stage is never reached [32a].

Both the quality and course of tuberculosis of the skin are generally independent of the processes in the inner organs, whereas the cutaneous symptoms of leprosy change in close correlation with the alterations of the bones and the nerves [82, 121].

The differences between the symptoms of tuberculosis and leprosy [84b, 89, 91, 102, 125, 146] may be attributed, in the first place, to the difference between the two pathogens and to their relation to the host tissues. The immunogenicity of *M. leprae* is weak and its stimulus upon the tissues is less effective than that of *M. tuberculosis* [32a, 54, 55, 83, 101, 108, 144]. A tolerance as marked as in the foci of lepromatous leprosy can never be found in tuberculosis of the skin. Moreover, *M. leprae* is considerably less resistant to the immune powers of the organism than *M. tuberculosis*.

ALLERGY TESTS

Investigating the antigenic mosaic of *M. leprae*, antisera against tissue separated *M. leprae* showed the presence of five detectable antigens, but two of these cross-reacted with a number of other mycobacterial species. Chromatographic separation of the antigens resulted in a number of fractions, some of which gave immunoprecipitates when tested against the anti-lepra serum. Few of the fractions were able to elicit hypersensitivity in the homologously sensitized animals [103a]. The heat-resistant polysaccharide antigen fraction of *M. leprae* is less specific, it forms a precipitate with BCG and with *M. microti* antisera, too, whereas the heat-sensitive protein antigen fraction reacts only with rabbit serum produced against leprous lymph nodes [1]. The allergy against the bacterial protein (indicated by the Fernandez reaction; see below) is much weaker than found with tuberculin [45, 58, 83, 89]. Consequently it seems unlikely that *M. leprae* would contain a toxin corresponding to tuberculin [83]. The bacterial allergy characteristic of tuberculosis is absent in leprosy and so is the hypersensitivity to the components of the bacterial body (Koch's phenomenon). The strong antibacterial mechanism in tuberculoid leprosy cannot be examined, owing to the failure to obtain a pure bacterial suspension [133b, 134, 144]. It may only be supposed that it corresponds to the cell-mediated immune mechanism operating in tuberculosis.

Lepromin test is a skin test of tuberculin type which indicates delayed hypersensitivity to *M. leprae* in patients with leprosy. Lepromin is an extract of skin nodules containing *M. leprae* from patients with lepromatous leprosy and is injected intracutaneously (0.1 ml); the positive reaction consists of a delayed-type inflammatory nodule, appearing in 1 to 2 weeks, maximal after 3 to 4 weeks, and then disappearing slowly [17a, 133a, b].

This late reaction is called *Mitsuda reaction* [98a, b, c]; histologically it corresponds to tuberculoid leprosy: the nodule contains an accumulation of epitheloid and giant cells with lymphocytes and occasionally caseation. In lepromin beside *M. leprae* the tissue elements also act as antigens [141], and the reaction is therefore not identical with the tuberculin tests [52, 89]. Its mechanism corresponds mainly to accelerated tubercle formation which develops in a spectacular manner around the *M. tuberculosis* reintroduced into the guinea pig already infected by the same bacterium [52]. The Mitsuda reaction can be elicited only with suspensions containing intact bacterial bodies [77]. Since the bacterium content of the different lepromin preparations is highly variable, its standardization would be desirable [19]. WHO recommends the use of the 1 : 8 dilution of a standard preparation containing 160 million bacterial cells per ml [59]. The reaction can be more accurately evaluated by microscopic reading [111].

The positive reaction indicates antibacterial resistance: it occurs in tuberculoid leprosy of good defence mechanism, whereas it is negative in the completely anergic lepromatous form, it is weakly positive in borderline-tuberculoid, and negative in borderline-lepromatous variants [35, 44, 58, 89, 101, 111, 115, 117, 142]. Thus the test is of diagnostic and prognostic importance in distinguishing the two polar variants of the disease [148]. Its specificity is reduced [76b, 111, 118e] by the finding that the similarly prepared extracts of normal skin may also produce a positive reaction which is, however, weaker [38, 76a, 84a]. Repeated lepromin injections or BCG inoculation may turn a negative Mitsuda reaction into positive [3, 9, 13b, 16, 28, 32c, 35, 84a, 126], and in tuberculous persons and even in healthy adults, it might often be positive [35], though in healthy children it is generally negative [22, 58, 60]. Oral and intradermal routes of vaccination induce equivalent lepromin positivity [9, 92, 96]. Its chief diagnostic value consists in its positivity excluding lepromatous leprosy, although a negative test does not prove the reverse. The role of the individual fractions of *M. leprae* could not yet be examined so far, since no pure cultures are available [33a, b, 79, 88, 160].

Fernandez reaction [45]. This is the early stage of the lepromin reaction in which an indurated nodule appears 24–48 h after injection of an extract containing *M. leprae* into patients with tuberculoid leprosy. The reaction indicates delayed-type hypersensitivity to the protein fractions of *M. leprae* [13a, 19, 89, 115, 134, 143] in cases in which lymphocyte transformation would normally be positive [115]. The Fernandez reaction is always negative in lepromatous leprosy, indicating lower resistance together with anergy [115]. Unlike the Mitsuda reaction, the Fernandez reaction can be abolished by repeated injections of the bacterial proteins. Therefore it is regarded as corresponding to the tuberculin reaction in tuberculosis [13a, 89, 143, 144]. The strength of the reaction can be increased by using Dharmendra's bacterial component [134]. The Fernandez reaction is diagnostically less important than the Mitsuda reaction.

The study of the lepromin reaction in normal and tuberculous individuals and, inversely, BCG trials in leprous regions and on leprosy patients has brought surprising results. Besides the hypotheses which still await proving — e.g. antagonism of tuberculosis and leprosy [31, 84b, 102] — important theoretical and (particularly in leprosy) practical results have been obtained [13b, 28, 58]. It has been shown that the lepromin reaction is frequently positive in patients suffering from tuberculosis, moreover, lepromin tests turn out positive even in healthy (non-tuberculous and non-leprous) individuals [14, 47, 60], particularly in tuberculin-positive healthy persons. Remarkably, the same has been observed in countries free of leprosy [30, 60, 126, 158]. Not only natural tuberculous infection but also vaccination may induce lepromin positivity or increase the strength of a weak Mitsuda reaction [29, 43, 99]. This effect is, however, not mutual, since the tuberculin reaction is not significantly influenced by either forms of leprosy; there is no marked tuberculin allergy in leprosy [84a, 90].

The obvious explanation of lepromin positivity in tuberculin-positive persons is supplied by the fact that the two *Mycobacteria* share some common or related antigens. Tuberculin-positive individuals are allergic to both tuberculin and the bacterial body and possess also acquired immunity. Thus the lepromin introduced into the sensitized skin of tuberculous persons meets, owing to the similarity between tuberculous and tuberculoid leprous tissues [61, 63, 92] similar conditions as in the skin of patients suffering from tuberculoid leprosy. Contrarily, this state of reactivity is absent in lepromatous leprosy as well as in subjects (mostly children) who have not yet been in contact with *M. tuberculosis*.

There is no evidence that leprous infection could start some kind of 'isopathic reaction' (a special foam cell reaction not containing bacilli) or an immune process against tuberculous material (tuberculin, living BCG) or some other substances (Indian ink, Leishmania parasites, peptone, milk) [64a, 69, 75, 128a, 129a, b, 130]. However, the isopathic phenomenon elicited with BCG can help to detect all types of latent leprosy infections [117a].

These processes upon which the positivity of the lepromin test is based serve the protection of the organism since the lepromin-positive healthy persons are either not attacked by leprosy or the disease takes a less severe course in them [10, 32a, 58, 89]. The ability of BCG to convert the lepromin action into positive has supplied a theoretical basis for BCG immunization in the control of leprosy, which is justified by practical results [13b, 19, 28, 77, 102]. It may be supposed that even if it is not yet generally accepted the cellular immune processes induced by BCG may produce an accelerated reaction and, consequently, a more effective protection against a subsequent leprous infection. BCG immunization may be beneficial particularly in persons, mainly children, who live in as leprous environment [22, 58]. It would be highly justified to initiate screening tests for persons reacting weakly and to develop prophylactic measures including vaccination for them. Observations suggesting that BCG vaccination of patients suffering from lepromatous leprosy may initiate a tendency to shift the clinical and histological picture towards the picture of the tuberculoid form are promising [128].

SEROLOGY

In leprosy as well as in tuberculosis the immunological status may be assessed based, in the first place, on the clinical symptoms, histological signs and on the course of the illness. The laboratory findings are of little importance and the components of the serum show no changes of diagnostic value [6, 20, 27, 80].

Since no satisfactory *M. leprae* preparations are available, fractions prepared from *M. tuberculosis* utilized in tuberculosis serology have been introduced as antigen in the serology of leprosy with considerable success. The antigenic properties of the corresponding fractions of *M. leprae* and *M. tuberculosis* have much in common [5, 60, 100, 115, 127, 134, 144, 152, 154]. Antibodies can be demonstrated against mycobacterial proteins and, particularly, against polysaccharides [35, 89]. The same methods are used as in tuberculosis, e.g. C fixation, precipitation, agglutination. An increase in the IgG, IgA and IgM levels [27] and in the C levels [135, 159], and the appearance of cryoglobulins [20, 133b] have been observed in lepromatous leprosy and in connection with the erythema nodosum symptom. Recently it has been shown that the immunoglobulins change parallel in lepromatous and tuberculoid leprosy; the IgG, IgM and IgA levels are elevated in both. The IgA level is especially high if the illness is of prolonged course. In regression due to therapeutical interventions the IgM level declines while the IgA level remains high [139]. Cryoglobulins consisting of IgG and IgM compo-

119

nents can be isolated mainly from lepromatous cases. The IgM fractions of leprous sera have shown an anti-γ-globulin activity [20]. The sera of leprosy patients may also contain C-reactive protein. The precipitation line of coeruloplasmin has been found enhanced in a number of cases, and sometimes haptoglobin has been found increased [80].

The frequency of positive serological reactions is more frequent and stronger in lepromatous leprosy than in tuberculoid leprosy [89, 121, 149, 154]. Moreover, the serological positivity is much more frequent and stronger than in any forms of tuberculosis [85, 89, 136, 141, 152]. Cross-reactions can also be demonstrated between *M. leprae* and Stefansky's *M. lepraemurium* the bacterium causing rat leprosy. This permits a quantitative comparison of the humoral antibodies in leprosy patients by indirect immunofluorescence techniques, using the smear of either *M. leprae* or *M. lepraemurium* as antigen [95, 96]. The presence of antibodies in leprosy sera has been confirmed by the action of minced rat lepromas or by the effect of bacteria obtained by ultracentrifugation from the lepromas on guinea pig ileum sensitized by such sera [96]. Leprosy antigen produces strong cross-sensitivity in intracutaneous test with the so-called photochromogenic atypical Mycobacteria [21]. Antibodies have been demonstrated also against other related antigens [140]. As a result of the above facts, the serological reactions are scarcely specific for leprosy, and the situation is further complicated by the positive results obtained with syphilitic lipid antigens [133b] which, at least partly, should be considered as biologically false positive results. The relatively high frequency of Australia (hepatitis B) antigen in leprous sera cannot be attributed to the disease; the occurrence of this antigen is similarly high in the general populations of the areas afflicted by leprosy [138]. Due to the extensive tissue destruction, non-organ-specific autoantibodies (rheumatoid factor, anti-thyroglobulin and anti-nuclear antibodies) occur more frequently but in lower titres than in control populations, particularly in the lepromatous form. The fact that in South-East-Asian patients the prevalence of autoantibodies is high seems to be suggestive of a difference in immune response [113]. There is a serologic similarity of the lepromatous form with both SLE and rheumatoid arthritis [19], and thus these, too, should be considered as non-specific reactions. The humoral antibodies could be hardly connected with the effective immune processes in leprosy [6].

THERAPY

Dapsone (diaminodiphenyl sulphone) is the drug of choice [23]. It is effective in all varieties of leprosy, and if given with due care, relatively free from severe side effects. It can safely be given by mouth and over long periods, it induces resistance very rarely, and is very cheap. The two basic principles of Dapsone therapy are [67]: (*i*) to start with small doses and to increase them slowly; (*ii*) to maintain an optimum dose which is not larger than necessary. Length of treatment depends on the type of leprosy [66]. Recently acetyl derivatives have been introduced; these are repository sulphones, the intramuscular injection being effective for over 2 months. The second-line drug recommended for routine use is thiambutosine, a complex diphenylthiourea which is given to patients exhibiting intolerance to Dapsone, precocious neuritis, or acute psychosis. Long-acting sulphonamides have a certain action in leprosy but possess no real advantages over Dapsone [23]. Several other drugs are occasionally employed in leprosy, and others are at present under investigation, e.g. a riminophenazine compound (clofazimine) which has the unique property of being effective also as an anti-inflammatory agent. Antibiotics include cycloserine and terramycin, but the most effective by far is rifampicin. The acute exacerbation of lepromatous leprosy responds to antimonials such as tartar emetic and stibophen or to antimalarials. Patients suffering from persistent exacerbation will need corticosteroids. Repeated infusions of allogeneic lymphocytes [87a] and transfusion of whole blood from Mitsuda positive donors [6a] brought about improvement of the lepromatous leprosy patients. The surgical complications cannot be considered here in detail. Physiotherapy, vocational training, the treatment of the psychological accompaniments, the provision of sympathetic care and understanding, the avoidance of social dislocation and the evils of institutionalization are part of the modern therapy of leprosy [23].

REFERENCES

1. Abe, M.: *Int. J. Leprosy* **38**, 113 (1970).
2. Abe, M., Minagawa, F., Yoshino, Y. and Okamura, K.: *Int. J. Leprosy* **40**, 107 (1972).
3. Acuri, P. B. and Puga, G.: *Leprologia* **13**, 125 (1968).
4. Ali, P. M.: *Indian J. Publ. Hlth.* **10**, 145 (1966).
5. Almeida, de, J. O.: *Bull. Wld Hlth Org.* **42**, 673 (1970).
6. Almeida, de, J. O., Bechelli, L. M., Bullock, W. E., Convit, J., Guinto, R. S., Han, H., Rees, R. J. W., Shepard, C. C., Szemberg, A., Talwar, G. P. and Turk, J. L.: *Bull. Wld Hlth Org.* **43**, 879 (1970).
6a. Almeida Goncalves, J. C. and Custodio, J.: *Leprosy Rev.* **46**, 15 (1975).
7. Anderson, W. A. D.: *Pathology.* Mosby, St. Louis 1966, p. 234.
7a. Antia, N. H. and Khanolkar, S. R.: *Int. J. Leprosy* **42**, 28 (1974).
8. Aquino, T. I. and Skinses, O. K.: *Int. J. Leprosy* **38**, 134 (1970).
9. Azulay, R. D., Kahn, H., Scorzelli, A. and Meyerheim, R.: *Int. J. Leprosy* **39**, 508 (1971).
10. Baccareda-Boy, A., Bertamino, R. and Farris, G.: *Derm. int.* *(Philad.)* **6**, 224 (1968).
10a. Balina, L. M., Fliess, E. L. and Cardama, J. E.: *Int. J. Derm.* **13**, 300 (1974).
11. Barbieri, T. A. and Correa, W. M.: *Int. J. Leprosy* **35**, 377 (1967).
11a. Barnetson, R. Stc., Bjune, G., Pearson, J. M. H. and Kronvall, G.: *Brit. med. J.* **iv**, 435 (1975).
12. Basset, A.: *Acta leprol.* *(Genève)* **40**, 35 (1970).
13a. Bechelli, L. M.: *Acta leprol.* *(Genève)* **25**, 1 (1966).
13b. id., *Erg.-Werk zu J. Jadassohns Handbuch der Haut- und Geschlechtskrankheiten.* Vol. IV/1B. Ed. by Röckl, H. Springer, Berlin 1970, p. 332.
14. Beiguelman, B.: *Bull. Wld Hlth Org.* **37**, 461 (1967).
15. Beiguelman, B. and Barbieri, T. A.: *Cienc. Cult.* *(Sao Paulo)* **17**, 304 (1965).
16. Beiguelman, B., Quagliato, R. and Camargo, D. P.: *Int. J. Leprosy* **33**, 795 (1965).
17a. Bergel, M.: *Lepro* *(Tokyo)* **37**, 291 (1968).
17b. id., *Ther. Gegenw.* **110**, 1472 (1971).
18. Binford, C. H.: *Lab. Invest.* **11**, 942 (1962).
19. Binford, C. H., Convit, J., Iyer, C. G. S., Shepard, C. C., Torsuev, N. A. and Yoshie, Y.: *Wld Hlth Org. techn. Rep. Ser. No. 459* (1970).
20. Bonomo, L. and Dammaco, F.: *Clin. exp. Immunol.* **9**, 175 (1971).
21. Bovornkitti, S., Ramasutra, Th. and Chantarakul, N.: *J. med. Ass.* *(Thailand)* **53**, 338 (1970).

22. Brown, J. A. K. and Stone, M. M.: *Brit. med. J.* i, 7 (1966).
23. Browne, St. G.: In *Dermatology in General Medicine.* Ed. by Fitzpatrick, B., Arndt, K. A., Clark, W. H., jr., Eisen, A. Z., van Scott, E. J. and Vaugham, J. H. McGraw-Hill, New York 1971, p. 1549.
24*a*. Bullock, W. E.: *Clin. Res.* **14**, 337 (1966).
24*b*. id., *New Engl. J. Med.* **278**, 298 (1968).
24*c*. Bullock, W. E., Callerame, M. L. and Panner, B. J.: *Amer. J. trop. Med. Hyg.* **23**, 78 (1974).
24*d*. ibid., **23**, 81 (1974).
25. Bullock, W. E., jr. and Fasal, P.: *J. Immunol.* **106**, 888 (1971).
26. Bullock, W. E., Fields, J. P. and Brandriss, M. W.: *New Engl. J. Med.* **287**, 1053 (1972).
27. Bullock, W. E., Ho, Min-Fu and Chen, Mei-Jan: *J. Lab. clin. Med.* **75**, 863 (1970).
28. Campos, N. S.: *Rev. bras. Leprol.* **36**, 37 (1969).
29. Campos, N. S., Leser, W., Quagliato, R., Bechelli, R. and Rotberg, A.: *Rev. bras. Leprol.* **30**, 3 (1962).
30. Campos, N. S. and Lobo, O. P.: *Rev. bras. Leprol.* **32**, 23 (1964).
31. Choussinand, R.: *Leprosy Rev.* **24**, 90 (1953).
32*a*. Cochrane, R. G.: In *Ciba Foundation Symposium on Experimental Tuberculosis. Bacillus and Host. With an Addendum on Leprosy.* Ed. by Wolstenholme, G. E. W. and Cameron, M. P. Churchill, London 1955, p. 355.
32*b*. id., *Leprosy in Theory and Practice.* Wright, Bristol 1959.
32*c*. id., *Int. trop. Med.* **1**, 1 (1961).
32*d*. id., *Leprosy Rev.* **36**, 189 (1965).
33*a*. Choucroun, N.: *C. R. Acad. Sci.* **229**, 145 (1949).
33*b*. id., *Amer. Rev. Tuberc.* **56**, 710 (1949).
34. Cline, M. J.: *Infect. Immunol.* **2**, 156 (1970).
35. Convit, J., Dharmendra., Guinto, S., Hanks, J. H., Laviron, P. and Rees, R. J. W.: *Wld Hlth Org. techn. Rep. Ser. No. 319* (1966).
36. Convit, J., Lapenta, P., Ilukevich, A. and Imaeda, T.: *Int. J. Leprosy* **32**, 136 (1964).
37. Cooper, M. D., Gabrielsen, A. E. and Good, R. A.: *Ann. Rev. Med.* **18**, 113 (1967).
38. Davey, T. F. and Drewett, S. E.: *Leprosy Rev.* **29**, 197 (1958).
39*a*. Dharmendra: *Indian J. med. Res.* **30**, 1 (1942).
39*b*. id., *Leprosy in India* **14**, 122 (1942).
40. Dierks, R. E. and Shepard, C. C.: *Proc. Soc. exp. Biol.* (*N. Y.*) **127**, 391 (1968).
41. Drutz, D. J., Chen, T. S. N. and Lu, W. H.: *New Engl. J. Med.* **287**, 159 (1972).
41*a*. Dutta, R. N. and Saha, K.: *Indian J. med. Res.* **61**, 1758 (1973).
42. Dwyer, J. M., Bullock, W. E. and Fields, J. P.: *New Engl. J. Med.* **288**, 1036 (1973).
43. Epstein, W. L.: *Progr. Allergy* **11**, 36 (1967).
44. Escande, J. P.: *Nouv. Presse méd.* **3**, 461 (1974).
45. Fernandez, J. M. M.: *Int. J. Leprosy* **8**, 1 (1940).
46. Fernandez, J. M. M. and Castro, M. O.: *Rev. argent. Dermat.* **25**, 435 (1941).
47. Furtado, T. A. and Schulz, K. H.: *Rev. bras. Leprol.* **33**, 75 (1965).
48. Gajl-Peczalska, K. J., Lim, S. D., Jacobson, R. R. and Good, R. A.: *New Engl. J. Med.* **288**, 1033 (1973).
49*a*. Gaugas, J. M.: *Brit. J. exp. Path.* **48**, 417 (1967).
49*b*. id., *Nature* **220**, 1246 (1968).
49*c*. Gelber, R. H., Drutz, D. J., Epstein, W. V. and Fasal, P.: *Amer. J. trop. Med. Hyg.* **23**, 471 (1974).
50. Godal, Z. and Rees, R. J. W.: Cited by Almeida, J. O. et al.: *Bull. Wld Hlth Org.* **43**, 879 (1970).
51. Godal, T., Rees, R. J. W. and Lamvik, J. O.: *Clin. exp. Immunol.* **8**, 625 (1970).
52. Goihman-Yahr, M., Raffel, S. and Ferraresi, R. W.: *Int. Arch. Allergy* **36**, 450 (1969).
53. Guinto, R. S. and Mabalay, M. C.: *Int. J. Leprosy* **30**, 278 (1962).
54. Hadler, W. A.: *Leprosy Rev.* **36**, 171 (1965).
55. Haensch, R. and Schmalbruch, H.: *Arch. derm. Forsch.* **241**, 179 (1971).
56. Han, S. H , Weiser, R. S., and Tseng, J. J.: *Int. J. Leprosy* **39**, 719 (1972).

57. Han, S. H., Weiser, R. S., Tseng, J. J. and Kau, S. T.: *Int. J. Leprosy* **39**, 715 (1972).
58. Hanks, J. H.: *Ciba Foundation Symposium on Experimental Tuberculosis*. Churchill, London 1955, p. 364.
59. Hanks, J. H., Abe, M., Nakayama, T., Tuma, M., Bechelli, L. M. and Dominguez, V. M.: *Bull. Wld Hlth Org.* **42**, 703 (1970).
60. Hinden-Leizinger, M.: *Dermatologica (Basel)* **140**, Suppl. 2, 35 (1970).
61. Hirano, N.: *Lepro (Tokyo)* **32**, 83 (1963).
61a. Hokama, Y., Su, D. W. P., Skinsnes, O. K., Kim, R., Kimura, L. and Yanagihara, E.: *Int. J. Leprosy* **42**, 19 (1974).
62. Imaeda, T., Convit, J., Ilukevich, H. and Lapenta, P.: *Int. J. Leprosy* **30**, 395 (1962).
63. Innami, S.: *Lepro (Tokyo)* **37**, 331 (1968).
64a. Job, C. K.: *Int. J. Leprosy* **37**, 365 (1969).
64b. id., *J. Path. Bact.* **17**, 75 (1974).
65. Jonquires, S. L., Melamed, J. and Manzi, R. O.: *Int. J. Leprosy* **31**, 1 (1963).
66. Jopling, W. H.: *Brit. J. Hosp. Med.* **43** (1974).
67. Jopling, W. H. and Harman, R. R. M.: In *Textbook of Dermatology*. 2nd ed. Vol. 1. Ed. by Rook, A. J., Wilkinson, D. S. and Ebling F. J. G. Blackwell, Oxford 1972, p. 680.
68. Jopling W. H. and Morgan-Hughes, J. A.: *Brit. med. J.* **ii**, 799 (1965).
69. Kanaar, P.: *Derm. int. (Philad.)* **6**, 11 (1967).
70. Karat, A. B. A.: *Leprosy Rev.* **38**, 97 (1967).
71. Katz, St. I., De Betz, B. H. and Zaias, N.: *Arch. Derm.* **103**, 358 (1971).
72. Khanolkar, V. R.: In *Leprosy in Theory and Practice*. 2nd ed. Wright, Bristol 1964, p. 125.
73. Kirchheimer, W. F. and Storrs, E. E.: *Int. J. Leprosy* **39**, 692 (1971).
74. Klingmüller, V.: In *Erg.-Werk zu Handbuch der Haut- und Geschlechtskrankheiten*. Vol. X/2. Springer, Berlin 1930, p. 1.
75. Kooij, R.: *Dermatologica (Basel)* **135**, 42 (1967).
76a. Kooij, R. and Gerritsen, Th.: *Int. J. Leprosy* **24**, 171 (1956).
76b. id., *Dermatologica (Basel)* **116**, 1 (1958).
77. Kooij, R. and Rutgers, A. W. F.: *Int. J. Leprosy* **26**, 24 (1956).
78. Kopyeva, T. N.: *Arkh. Path. (Moscow)* **34**/4, 35 (1972).
79. Kováts, F. and Sipos, K.: In *Allergiya i allergicheskie zabolevaniya* (Allergy and allergic diseases.) Ed. by Rajka, E. Akadémiai Kiadó, Budapest 1966, p. 627.
80. Kulagin, P. P.: *Vestn. Derm. Vener. (Moscow)* **44**, 64 (1970).
81a. Kunal Saha, K. and Mittal, M. M.: *Clin. exp. Immunol.* **6**, 969 (1970).
81b. ibid., **8**, 901 (1971).
82. Languillon, J.: *Méd. trop. (Madr.)* **26**, 115 (1966).
83. Leider, M.: *Med. Clin. N. Amer.* **49**, 817 (1965).
84a. Leiker, D. L.: *Int. J. Leprosy* **36**, 52 (1968).
84b. id., *Prax. Pneumol.* **18**, 816 (1964).
85. Levine, M.: *Proc. Soc. exp. Biol. (N. Y.)* **76**, 171 (1951).
86. Levy, L., Fasal, P. and Murray, L. P.: *Arch. Derm.* **100**, 618 (1969).
87. Lim, S. D., Fusaro, R. and Good, R. A.: *Clin. Immunopathol.* **1**, 122 (1972).
87a. Lim, S. D., Kiszkiss, D. F. and Choi, Y. S.: *Birth Defects Orig. Art. Ser.* **11**, 244 (1975).
87b. Lim, S. D., Kiszkiss, D. F. and Jacobson, R. R.: *Infection Immunity* **9**, 394 (1974).
88. Lindemayr, W.: *Wien. klin. Wschr.* **75**, 761 (1963).
89. Lowe, J.: In *Ciba Foundation Symposium on Experimental Tuberculosis*. Churchill, London 1965, p. 344.
90. Lowe, J. and McNulty, F.: *Leprosy Rev.* **24**, 6 (1953).
91. Lurie, M. B.: In *Ciba Foundation Symposium on Experimental Tuberculosis*. Churchill, London 1955, p. 340.
92. Maeda, M. and Nakamura, K.: *Lepro (Tokyo)* **34**, 294 (1965).
93. Mehra, V. L., Talwar, G. P., Balakrishnan, K. and Bhultani, L. K.: *Clin. exp. Immunol.* **12**, 205 (1972).
94. Mendes, E., Raphael, A., Mota, N. G. S. and Mendes, N. F.: *J. Allergy clin. Immunol.* **53**, 223 (1974).

94a. Meneghini, C. L., Angelini, G., Lospalluti, M. and Trimigliozzi, G.: *Trans. St. John's Hosp. Derm. Soc.* **60**, 91 (1974).
95. Merklen, F. P. and Cottenot, F.: In *XIII. Congr. Int. Derm.* Springer, Berlin 1968, p. 1305.
96. Merklen, T. P., Cottenot, F. and Potier, J. C.: *Int. J. Leprosy* **39**, 565 (1971).
97. Merklen, F. P., Renoux, M. and Brichoux, M.: *Bull. Soc. franç. Derm. Syph.* **69**, 876 (1962).
98a. Mitsuda, K.: *Jap. J. Dermatol.* **11**, 47 (1911).
98b. ibid., **13**, 265 (1913).
98c. ibid., **27**, 709 (1927).
99. Montestruc, E.: *Courrier* **11**, 497 (1961).
100. Montestruc, E., Gernez-Rieux, C. and Tacquet, A.: In *Proc. 6th Int. Congr. Leprosy, Madrid 1953*, p. 871.
101. Montgomery, H.: *Dermatopathology.* Vol. 1. Harper and Row, New York 1967, p. 433.
102. Müller, R. W.: *Tuberk.-Arzt* **16**, 595 (1962).
103. Nakamura, K. and Hisai, S.: *Lepro (Osaka)* **39**, 7 (1970).
103a. Nath, I., Curtis, J., Bhutani, L. K. and Talwar, G. P.: *Clin. exp. Immunol.* **18**, 81 (1974).
103b. Navalkar, R. G.: *Z. Tropenmed. Parasit.* **24**, Suppl. 1, 66 (1973).
104. Nelson, D. S., Nelson, M., Thurston, J. M., Waters, M. T. R. and Pearson, J.: *Clin. exp. Immunol.* **9**, 33 (1971).
105. Newell, K. W.: *Bull. Wld Hlth Org.* **34**, 827 (1966).
106. Nishimura, S.: *Lepro (Tokyo)* **32**, 1 (1963).
107. Nishiura, M.: *Int. J. Leprosy* **28**, 357 (1960).
107a. Okada, S., Nakai, E. and Narita, M.: *Int. J. Leprosy* **42**, 33 (1974).
108. Orfanos, C.: *Hautarzt* **17**, 459 (1966).
109. Paradisi, E. P., de Bonaparte, Y. P. and Morgenfeld, M. C.: *Lancet* i, 308 (1968).
110. Pares, Y.: *Acta leprol. (Genève)* **40**, 3 (1970).
111. Pearson, J. M. H., Petit, J. H. S., Siltzbach, L. E., Ridley, D. S., D'Arcy Hart, P. and Rees, R. J. W.: *Int. J. Leprosy* **37**, 372 (1969).
112. Pedley, J. C.: *Leprosy Rev.* **41**, 167 (1970).
113. Petchclai, B., Chuthanondh, R., Rungruong, S. and Ramasoota, T.: *Lancet* i, 1481 (1973).
114. Pfaltzgraff, R. E.: *Leprosy Rev.* **38**, 15 (1967).
115. Potier, J. and Foucault, J. T.: *Quest. Med.* 1755 (1971).
116. Ptak, W., Gaugas, J. M., Rees, R. J. W. and Allison, A. C.: *Clin. exp. Immunol.* **6**, 117 (1969).
116a. Quismorio, F. P., Rea, Th. H., Levan, N. E. and Friou, G. J.: *Arch. Derm. (Chic.)* **111**, 331 (1975).
117. Raffel, S.: *Immunity.* 2nd ed. Appleton-Century-Crofts, New York 1961, p. 412.
117a. Rao, B. N., Satyanarayana, B. V., Venkatarathnam, G. and Reddy, C. R. R. M.: *Dermatologica* **150**, 169 (1975).
118a. Rees, R. J. W.: *Nature*, **211**, 657 (1966).
118b. id., *Bibl. tuberc. (Basel)* **189** (1970).
118c. id., *Leprosy Rev.* **41**, 136 (1970).
118d. ibid., **41**, 154 (1970).
118e. id., *Postgrad. med. J.* **46**, 486 (1970).
119. Rees, R. J. W. and Weddel, A. G. M.: *Trans. roy. Soc. trop. Med. Hyg.* **64**, 31 (1970).
120. Rees, R. J. W., Weddel, A. G. M., Palmer, E. and Pearson, J. M. H.: *Brit. med. J.* iii, 216 (1969).
120a. Reis, A. P., Maia, F., Reis, V. F., Andrade, I. M. and Campos, A. A. S.: *Lancet* ii, 1384 (1974).
121. Richter, R.: In *Dermatologie und Venerologie.* Ed. by Gottron, H. A. und Schönfeld, W. No. 5. Part 1. Thieme, Stuttgart 1963, p. 497.
122. Ridley, D. S.: *Leprosy Rev.* **40**, 77 (1969).
123a. Ridley, D. S. and Jopling, W. H.: *Leprosy Rev.* **33**, 119 (1962).
123b. id., *Int. J. Leprosy* **34**, 255 (1966).
124. Rojas-Espinosa, O., Mendez-Nayarrete, T. and Estrada-Parra, S.: *Clin. exp. Immunol.* **12**, 215 (1972).

125. Rollier, R. and Chenebault, J.: *Acta leprol. (Genève)* **27**, 88 (1967).
126. Rosenberg, J., Campos, N. S. S., Aun, J. N. and Rocha, D. M. C.: *Int. J. Leprosy* **28**, 271 (1960).
127. Ruge, H.: *Med. Welt (Stuttg.)* **17**, 2620 (1966).
128. Ruscher, H., Faye, J., Bloc, G. and Diouf, S.: *Bull. Soc. méd. Afr. Noir lang. franç.* **17**, 27 (1972).
128a. Sagher, F.: *Lepr. Rev.* **30**, 138 (1959).
129a. Sagher, F., Kocsard, E. and Liban, E.: *Int. J. Leprosy* **24**, 344 (1952).
129b. id., *Arch. Derm.* **70**, 631 (1954).
130. Sagher, F., Liban, E., Zuckerman, A. and Kocsard, E.: *Int. J. Leprosy* **21**, 459 (1953).
131. Saha, K. and Mittal, M. M.: *Clin. exp. Immunol.* **8**, 901 (1971).
132. Saul, A., Rodriguez, O. and Novales, J.: *Int. J. Derm.* **9**, 137 (1970).
133a. Schmidt, H.: *Hautarzt* **20**, 271 (1969).
133b. id., In *Erg.-Werk zu J. Jadassohns Handbuch der Haut- und Geschlechtskrankheiten.* Ed. by Röckl, H. Vol. IV/1B. Springer, Berlin 1970, p. 520.
134. Schuppli, R.: *Schweiz. med. Wschr.* **97**, 307 (1967).
135. Seitz, E. W., Dierks, R. E. and Shepard, C. C.: *Int. J. Leprosy* **36**, 400 (1968).
136. Sheagren, J. N., Block, J. B., Trautman, J. R. and Wolff, S. M.: *Ann. intern. Med.* **70**, 295 (1969).
137. Shepard, C. C.: *Int. J. Leprosy* **30**, 291 (1962).
138. Shwe, T. and Zuckerman, A. J.: *J. clin. Path.* **25**, 401 (1972).
139. Sirisinha, S., Charupatana, C. and Ramasoota, T.: *Proc. Soc. exp. Biol. Med. (N. Y.).* **140**, 1062 (1972).
140. Skinses, O. K.: *Int. J. Leprosy* **38**, 203 (1970).
141. Sushida, K. and Hirano, M.: *Lepro (Tokyo)* **30**, 81 (1961).
142. Talwar, G. P., Krishnan, A. D., Mehra, V. L., Blum, E. A. and Pearson, J. H.: *Clin. exp. Immunol.* **12**, 195 (1972).
143. Taylor, C. E.: *Proc. 12th Int. Congr. Derm., Washington 1962.* **1**, 793 (1962).
144. Taylor, C. E. and Hanks, J. H.: *Int. J. Leprosy* **30**, 465 (1962).
145. Thomas, M. and Job, C. K.: *Brit. med. J.* **iii**, 390 (1972).
146. Tisseuil, J.: *Bull. Soc. franç. Derm. Syph.* **69**, 22 (1962).
147. Tran-Van-Bang: *Münch. med. Wschr.* **103**, 1499 (1961).
148. Turiaf, J., Brocard, H., Battesti, J. P., Gallouedec, C. H. and Basset, F.: *Presse méd.* **79**, 1459 (1971).
149. Turk, J. L.: *Proc. roy. Soc. Med.* **64**, 942 (1971).
150. Turk, J. L. and Path, M. R. C.: *Brit. med. J.* **iii**, 363 (1970).
151a. Turk, J. L. and Waters, M. F. R.: *Lancet* **ii**, 436 (1968).
151b. ibid., **ii**, 243 (1969).
151c. id., *Clin. exp. Immunol.* **8**, 363 (1971).
152. Ulrich, M., Pinardi, M. E. and Convit, J.: *Int. J. Leprosy* **37**, 22 (1959).
153. Valdimarsson, H., Holt, L., Riches, H. R. C. and Hobbes, J. H.: *Lancet* **i**, 1259 (1970).
154. Vinogradova, O. V.: *Vestn. Derm. Vener. (Moscow)* **42**, 44 (1968).
155. Wade, H. W.: *Int. J. Leprosy* **18**, 373 (1950).
156. Waldorf, D. S., Sheagren, J. N., Trautman, J. R. and Block, J. B.: *Lancet* **i**, 773 (1966).
156a. Waters, M. F. R. and Helmy, H. S.: *Leprosy Rev.* **45**, 299 (1974).
157. Weddel, A. G., Palmer, E. and Rees, R. J. W.: *J. Path. Bact.* **104**, 77 (1971).
158. Weiss, D. W. and Wells, A. Q.: *Amer. Rev. resp. Dis.* **82**, 339 (1960).
159. Wemambu, S. N. C., Turk, J. L., Waters, M. F. R. and Rees, R. J. W.: *Lancet* **ii**, 933 (1969).
160. Wilkinson, F. F., Rinaldi, P. and Gogo, J.: *Int. J. Leprosy* **30**, 957 (1962).
161. Wolcott, R. R.: *Int. J. Leprosy* **15**, 380 (1947).

CHAPTER 75

MYCOTIC ALLERGY

by

I. TÖRÖK and E. FEJÉR

INTRODUCTION

Research into mycotic allergy was started with the investigations of Plato [170] in 1902, that is, prior to the discovery of serum allergy. The recognition that some mycotic infections manifested themselves not only in local phenomena but also affected the whole organism was of great importance. Further relevant experimental and clinical examinations were carried out by Bloch and Jadassohn [3, 91]. Since that time several research workers have studied the altered reactivity of the organism. Their investigations have led not only to revealing some important and unsolved problems of dermatology (mycotic dyshidrosis, eczema, mycids and bacterids, etc.) but also have had a great importance from the aspect of general pathology because they represent a modern immunobiological approach — in contrast to the old morphological one. The growing incidence of mycotic diseases in general (especially the mycoses of the feet, the nails, and the female genitals) and of the allergic diseases of mycotic origin in particular have directed renewed attention to the allergic (immunological) aspects of mycotic diseases.

Mycotic allergy means an altered reactivity of the organism due to repeated contact with fungi. As allergic reactions in general, those of mycotic allergy are highly variable.

The antigen is the whole fungus or one of its components. Under the effect of the antigen, antibodies are produced and different types of cells (macrophages, leukocytes, lymphocytes) are stimulated. The allergic and immunological manifestations are due to this complex defense mechanism of the organism.

Mycotic immuno-allergic symptoms may be elicited by dermatophytes, yeast-like fungi and moulds.

DERMATOPHYTOSES

The aetiological agents of dermatophytoses have the common property of affecting primarily the skin and its keratin-containing formations: the horny layer, the hair follicles, the hair and the nails (keratophilia). Bloch [23a] was the first to mention the peculiarities of skin reactivity, furthermore, the importance of the interactions between the organism and the pathogenic agent. These interactions explain why the same pathogenic agent may elicit different clinical symptoms, and why different fungi may induce similar diseases. According to Bloch, dermatomycosis induced by the rubbing of guinea pigs with *Trichophyton (Achorion) quinckeanum* generally lasts about 3 weeks and usually heals spontaneously. Overcoming of the infection results in an altered specific immunobiological reactivity of the experimental animal, in so far as its skin reacts to a second injection (reinoculation) with an altered accelerated reaction. The secondary infection usually lasts for 10–12 days. After repeated infections an immune state will develop not only against the strain used for the first inoculation but also against other antigenically related dermatophytes. This phenomenon, called Bloch phenomenon, has been reproduced by other research workers [53, 186]. The intracardiac injection of the spore suspension of a dermatophyte has elicited haematogenous dermatomycosis [190]. Immunological alterations may be associated with haematogenous mycoses. According to recent observations, certain dermatophytes may also attack internal organs under particular conditions. Aravijskij [2b] has reported on a lethal, systemic *Tr. violaceum* infection; the pathogenic agent was demonstrated in the cerebrospinal fluid and in the brain. Another of his patients died of meningitis favosa caused by *Tr. (A.) schönleinii*, but the site of penetration could not be revealed. A fatal *Tr. rubrum* infection was observed by Okudaira [158] in Japan. Systemic dermatophytoses are thought to be due to a decreased fungistatic activity of the serum.

The fungistatic activity of the serum was first examined in dermatophytoses by Ayers and Anderson [5] in 1934. According to these authors the sera of their trichophytin-positive patients inhibited the growth of fungi *in vitro.* The sera of healthy individuals showed no such inhibitory effect. Other authors published similar results [93b, c, 101a, b, 166]. Lorincz et al. [132] have demonstrated that the fresh, normal human serum also contains a dialysable water-soluble, unstable factor (not of γ-globulin character), which plays an important role in the inhibition of the growth of fungi. Roth et al. [189] have suggested that the fungistatic capacity of the serum is the outcome of the complex effect of several factors resulting in the inhibition of the metabolic activity of dermatophytes [189]. A decreased antifungal activity of the serum was demonstrated in dermatomycoses due to *Tr. rubrum.* The mechanism of the fungistatic effect of the human serum is not quite clear.

Another factor found in the sera of patients with chronic dermatophytic infections is the serum blocking factor. It has been shown by *in vitro* leukocyte adherence that the serum of chronically infected children specifically blocked the activity of their own leukocytes or the leukocytes of other patients with the same species of infecting organism [236a]. Reactivity to tuberculin was not blocked by the patients' sera.

In the course of infection dermatophytes produce proteolytic enzymes with keratolytic activity termed keratinases. Besides enabling the fungus to penetrate, these enzymes also play a role in allergic reactions. Guinea pigs sensitized by cutaneous infection (*Tr. mentographytes* var. *granulosum*) developed delayed-type cutaneous hypersensitivity, the most intense reaction being to the heat-inactivated keratinase II [70]. No humoral antibodies to keratinases have been detected. Guinea pigs immunized with active keratinases developed first dermal reactivity, then humoral antibodies, to the keratinases [70]. Serum γ-globulin from immunized guinea pigs also inhibited the proteolytic activities of the keratinases. Fluorescent-antibody studies have shown that keratinase II is produced during infection and there is a local reaction at the infection site (perifollicular pattern of green fluorescence at the level of the external root sheath of the hair follicle) [32]. In previously infected guinea pigs, keratinase II elicited a stronger cutaneous reaction than keratinase I [70], however, *in vitro*, cells from such guinea pigs incubated with keratinase I had lower migration indices, measured by capillary tube migration test, than those incubated with keratinase II [46a]. At the same time trichophytin did not cause any significant inhibition of migration.

Experimental trichophytosis induces an immune response also in man. The immunity may have different degrees from an accelerated reaction to complete immunity. The degree of allergy or immunity depends on several factors, such as the virulence of the strain of fungus, the quantitative and qualitative conditions of antibody production, the extension and depth of the process, the intensity of the inflammatory reaction, the number of primary foci, etc. [23b, 52d]. Repeated inoculations result in a cumulative immunological effect.

The experimental results tally with the clinical experiences: the deep, intensive, suppurative inflammations caused by Tr. mentagrophytes, Tr. verrucosum, and Tr. violaceum (trichophytia profunda) induce a strong allergic state, the processes heal quickly and there is a tendency to spontaneous healing. Further attacks and reinfections usually do not occur after healing, suggesting the existence of an immune state. The dermatophytes that do not elicit considerable inflammatory reactions and rather induce chronic, dry, desquamating lesions (first of all, Tr. rubrum) sensitize poorly and lead to hardly any immunity. Desai et al. [41] succeeded in reinfecting the region of a previous infection with Tr. rubrum, indicating the absence of local immunity.

Immunological responses to experimental dermatophyte infections have been shown to have the following in common [77a]: (i) during infection the host acquires a gradually increasing resistance to infection; (ii) sites of reinfection in immune animals closely resemble the original infectious lesion, but resolve more rapidly and the fungus is difficult to demonstrate; (iii) the acquired immunity crosses species lines (i.e. infection with Tr. mentagrophytes produces immunity also to Tr. rubrum and other dermatophytes); (iv) delayed-type reactivity to trichophytin appears at approximately the same time as does resistance to reinfection.

Recent animal experiments and clinical observations have suggested that the acquired immunity to dermatophyte infections is not complete, but relative.

TRICHOPHYTIN

Different types of fungal antigens are responsible for sensitization. Trichophytin is used for the examination of allergy against dermatophytes. Trichophytin is, at least partially, present in each dermatophyte. The trichophytin skin test is therefore group-specific, and the results give no answer to the question whether the sensitivity is induced by Microsporum, Trichophyton, or Epidermophyton. The qualities of the applied antigen play a decisive role in the specificity of the reaction. Stuka and Burell [212] using agar-gel diffusion method have shown that the quality of the antigen depends on the age of the mycelia and on the nitrogen concentration of the culture medium. Young mycelia have proved to be more antigenic.

Trichophytin is produced usually from virulent Tr. mentagrophytes strains of good antigen-producing capacity.

For trichophytin production fungi are cultivated in liquid media and extracted by means of physical and/or chemical procedures. The product thus obtained is inevitably contaminated by components of the culture medium (peptone, glucose). Since these impurities of protein nature may sensitize themselves, they must be removed, which is usually done by dialysis. The original Trockentrichophytin (TTR) of Bloch is a fine yellow powder with a minimum protein content (0.01–0.1 per cent). In order to eliminate the contaminants, recently synthetic culture media have been used, primarily the medium of Rippel and Lehmann, containing glucose, glycine and inorganic salts; sometimes the composition of the medium is slightly modified. The trichophytin gained in this way is further purified. Antibiotics added to the culture medium inhibit the trichophytin production.

The purified antigen is a nitrogen-containing water-soluble polysaccharide [24]. Trichophytin itself is thermostable, preserves its effectiveness for several years and is precipitable by absolute methanol.

Recent immunoelectrophoretic and agar diffusion methods have allowed the identification of several antigenic components of dermatophytes, thus antigenic polysaccharide, protein and lipid fractions have been isolated. The immuno-logically active material purified and demonstrated was galactomannan peptide of approximately 40,000 molecular weight [38]. Bishop et al. [18] have further decomposed the nitrogen-free polysaccharides into galactomannan I, galacto-mannan II, and glucan fractions. Grappel et al. [71] have compared these fractions by means of gel diffusion and complement fixation in different species. They demonstrated significant differences in the quantitative rates of monosaccharides and also in their fine chemical structure. Most research workers presume polysac-charides to be responsible for the antigenicity of trichophytins [20, 24, 25, 86, 238], but there is no agreement whether the specific role [10, 38, 88, 96] is played by the nitrogen-free polysaccharide [18, 71] or by the polysaccharide–nitrogen complex. The purified polysaccharide of trichophytin being a hapten, has proved to be the most specific serologically and in skin tests. The protein fraction often elicits a positive but less specific skin reaction. The lipid fraction is the least active [86, 222].

TRICHOPHYTIN ALLERGY

Plato and Neisser [152] administered trichophytin subcutaneously to patients suffering from trichophytia profunda and thus elicited local and systemic reac-tions. This was the first step in the recognition of trichophytin allergy. The reaction was considered to be highly specific, for it was observed only in tri-chophytia profunda. In superficial mycoses it could be observed only if a severe local inflammation had been elicited with an irritant or the affected area had been X-ray irradiated. The allergic reaction usually developed as early as on the 7–8th day after the infection and could be elicited for a long time after healing. It has since become known that superficial processes also give rise to hypersensitivity and fungal allergic disease.

The earlier methods of applying trichophytin for diagnostic purposes (sub-cutaneous test, patch test, rubbing test, ophthalmo-reaction etc.) are no longer used today. The intracutaneous method has proved best since it is very sensitive and allows an exact dosage: 0.1 ml of a 1 : 10–1 : 20 dilution of commercial preparations (Trichophytin, Trichosan, etc.) is usually administered. The severity of the reaction is read off after 15–20 min, 24 h and 48 h. In cases of strong hypersensitivity the use of higher dilutions (1 : 1,000–1 : 10,000) seems to be advisable [127]. The patch test with concentrated trichophytin yields a positive reaction only in highly allergic subjects [214]. To avoid severe shock in sensitized subjects trichophytin must not be administered intravenously.

Two reaction types may be observed in connection with the intradermal tricho-phytin test:

1. The tuberculin-type (delayed-type) reaction after 24–48 h is the most frequent (Fig. 75-1).

2. The immediate-type reaction (after 15–20 min), is less frequent (3–4 per cent). This reaction type occurs mainly in *Tr. rubrum* infections of patients with atopy [39].

Both reaction types may be accompanied by focal and systemic reactions. In the case of a severe allergy the delayed-type reaction may be vesicular, vesiculo-

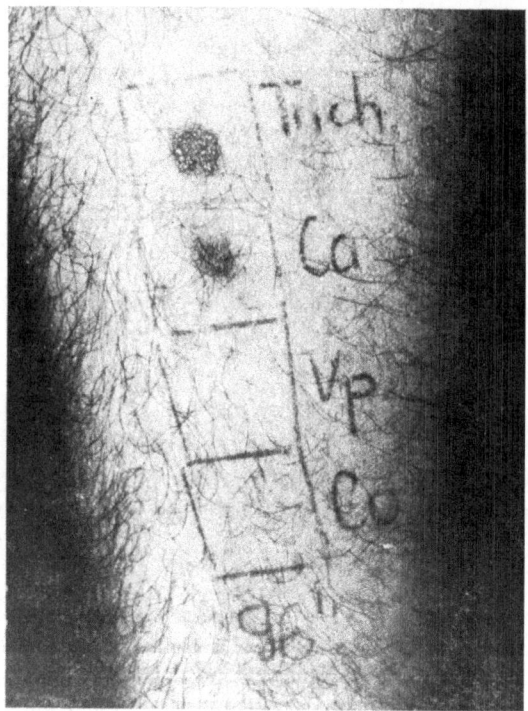

Fig. 75-1. Delayed, tuberculin-type reactions. A positive 96-hour intracutaneous test to trichophytin and candidin in mycotic eczema. Vp, mixed moulds; Co, control

pustular or eczematoid; even tissue necrosis may occur. The character of the reaction is sometimes similar to the spontaneous allergic exanthems (isomorphous reaction) (Fig. 75-2). More severe reactions may be observed near the mycotic processes (regional hypersensitivity). As a result of serial injections of the antigen the symptoms of hypersensitivity may recede (therapeutic desensitization).

The delayed-type reaction may be missing or very mild presumably due to the quick absorption of the antigen, and in such cases only manifestations of the immediate-type response are seen, yet immediate and delayed-type reactions may also occur together. The immediate-type reaction usually occurs in a phase of the allergic processes when skin sensitizing antibodies (reagins of the IgE class) appear in the blood. This can be established by passive transfer (Prausnitz–Küstner method). The delayed-type reaction usually precedes the immediate one [98]. Both reactions are specific, but different antigen components of trichophytin are supposed to be responsible for their induction [98]. A correlation has been found between the infecting species and the type of reaction [77a]: in 47 per cent of *Tr. rubrum* patients only immediate-type reaction was obtained,

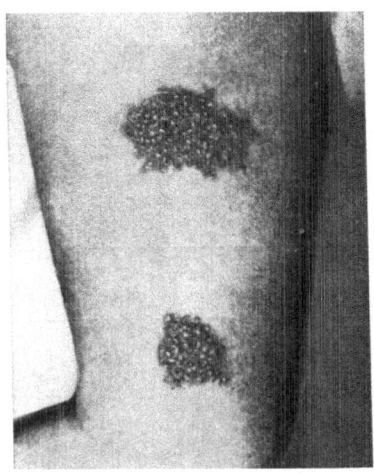

Fig. 75-2. Isomorphous skin reaction after i.c. injection of trichophytin in children suffering from trichophytia profunda

in 12 per cent only delayed, and in 12 per cent both; for *Tr. mentagrophytes* patients the percentages were 0 per cent, 79 per cent and 7 per cent, respectively. This indicates a species-dependent difference in antigenic fractions responsible for immediate and delayed hypersensitivity. The immediate-type urticarial reactions have to be treated carefully, for the administration of a minute quantity of trichophytin may induce a severe shock [109, 163a, d, 179b, d]. In connection with an immediate-type reaction generalized urticarial exanthems may also occur.

In sensitized subjects a focal reaction may be induced by trichophytin injection; this means that the primary mycotic focus and its surroundings, furthermore, the secondary exanthems and the healed trichophytin reactions may flare up. The trichophytin injection may sometimes provoke secondary exanthems, mycids, etc. A systemic reaction (fever, shivering, malaise etc.) occurred earlier, mostly when concentrated and not sufficiently purified fungal extracts were applied. Such side-effects are rare if purified polysaccharide antigens are used.

According to earlier observations only deep inflammatory processes due to highly sensitizing fungi like *Tr. mentagrophytes, Tr. quinckeanum* were accompanied by trichophytin allergy. Hypersensitivity only develops if the antigen penetrates into deeper layers [186]. Superficial processes such as interdigital and dyshidrotic foot mycoses, nail mycoses and also the mycoses of the female genitals may give rise to hypersensitivity because of continuous absorption of fungal antigens. Graffenried [62] was the first to demonstrate trichophytin allergy in connection with foot mycoses, and it has since turned out that such processes are the most frequent sources of mycotic allergy in adults—because foot and nail mycoses have become extremely widespread. The sensitizing effect of the different dermatophytes is shown in Table 75–I.

TABLE 75-I

Trichophytin allergy (delayed-type reactions) in dermatomycoses due to different dermatophytes
(after Lewis and Hopper) [120]

No. of cases	Fungal species	Negative reactions	Dubious reactions	Positive reactions			Per cent positive reactions
				+	+ +	+ + +	
39	*M. canis*	4	5	15	14	1	76
48	*M. audouinii*	18	15	8	7	0	31
10	*Tr. schönleinii*	7	1	2	—	—	20
50	*Tr. rubrum*	25	13	8	2	2	24
88	*Tr. mentagrophytes* var. *interdigitale*	13	12	35	23	5	71
6	*Tr. violaceum*	3	—	2	1	—	50
4	*M. gypseum*	—	1	1	2	—	75
4	*Tr. niveum*	1	—	—	3	—	75
3	*E. floccosum*	1	1	1	—	—	76
2	*Tr. tonsurans*	—	—	1	1	—	100

Like tuberculin, trichophytin is also a 'passive antigen'. It is suitable for the demonstration of the allergic state and also for specific desensitization, but it has usually no sensitizing power of its own. Immunization needs a rather expressed dermatophytic skin reaction to develop [186]. The most frequent fungal allergic diseases are in man elicited by epidermal foci [47g]. The dermatophytes sensitize the whole organism; this can be demonstrated in sensitized humans and experimental animals by shock phenomena elicited often by trichophytin itself, furthermore by inducing contraction in the uterus of sensitized guinea pigs by trichophytin (Schultz–Dale reaction). The involvement of the inner organs has been shown, e.g. by reinoculation of the same fungus into experimental animals which gave rise to lesions in internal organs (lungs, brain and liver) like mycotic granulomas, phlebitis and arteritis, furthermore, erythema nodosum-like lesions [84, 120, 121]. Complement-fixing and precipitating antibodies have been demonstrated in the sera of such animals, and a positive skin test has been observed with the polysaccharide antigen. In experimental animals the trichophytin allergy is usually milder than in man: the mucous membrane of the mouth generally does not react to trichophytin, but the conjunctiva does.

The specificity of the trichophytin allergy has been disputed. The overwhelming majority of investigators, including Bloch himself, insisted on the strict specificity of the reaction and on group specificity of dermatophyte, but there are contrary opinions, too, relying on positive reactions of seemingly healthy individuals. According to Götz and Thies [68a, b] diluted trichophytin elicited positive delayed-type skin reaction in 63 per cent of cases with skin lesions clinically not due to mycosis or tuberculosis. These seemingly non-specific reactions should, in our present opinion, be attributed partly to the toxic effect of concentrated and not sufficiently purified fungus extracts used earlier and partly to the effect of un-revealed or healed mycotic foci. Hypersensitivity may persist for several years. Some authors have observed positive reactions also in patients suffering from tuberculous skin lesions [4, 68a, b] and consequently questioned the specificity of the reaction, yet others disputed this correlation [139, 140]. The contradictory findings partly derive from frequent tuberculous and mycotic infections in adults with a consequent allergy against both of these pathogens. Therefore the adult age does not seem to lend itself for studying this problem. Fejér [52b,

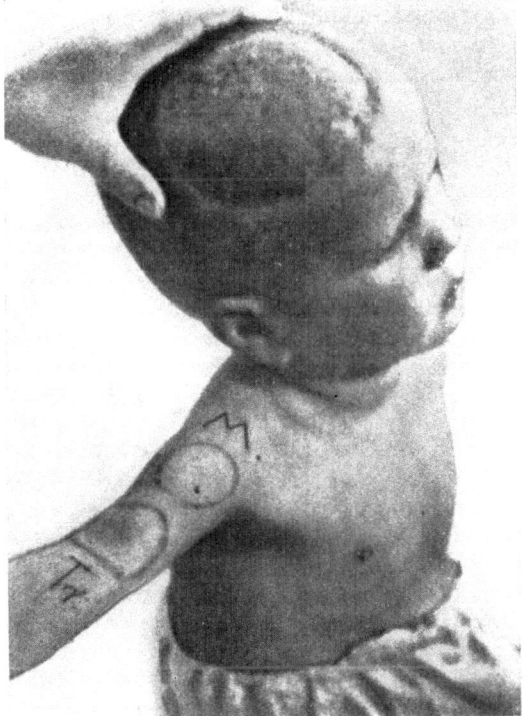

Fig. 75-3. Positive trichophytin reaction (Tr) of a 3-year-old boy suffering from trichophytia profunda. The Mantoux reaction (M) is negative

TABLE 75-II

*Comparative study of tuberculin allergy and trichophytin allergy**

Diagnosis	No. of cases	Tuberculin reaction		Trichophytin reaction	
		positive	negative	positive	negative
Skin tuberculosis, scrophuloderma	8	8	0	0	8
Trichophytia profunda	10	0	10	10	0
Different nonmycotic diseases of the skin	124	14	110	0	124
Total	142	22	120	10	132

* 600 children, repeated tests.

c, e, f, i, j] who has examined a large number of infants and children has suggested that trichophytin allergy and tuberculin allergy are completely independent specific phenomena (Fig. 75-3). Several authors have accepted this opinion [179, 233a]. Table 75-II shows that trichophytin reaction and tuberculin reaction do not show any parallelism.

False negative results were obtained in the case of processes accompanied by mild inflammation, in anergic state or upon therapeutic inhibition of intracutaneous reactions by corticosteroids, or high doses of antihistamine drugs.

Artificial sensitization and immunization

Efforts have been made to immunize with fungal extracts, although, according to the general opinion, only a skin disease elicited by a living fungal pathogen can immunize. Sensitization as well as immunization with dialysed protein-free trichophytin has been unsuccessful (probably due to its hapten character) [202, 233b]. Immunization of experimental animals has been attempted [40, 108], applying live vaccine prepared from *Tr. mentagrophytes*. As a result, delayed hypersensitivity developed against the fungus and the resistance to reinfection increased.

The resistance usually lasted for 30 days. A complete immunity, however, could not be achieved. Wharton et al. [239] injected a *Tr. rubrum* suspension into guinea pigs subcutaneously and obtained a short-term immunity. Topical application of fungal antigen to guinea pigs induced hypersensitivity as well as enhanced resistance to infection with the homologous fungus [108]. Ito and Kirita [85], who parenterally injected killed fungus material into guinea pigs, stated that the animals became transiently immune. They succeeded in demonstrating the presence of agglutinating, complement-fixing and precipitating antibodies in the blood. Trichophytin contact sensitivity was demonstrated in guinea pigs infected with *Tr. mentagrophytes* using a new inoculation technique [218d]. The inoculation method utilized an occlusive dressing to keep a high humidity in the inoculation site. A definite infection lasting for several weeks was thus produced. The provocative epicutaneous test was made with sodium lauryl sulphate and undiluted crude trichophytin from filtrates of broth medium. For the routine epicutaneous test purified trichophytin was used consisting of polysaccharide with attached peptides. The incidence of contact sensitivity increased with the number of infections; it was 55 per cent after the first infection, 80 per cent after the second and 91.5 per cent after the third one.

It has recently been shown that naturally infected subjects may have (i) acquired resistance to clinical reinfection, or (ii) humoral immunity with or without cell mediated immunity and be susceptible to infection [99a]. The antibodies produced to cell surface antigens of dermatophytes may cross-react with intercellular glycoprotein material of epithelial tissue [83a].

Flórián [55a, b], Dokudovskij [42] and Kielstein [110] immunized new-born calves against trichophytia profunda with a vaccine prepared from a *Tr. verrucosum* culture. Fifty per cent of the animals treated with the vaccine did not become ill when kept among infected animals, in 30–40 per cent the infection was very mild and only 10–20 per cent became manifestly ill.

Serial intracutaneous injections of trichophytin seemed to be effective for desensitizing certain patients suffering from mycosis [13, 52b, 117, 180, 218a]. Some authors, however, questioned the effectiveness of this therapy [56, 173, 233b]. The introduction of Griseofulvin as a causal therapy has decreased the practical value of desensitization, although Griseofulvin does not terminate the sensitized state.

The use of specific immunotherapy is, therefore, justified as an additional method [218e] in the treatment of superficial dermatomycoses in severe and persistent cases when other therapeutic measures have failed. The results have improved with the better quality of the vaccines. Treatment of trichophytiasis for 18 months brought complete healing in 56.4 per cent, that of candidiasis in 62.5 per cent [218e]. Failure sometimes results from inaccurate diagnosis, the disease not being primarily of mycotic aetiology.

Cross-reactions. Relationship between mycotic infections and penicillin allergy

Positive intradermal reaction can be elicited even with trichophytins prepared from dermatophytes differing from the sensitizing fungus (group antigen, group allergy). Basarab et al. [11a] showed that the glycopeptides from different dermatophytic species *(Tr. mentagrophytes, Tr. rubrum, M. canis)* are chemically similar and that they cross-react. In processes characterized by mild inflammation and weak hypersensitivity, e.g. superficial trichophytia, microsporia and favus, the skin tests carried out with the homologous antigen may yield weakly positive [3, 4, 152, 186] or even negative results. In the atypical microsporia characterized by a profound inflammation, furthermore, in animal favus positive reactions to trichophytin may occur in high percentages [4, 208]. There is no interrelation between trichophytin allergy and allergy to the antigens of yeasts indicating that yeasts form a separate antigen group [52, 139, 213a–d].

The correlation between the trichophytin allergy and the penicillin allergy has been investigated by several authors [26, 35, 52b, c, e, f, j, 68a, b, 177]. No positive reaction to penicillin occurred in children suffering from trichophytia

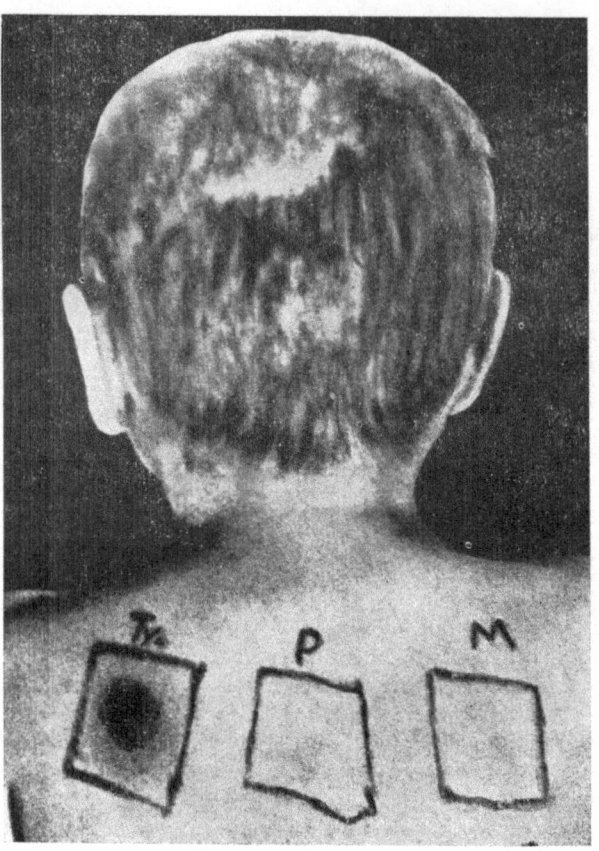

Fig. 75-4. Positive trichophytin reaction (Tr) of a boy
suffering from trichophytia profunda. The penicillin (P)
and the Mantoux (M) reactions are negative

profunda (Fig. 75-4) [52b, f, i, j]. In the series of Prochacki et al. [177] intracutaneous skin tests with penicilloyl-polylysine (PPL), a synthetic antigen, on
91 patients with active dermatomycosis showed a negative reaction in every case
except in actinomycosis. The joint occurrence of positive trichophytin and penicillin reactions in adults might be ascribed to sensitization to both antigens and
not to cross-reaction. A dermatophytic infection can usually be demonstrated
in the cases of trichophytin allergy, and in patients suffering from penicillin
allergy there is often a mould infection (Penicillium, Aspergillus, etc.) mainly in
foot and/or nail mycoses (Fig. 75-5). Mixed mycotic infections (dermatophyte
and moulds) on double-sensitized patients have been observed. Other authors,
however, have described cross-reactions [35, 36].

Penicillin allergy can be interpreted in different ways. Several authors attribute
it to the penicillin production of some dermatophyte or to assumed common
antigenic components in dermatophytes and penicillin [35]. The production of

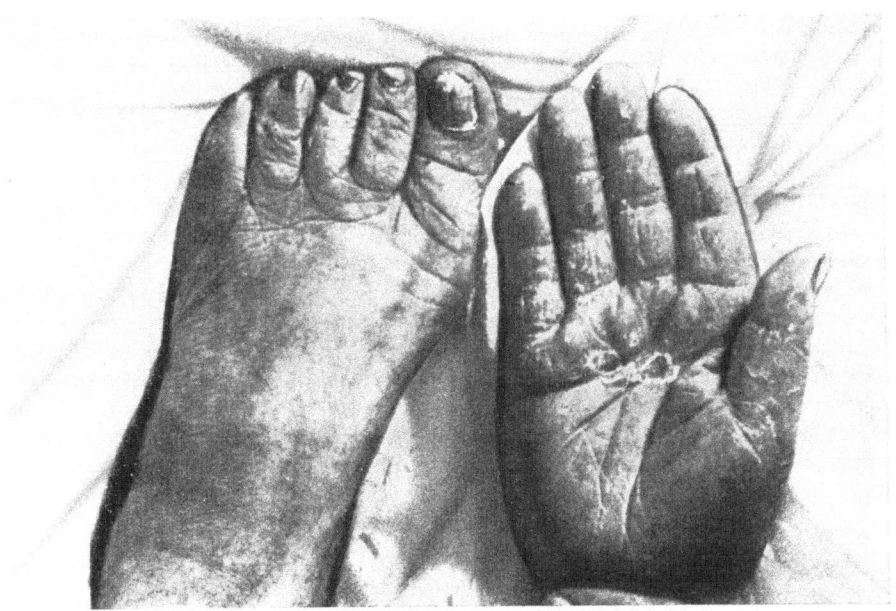

Fig. 75-5. Dyshidrosis lamellosa sicca elicited by penicillin. Onychomycosis of the left foot caused by Penicillium

antibiotics—including penicillin—by certain dermatophyte strains has been demonstrated [54, 165, 232]. Peck and Hewith [165] found penicillin production in 7 out of 12 dermatophyte strains, Úri [231] in 10 out of 20. Other investigators, however, could not reveal production of penicillin or any other antibiotic by *Tr. mentagrophytes* and by *Tr. mentagrophytes* var. *interdigitale* [187]. Schirren [195] has found no penicillin production by moulds in any of the scrapings of 500 patients suffering from foot mycosis.

It may be concluded that the cross-reaction between trichophytin and penicillin has not been completely clarified so far.

IMMUNOLOGICAL STUDIES IN DERMATOMYCOSES

Mycotic infections induce humoral and cell-mediated immune responses which may be studied with different immunological methods. Since these methods are complicated and the results are inconsistent, the immune serology of dermatomycoses has not been given too much attention. The production of humoral antibodies depends on the depth and extension of the process, on its duration, on the species of the pathogen, furthermore, on the reactive capacity of the infected organism. The quality of the antigen and the sensitivity of the applied methods also have a decisive influence on the results. Therefore, the use of stable antigen and standard methods would be very important. Several authors stress the importance of complex immunological examinations [8, 150, 197c].

The antibody response is less intensive in dermatophytoses than in deep processes. Among the different serological methods agglutination is not used in practice, probably because the conidium suspensions of hyphomycetes or its macroconidia are not suitable for this purpose. Kuroda [122] obtained positive complement fixation and precipitation, together with positive skin reaction, in the sera of patients suffering from mycogen dyshidrosis. Others could not reveal such antibodies [72, 146]. Fegeler [50] found the complement fixation non-specific in 24 per cent of dermatomycosis patients. The passive transfer of humoral antibodies from mycotic patients showing immediate-type trichophytin reactions was successful even with high dilutions of the sera (1 : 10–1 : 100), and with the application of very high dilutions of trichophytin (in certain cases with a dilution of 1 : 100,000) in the skin test [179e] (Fig. 75-6). In the sera of such patients a substance inhibiting trichophytin reaction was demonstrated after specific desensitization.

The antibodies induced by dermatophytic infection are partly group specific partly species-specific. The sera of rabbits infected with *Tr. rubrum* cross-agglu-

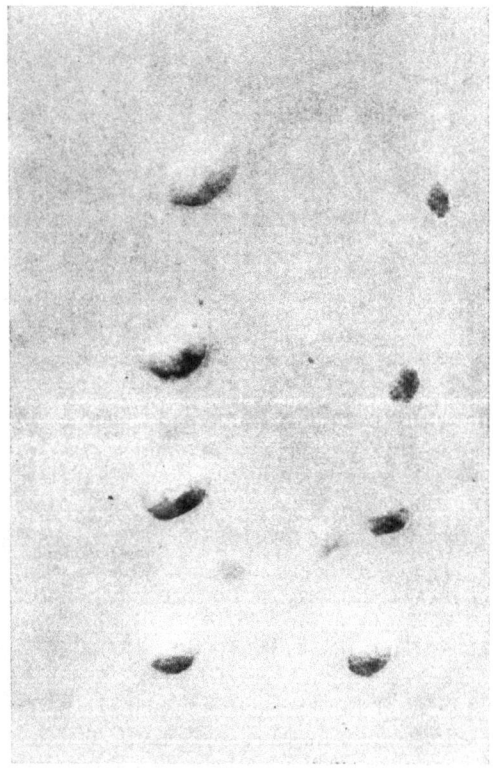

Fig. 75-6. Positive Prausnitz–Küstner transfer with 1 : 10–1 : 100 serum dilutions in a trichophytin-allergic patient (courtesy of E. Rajka)

tinate the spores of *Tr. mentagrophytes* [197a], furthermore give positive precipitation and C fixation tests with the polysaccharide fraction of different dermatophytes. Using the agar gel diffusion method, Pepys [168] tested serum samples from patients suffering from *Tr. rubrum* infection against antigens extracted from *Tr. rubrum* and *Tr. mentagrophytes* and thus demonstrated common antigens in these fungi. Walzer and Einbinder [237] found in the sera of mycotic patients antibodies against *Tr. rubrum* and *Tr. mentagrophytes*. In the sera of 12 patients with vasculitis of fungal allergic origin, Halmy and Pintye [77] observed gel precipitation with trichophytin antigen in 7 cases. Using the Ouchterlony agar gel precipitation method Paldrok [159] found the dermatophytes, especially those causing foot mycoses, *Tr. mentagrophytes, E. floccosum* and *Tr. rubrum* to be closely related serologically.

The positivity of different serological reactions, furthermore, the positivity of the trichophytin skin test and the serological reactions usually do not display any parallelism [10, 87, 203]. Specific antibodies could be demonstrated using the fluorescent antibody test in highly sensitizing primary processes (kerion celsi) [220a, 246]. Furthermore, an antibody of globulin character was found in the vessel wall in nodular vasculitis, while in other studies of similar lesions a trichophytin-like antigen could be demonstrated by an immune histological technique [10, 162, 218b, c].

The cellular defense of the patients can be investigated *in vitro* by the lymphocyte transformation test. Sensitized lymphocytes undergo blastic transformation in the presence of the sensitizing antigen. Blastic transformation was first used by Götz and Heitman [67] for the study of mycotic sensitization. Whenever the lymphocytes of patients suffering from tinea capitis were mixed with the trichophytin antigen, the lymphocyte transformation occurred in a significantly higher number than in the controls. Balogh et al. [9] observed a 6–35 per cent blastic transformation if the lymphocytes of patients with Trichophyton infection were treated with trichophytin antigen. This method seems to be more valuable for the establishment of mycotic allergy than the intracutaneous test; positivity is usually accompanied by the presence of serum precipitins. Pólay et al. [172] compared the results of the trichophytin skin tests with the lymphocyte transformation tests. Applying trichophytin antigens no close correlation could be demonstrated between the results of the lymphocyte transformation, the duration and extension of the disease and the skin test positivity. Similar results were obtained when patients with candidiasis were tested by candidin skin test and lymphocyte transformation.

According to other authors [77a] the positive lymphocyte transformation correlated with the presence of delayed hypersensitivity, but not with immediate-type cutaneous reactions. A positive lymphocyte transformation is only observed where there are manifest clinical symptoms of mycosis. However, in clinically active forms the [lymphocyte response may be absent; in this case possibility of a selective anergy has been suggested [77a]. Immunotherapy failed to influence the result of lymphocyte transformation in response to Trichophyton antigen [218e].

Other methods for the investigation of the cellular defense mechanisms include the thrombocytopenic and the basophil degranulation tests, furthermore, the macrophage migration inhibition and stimulation test. These methods are now used mainly in animal experiments, their clinical applicability not being sufficiently clarified.

MYCIDS (DERMATOPHYTIDS)

Mycids are secondary fungal allergic diseases accompanying primary mycotic processes. Their main characteristics are as follows:

1. Mycids are sterile eruptions where, unlike in the primary foci, the presence of the aetiologic agent cannot be demonstrated.
2. They are caused by the metabolic products of distant mycotic foci (or of the fungus itself) in the specifically sensitized tissue.
3. Primary mycoses are usually unilateral, the mycids, however, mainly occur in disseminated and symmetrical localization after a certain incubation period.
4. Two main pathological components should be present:
   (a) primary focus
   (b) induced mycotic allergy.
5. The spread of metabolic products of the fungi (or the fungi themselves) is mainly haematogeneous but lymphogenic regional manifestations may also occur. The symptoms of the 'id'-s are more or less different from those of the primary lesions. The differences may be morphological, mycological or immunobiological.
6. The mycids are of a transient character, they heal with the elimination of the primary focus.

The postulate of Peck [166] that the haemoculture must be positive is not valid for the majority of mycids. The collective name dermatophytid covers the fungal allergic diseases accompanying the dermatophytoses, including (i) trichophytids, (ii) microsporids, and (iii) favids.

TRICHOPHYTIDS

Trichophytids are allergic reactions of the sensitized skin elicited through the haematogenous route by metabolic products of the fungus, or by the fungus itself. Sometimes the pathogenic agent is decomposed in the skin and the trichophytid is induced by its decomposition products. The allergic mechanism is proved by the appearance of focal and/or systemic reactions following the introduction and by the latency period corresponding to the period necessary for developing the state of maximum allergy. In this state the administration of specific antigen (e.g. trichophytin) alone may elicit trichophytids or even cause the primary focus to flare up. The primary foci of trichophytids may consist not only of deep mycotic processes but also of superficial ones, above all, of the highly sensitizing foot and nail mycoses.

Non-specific components may also play a role in the induction of mycids in a mycotic allergic state. These are:

1. Exposure to the sun or ultraviolet irradiation. Scarlatiniform trichophytids were observed after a trichophytin injection and exposure to sunshine, furthermore, trichophytids could be induced experimentally by UV irradiation (Fig. 75-7) [73].
2. X-ray irradiation of the primary focus.
3. Non-specific microbial superinfection.
4. Chemical allergens and drugs.
5. Mechanical irritants.

The mechanical irritation of the primary focus may also play a role in the mobilization of the antigen; for example, in the case of a foot mycosis long walking may induce dyshidrosis-like mycids.

The trichophytids may assume a variety of forms. Peck's [166] classification, though not complete, summarizes well the manifestations of trichophytids mainly from the point of view of tissue localization.

I. *Epidermal trichophytids*:
    1. eczematoid (dyshidrotic)
    2. lichenoid
    3. parakeratotic
    4. psoriatic

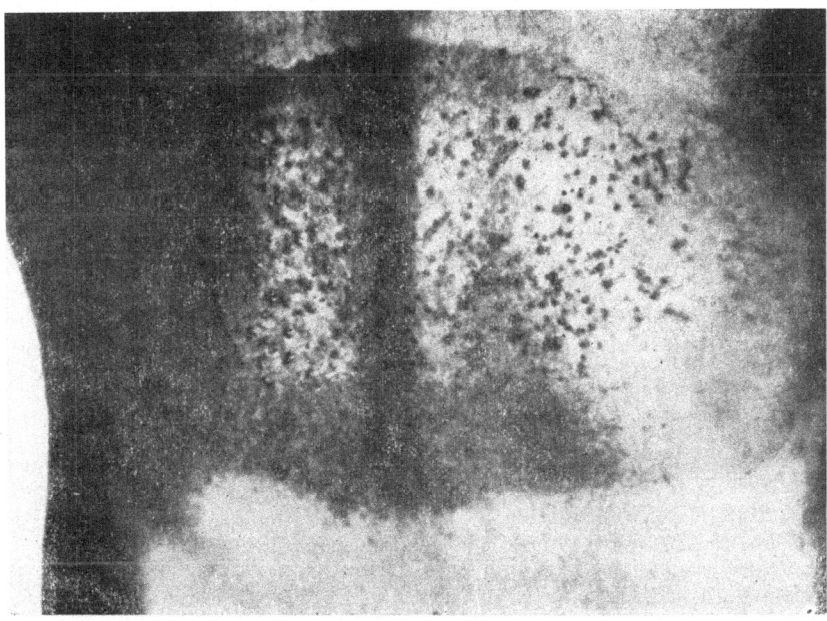

Fig. 75-7. Trichophytids in a skin area irradiated with an erythema-inducing dose of ultra-violet rays in a patient suffering from trichophytia profunda (courtesy of P. Gróf)

II. *Cutaneous trichophytids* (mainly localized in the stratum papillare):
   1. *Diffuse forms*
      (a) scarlatiniform exanthem
      (b) erythroderma
   2. *Circumscribed and disseminated forms*:
      (a) a follicular localization with a regular lichenoid character
      (b) not merely follicular localization: maculo-papular and vesicular exanthems
      (c) erysipelas-like
III. *Subcutaneous trichophytids* (erythema-nodosum-type subcutaneous nodules):
   1. acute forms with good healing tendency
   2. chronic forms with tissue disintegration
IV. *Vascular trichophytids*:
   1. venous trichophytid: phlebitis migrans
   2. capillary trichophytid: urticaria
   3. purpura

In addition to these, mycids occurring in the form of erythema exudativum multiforme, pityriasis rosea-like (Fig. 75-8), necrotizing varioliform [207], varicelliform, haemorrhagic lesions, and erythema annulare centrifugum [97] have been observed.

The fungus-free, dyshidrotic symmetrical hand eruptions (Fig. 75-9), accompanying foot mycoses as primary foci, have the greatest importance. Miescher [145] induced experimental dyshidrosis of hands by strong rubbing of an interdigital mycosis. Peck [166] elicited interdigital mycosis by the rubbing of epidermophyte into trichophytin-negative subjects. This procedure led to hypersensitivity within 10 days and sterile dyshidrotic epidermophytids occurred after 3 weeks.

Dyshidrotic trichophytid may occur near the primary focus as a regional localized mycid; far from the focus as a remote localized, and as generalized mycid.

Regional trichophytides are mainly found adjacent to foot and nail mycoses, on the toes, on the soles, and on the legs (Fig. 75-10).

Remote localized trichophytids occur simultaneously on both hands and assume an eruptive form; they include the dyshidrosis described by Tilbury-Fox in 1873 and to the 'pompholix' syndrome described by Hutchinson. Chronic, desquamating forms may also occur (Fig. 75-11). Dyshidrosis lamellosa sicca which is the summer desquamation of the hands and the palms is a variant of vesicular dyshidrosis.

Further forms of localized trichophytids are:

1. Symmetrical, small-papular mycids of the back of the hands occurring mainly in women. The primary foci are mostly mycoses of the feet and nails.

2. Eczematoid mycids on the flexor sides of the elbows and the knees; they occur either independently or associated with generalized trichophytids.

3. Localized eczematoid mycids may occur in any region of the skin, their most frequent localization being the back.

4. In some cases acne rosacea-like exanthems of the face have been observed which became symptomless after the healing of the primary focus or after specific desensitization.

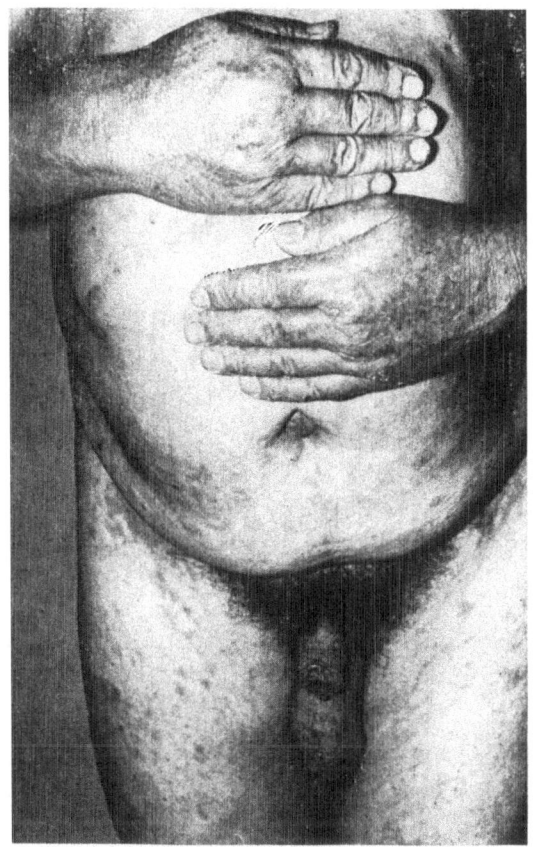

Fig. 75-8. Pityriasis rosea-like mycid associated
with erosio interdigitalis pedis

Generalized trichophytids may have a lichenoid or papular character (Figs
75-12 and 75-13). Rajka [179a] was the first to publish cases of scarlatiniform
and erythema exudativum multiforme-like mycids. The generalized forms mainly
accompany the more severe, extensive foot mycoses, which are sometimes combined with pyogenic infections or other irritations. They often occur during the
flare-up of the process in summer and are mostly characterized by a strongly
positive trichophytin reaction. In some cases the haemoculture was found to be
positive [124, 166]. They often occur along with the dyshidrotic mycids of the
extremities. In the case of a severe allergic state a trichophytin injection may also
elicit generalized eruptions, and sometimes shock symptoms, too.

Erythema nodosum trichophyticum (nodular cutaneous trichophytid) has
been described by several authors and is explained by fungi obliterating capillaries [23b, 186, 240]. This is a less frequent form of mycids occurring along with
trichophyta profunda of childhood or in connection with more severe foot mycoses.

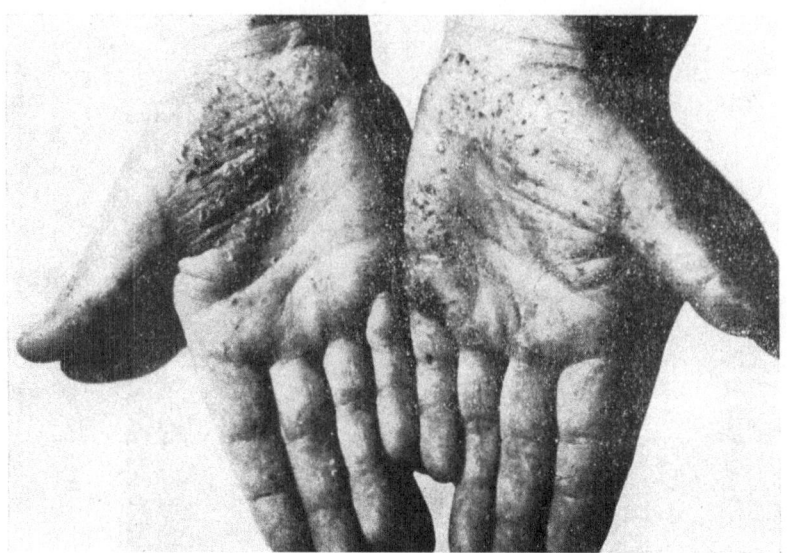

a

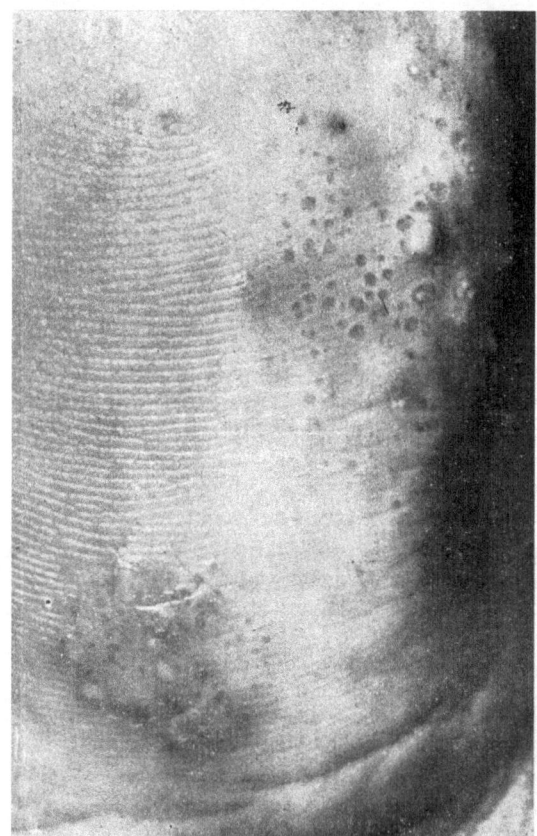

b

Fig. 75-9. *a* Dyshidrotic mycid of the palms associated with foot mycosis. *b* Deeply localized vesicles of a dyshidrotic mycid on the palms

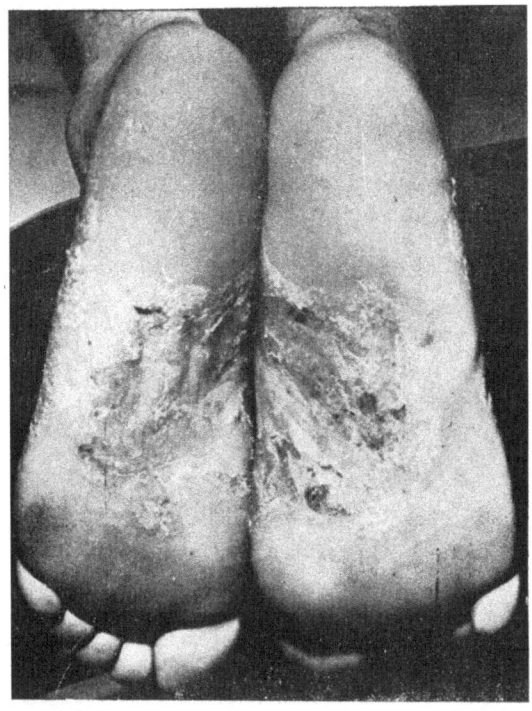

Fig. 75-10. Regional trichophytid on the soles.
Mycosis induced by *Tr. rubrum* was found on the
nails of the feet

Some chronic cases of urticaria may prove to be fungal allergic exanthems of mycid character. Urticaria following a trichophytin injection has also been observed. In a case of Waldbott and Ascher [235] there was an interdigital mycosis in the background of chronic, recurrent urticaria. An antimycotic treatment of the foot mycosis, furthermore specific vaccine therapy resulted in the healing of the mycid-like urticaria. Cases of thrombangiitis obliterans were also observed in connection with severe foot mycoses. On the basis of 80 per cent trichophytin positivity in these cases, some authors [82, 144, 221] suppose a causal relationship between the two processes. They assume the mycid character of some of these thrombangiitis cases, though, animal experiments do not always support this presumption [183]. Dermatophytin antigens may also play a role in the induction of allergic nodular vasculitis. Allergic vasculitis has been elicited experimentally by the reinoculation of *Tr. mentagrophytes* [87, 120]. Kulaga [119] could prove mycotic sensitization in 10 out of 76 cases of vasculitis. Balogh [7] revealed the presence of an established mycosis in 20 out of 31 cases of nodular vasculitis. In 17 of these 20 patients a positive trichophytin skin test was observed and antifungal antibodies were demonstrated in the sera of some patients.

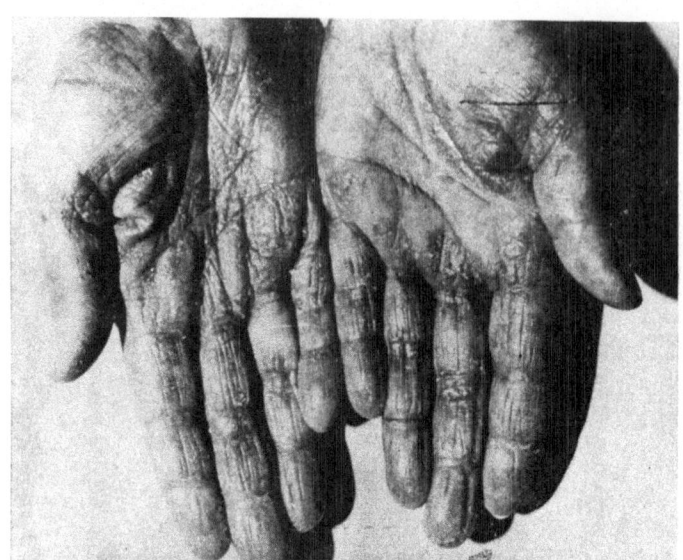

Fig. 75-11. Dry, desquamating dyshidrosis of the palms; the primary focus is the mycosis of the nails of the feet

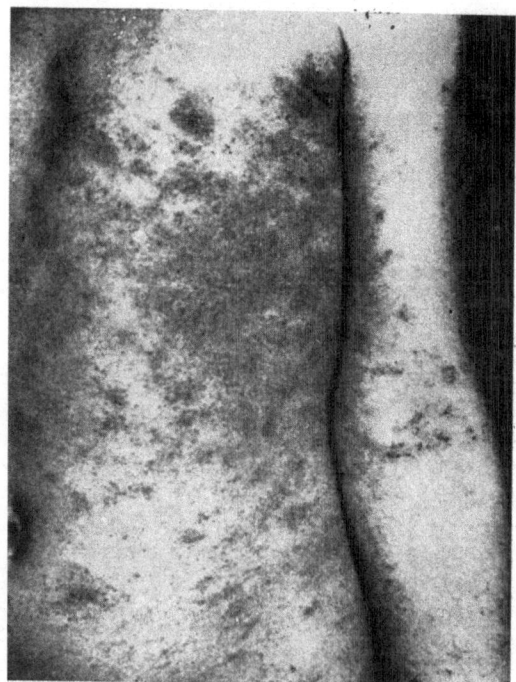

Fig. 75-12. Generalized lichenoid trichophytid in trichophytia superficialis capitis

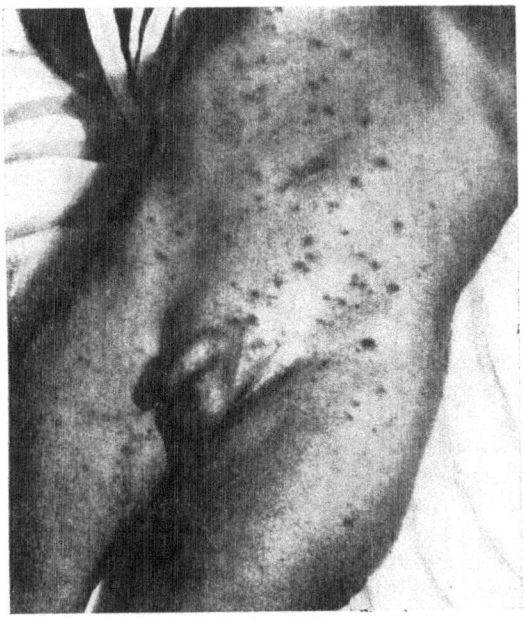

Fig. 75-13. Papular trichophytid in trichophytia
profunda

MICROSPORIDS

The superficial human microsporia *(M. audouinii)* has slight or no sensitizing effect and, therefore, does not induce mycids. More virulent strains, however, may induce deep inflammatory processes — as seen in the microsporia epidemic of Vienna of 1921–1924 — and may thus sensitize and lead to the development of mycids, mainly in the form of lichenoid or eczematoid id-reactions. These cases yield a positive reaction to microsporin (prepared from the homologous strain) as well as to trichophytin. *M. canis* and *M. gypseum* sensitize to a higher degree.

FAVIDS

Favids occur rarely. The favus capitis caused by *A. schönleinii (Tr. schönleinii)* usually does not sensitize, but the favus corporis cases induced by *A. quinckeanum (Tr. quinckeanum)* of animal origin are accompanied by a severe allergy, and favids may develop. In more than one half of these favus capitis cases Dostrovsky [43] has found a positive trichophytin reaction, suggesting differences in the virulence and sensitizing capacity of different strains.

YEAST ALLERGY
(CANDIDIDS OR LEVURIDS)

Yeasts may also induce hypersensitivity. The allergic symptoms elicited by yeasts are known as candidids (old names: levurid, oidiomycid, monilid, blastomycid). The pathogenesis of the candidids corresponds to that of other mycids. Its main components are:

1. The fungus-positive primary focus
2. The yeast allergy induced by the dissemination of the fungal products (or the fungus itself).

The fungal antigens rarely disseminate via a lymphatic pathway, more frequently via the blood circulation. Sometimes positive haemocultures can be obtained, mainly in connection with deeper processes [44, 95, 118].

Candida albicans, a facultative parasite, is the most frequent yeast inducing allergic symptoms. It is often present (10–50 per cent) in different regions of the body of healthy humans. It lives as a saprophyte in the mouth, in the intestinal tract and in the vagina. It is not a very virulent pathogen, its virulence depending on the general condition of the host. *C. albicans* is rarely the primary pathogenic agent in any disease, but associates with primary processes impairing the immune system. The following conditions predispose to candidiasis: single or multiple abnormalities of the endocrine system (diabetes mellitus, hypoparathyroidism, adrenocortical insufficiency), leukaemia, lymphoma, other tumours, long-term treatment with corticosteroids, antibiotics of a broad spectrum, immunosuppressants or oral anticoncipients. The Candida-endocrinopathy syndrome may be inherited as an antisomal recessive trait. In other subjects, the disease is associated with profound and occasionally fatal immunological deficiencies (e.g. Di George's syndrome). Defect in cell-mediated immunity has subsequently been verified [10a, 30]. Predisposition to Candida infection may be genetically determined [238a].

As almost everybody has been infected with *C. albicans*, it is hard to tell whether a positive skin test or circulating antibodies indicate an active process. It is, therefore, advisable to carry out different serological tests simultaneously establishing yeast allergy and to compare the results with those of the skin test, culture test and clinical symptoms [199a]. *C. albicans* has been shown to have 78 known antigenic components [4a, 199b].

The following antigens have been prepared from yeast—mainly from *C. albicans*—for purposes of skin tests and serological reactions: (i) cell-free filtrates, and (ii) vaccines containing Candida cells. Opinions differ as to whether the filtrate [103] or the corpuscular vaccine [123] is more specific in the skin test.

The cell wall of Candida contains polysaccharides (glucan and mannan), proteins and about 1 per cent lipids (phospholipid and sterols) [199c]. Most of the authors hold one of the polysaccharide fractions (mannan) responsible for antigenicity and immunogenicity; this has been found in the superficial layers of the cell wall. Glucan, which is sited deeply, is not immunogenic [19, 60, 96, 215, 225]. An endotoxin called canditoxin has been extracted from *C. albicans* by Japanese authors. It is an antigen of protein nature. Its role in the pathogenesis of candidiasis has not been clarified [90].

The relationship between the antigens of different yeast strains results in cross-reactions between the genera Candida, Trichosporon, Rhodotorula, Torulopsis, Saccharomyces, Cryptococcus, etc. [29a, 149, 209].

According to Biquet et al. [17] and Tsuchiya et al. [230] C. albicans is antigenically homogeneous whereas Hasenclever and Mitchell [80] have distinguished, by means of the tube agglutination test, two serological groups: (i) C. albicans A identical with C. tropicalis and (ii) C. albicans B identical with C. stellatoidea.

CANDIDIN SKIN TEST

The different Candida extracts are group-specific, i.e. the candidin skin test is positive in every process induced by yeast. Candidin is usually applied intracutaneously undiluted or in a 1 : 10 dilution. The skin test is the more specific the more purified the antigen and the higher its dilution. Three reaction types may be observed:

1. Urticarial, immediate-type reaction (to be read after 10–20 min)
2. Delayed (tuberculin-type) reaction (after 24–48 h)
3. Eczematoid delayed-type reaction (after 5–7 days).

Crounse [37] has claimed that the skin-reactive extract made from C. albicans by gel filtration may be separated into two glycoprotein fractions. The fraction of a higher molecular weight elicits pustule formation in the human skin, the other fraction induces erythema. Török and Flórián [227] applied four different antigens in the intradermal test. The reaction was the most specific when an antigen prepared by alkaline disintegration and trichloroacetic acid extraction was used. By epicutaneous application of live C. albicans positive result was obtained in 80 per cent regardless of the clinical diagnosis [228]. C. albicans could be isolated from 43 per cent of the positive cases. Presumably, the positive test in the remaining cases indicated postinfectious state and was independent of the actual skin disease. The epicutaneously applied live C. albicans and the intradermal test with Bencard's antigen yielded identical results in 78 per cent. From the histological examination of the epicutaneous reactions it was concluded that the keratinous layer was the first barrier against further penetration of the pathogen. The phagocytic leukocytes and the perivascular lymphocytes in the connective tissue formed the second and third protective mechanisms, respectively.

The intracutaneous test is positive in 15–48 per cent of healthy individuals. At the same time, several authors have observed a negative intracutaneous test with the C. albicans antigen in chronic mucocutaneous candidiasis [29, 30, 39, 111, 129]. According to Holti [85] the positivity of intracutaneous tests gradually increases from 14 to 83 per cent in seemingly healthy individuals aged from 10 to 50 years. Korossy et al. [116] observed a high percentage (53.1) of positivity with a C. albicans antigen in cases of nodular vasculitis and erythema induratum (Bazin). These reactions in themselves do not indicate an aetiological relationship because they may be due to previous sensitization. The intracutaneous test carried out with C. albicans very frequently yields both immediate and delayed-type reactions in diseases of polyaetiological origin [115]. The purified polysaccharide fraction of *C. albicans* elicits immediate-type reaction, whereas the purified protein extract elicits both immediate and delayed-type reactions [46b, 100, 201]. Positive transfer test was obtained with the cytoplasmic proteins [131b].

Nowakowski et al. [156] have found *C. albicans* in 78 per cent of children suffering from bronchial asthma. In 35 out of 47 asthmatic children an immediate reaction was observed with candidin. The agglutinin titre reached 1 : 320, but there was no correlation between the positive culturing, the agglutinin titre and the skin test positivity. In view of the above data the candidin skin test is of very little diagnostic value. Šikl et al. [201] examined the skin reactivity of 35 patients suffering from asthma bronchiale. At the same time inhalation tests and agar-gel precipitation tests were performed. The antigens applied in the tests were prepared from three different Candida species. The skin test and the inhalation tests made no distinction between the different species, whereas in the agar-gel precipitation tests there was some divergence between the different antigens.

THERAPEUTIC APPLICATION OF CANDIDIN

The vaccination results are very variable and are similar to those of trichophytin treatment in dermatophytoses. Some authors have found the vaccine treatment successful in dyshidrosis due to yeast [12, 52g, i, 75, 104, 105, 116]. Vaccination of patients suffering from dyshidrosis candidamycetica with the polysaccharide antigen of *C. albicans* made the majority of patients free of symptoms. At the same time the intradermal test remained positive and the agglutination and the precipitation titres did not change. The IgG and IgM levels in the serum doubled [76]. In rabbits immunized with *C. albicans* the antibody proved to be the IgG type [60]. Duperrat et al. [46] succeeded in desensitizing patients suffering from chronic urticaria due to candida allergy. Nevertheless, the wide use of vaccination is not justified.

IMMUNOLOGICAL ASPECTS

The defense mechanism of the organism against the lesion caused by *C. albicans* has both cellular and humoral factors. The humoral factors are circulating antibodies, namely, agglutinins, precipitins and C fixing antibodies. High-titre antibodies can be demonstrated mainly in extensive deep processes. Low titres occur in a high per cent of healthy subjects. Agglutinins are present in both the IgM and IgA fractions, whereas precipitins and C fixing antibodies only, and immunofluorescent antibodies mainly, in the IgG fraction [148a]. The IgA antibodies protect the mucous membranes. In Candida granuloma the IgA level of the saliva may be low or IgA may even be missing [30, 48].

The sera of normal individuals contain a factor inhibiting *in vitro* growth of *C. albicans*. This factor, protein in nature, is known as Louria's Candida lethal factor [134]. It migrates in the α- and β-globulin fractions, is thermostable and dialysable. Its level decreases or the factor is even missing in the sera of patients suffering from systemic and chronic mucocutaneous candidiasis, furthermore in diabetes, in diseases of the liver and in leukaemia. Its clinical importance has not been fully clarified. Subsequently, Louria et al. [137] have shown that Candida cells are not killed by the serum factor. The cells aggregate and pseudo-mycelia are formed. Another serum factor of IgG nature discovered by the same authors, prevents the cells from being aggregated.

Serological methods

Low-titre agglutinin (1 : 10–1 : 80) can be found in 22 to 64 per cent of healthy individuals [21, 138, 155, 184, 197b, 226, 243], but in candidiasis the titre varies between 1 : 160 and 1 : 5,120. According to several authors, titres higher than 1 : 160 should be regarded as positive [1a, 34a, b, c, d, 106, 175, 197b, 220]. Tomšíková and Seeliger [224] showed in Candida infections an increase in the IgM antibodies followed by a similar increase in IgG antibodies. But they could not draw any diagnostic conclusions concerning candidiasis from the presence of these immune substances. C. albicans gives cross-reactions with other species of Candida, e.g. Cryptococcus neoformans, Blastomyces dermatitidis, Histoplasma capsulatum and Saccharomyces cerevisiae. In superficial candidiasis of the skin and of the mucous membranes the agglutination test is not reliable for making the diagnosis [39, 58, 150, 175, 226].

The passive haemagglutination test is more sensitive than the agglutination test, but it should be applied combined with other serological methods [184]. In this test specific antibodies agglutinate sheep red blood cells sensitized with fungal antigens. Müller [148] has claimed that the passive haemagglutination test is specific in the differential diagnosis of candidiasis.

C fixation test is often negative in localized candidiasis. The test is usually considered as positive if the titre is 1 : 8–1 : 16 or higher [39, 65, 174, 197]. There are different opinions on the value of the reaction. Some authors attribute little value to this reaction because of its non-specificity [58, 105, 171], while others regard it as specific, provided an adequate antigen is applied [164, 199]. Török [226] showed positive C fixation reaction in 50 per cent in processes of the skin and the mucous membranes, but only in 30 per cent in vaginal candidiasis. Of antigens prepared by four different methods the one produced by freezing and thawing of C. albicans proved to be the most specific [227]. The C fixation test was positive in some cases of Leiner's disease as well [89]. A cross-reaction has been observed with some Histoplasma, Blastomyces, Coccidioides and Geotrichum species. The diagnostic value of the C fixation test is similar to that of the agglutination test.

Precipitation test is carried out in agar gel and in liquid media. The gel precipitation is positive in systemic candidiasis and in septicaemia; it is usually negative in superficial candidiasis [101b, 198, 205, 220, 226]. Using mannan, cytoplasmic and culture filtrate antigens obtained from C. albicans Stanley et al. [206] succeeded in demonstrating positive gel precipitation even in superficial candidiasis (vulvovaginitis candidomycetica). Precipitation in liquid medium is more useful in such processes [8]. Cross-reaction could be observed with other strains of Candida, with Chladosporium, Hormodendron, Nocardia, etc. Bläker et al. [21] showed that in patients capable of immune response there was a marked increase in C. albicans precipitins in the course of candidiasis. Cytostatics did not suppress antibody formation. Because of the duration of the disease or for compensatory reasons, antibody concentrations were especially high in patients with chronic granulomatous candidiasis and partial cell-mediated immune defects. These findings suggest [21] that candidiasis can be diagnosed serologically as long as the immune response of the patient is intact. Immunological diagnosis fails if, due to severe primary or secondary disturbance of antibody formation, the immune response is imparied. Biological false positive reaction apparently can occur as a result of an increased responsiveness, e.g. in bronchial asthma of children or hypergammaglobulinaemia in neutropenia. Stickle et al. [210] found immune diffusion combined with latex agglutination to be reliable in the diagnostics of systemic candidiasis. Precipitins were most often found in sera with high agglutinin titres [1a]. Possible functions of precipitins include prevention of dissemination of the infection, formation of immune complexes and suppression of cell-mediated immunity [4a].

Lehner [128] has examined 244 sera and salivas by means of quantitative immunofluorescence. In 85 per cent the titre exceeded in 1 : 16 in sera of patients

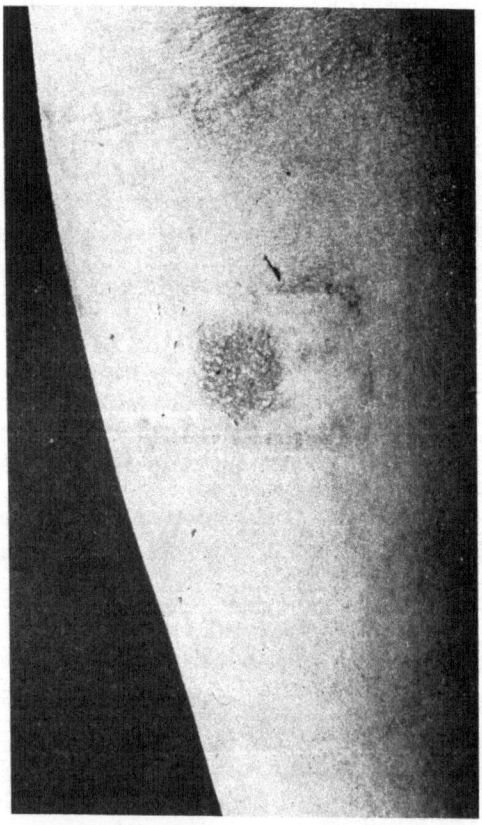

Fig. 75-14. Positive epicutaneous test with living *C. albicans*

suffering from candidiasis. The antibody titre of healthy individuals was below 1 : 8. Comaish et al. [33] published similar results. Autofluorescence may interfere with the evaluation of the results. The fluorescent antibody technique is a method enabling rapid identification of Candida in skin and nail scrapings [172a].

Immunobiological procedures may be used for the differentiation of Candida species [80, 125, 174, 192]. Quick determination has been performed by the fluorescent antibody technique [40a, 63, 66, 102, 107, 128]. This is, however, often disturbed by cross-reactions.

Biquet et al. [16] succeeded in demonstrating 9 antigenic fractions in *C. albicans* with immunoelectrophoresis. Two of these were species-specific. Other authors have also used this method for demonstrating differences between *C. albicans* strains [192, 219].

C. albicans extracts have been used for the demonstration of delayed hypersensitivity by means of lymphocyte transformation [58a, 59, 131a]. The *in vitro* stimulation of lymphocytes by the specific antigen is independent of the circulating antibodies, but shows a correlation with hypersensitivity. Folb and Trounce [57] observed blast transformation in a high per cent of lymphocytes from patients suffering from candidiasis. The blast transformation rate was significantly lower if the patients had been treated with corticosteroids and/or immunosuppressive substances; at the same time the circulating antibody level did not change. Balogh et al. [9] observed 20–48 per cent transformation with Candida antigen in candidiasis. Several authors have demonstrated a normal humoral defense mechanism in mucocutaneous candidiasis besides negative

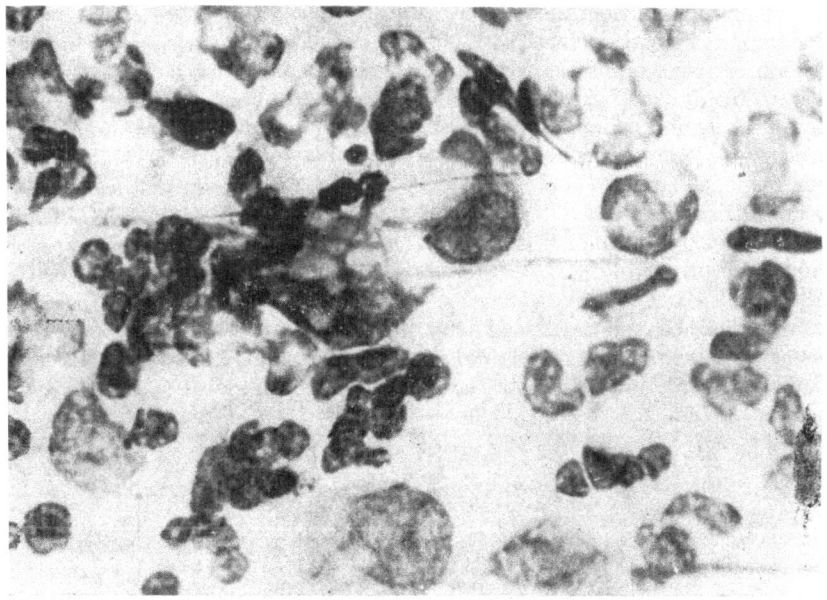

Fig. 75-15. Lymphoblasts in a smear prepared from positive epicutaneous test induced by *C. albicans*

lymphocyte transformation [209, 111]. Pöhler [175] performed lymphocyte transformation tests in 86 cases of mucocutaneous candidiasis and 14 control subjects, using candidin, trichophytin and aspergillin antigens containing the polysaccharide-nitrogen complex. The test was consistently positive with the homologous antigen and negative with the heterologous ones. The control tests were negative. Pöhler demonstrated a close relationship between the severity of the clinical picture and the lymphocyte transformation rate. Flórián and Török [56] demonstrated lymphoblasts in the positive epicutaneous reaction induced by living *C. albicans* (Figs 75-14 and 75-15).

Comparative experiments with the different serological reactions have been carried out using different antigens, in order to eliminate non-specific reactions [185, 217, 219, 223].

According to recent investigations, in patients with mucocutaneous candidiasis a significant correlation exists between skin test size and *in vitro* lymphocyte transformation. However, there is no quantitative correlation between either skin test size or lymphocyte transformation when compared to migration inhibition factor production. These findings suggest that possibly separate populations of cells are involved in blast cell transformation and soluble mediator production. Specific anti-Candida-precipitating antibody levels appear to be independent of the degree of lymphocyte transformation, indicating that the B cells' responsiveness is not related to the reaction of lymphocytes [15a].

Immunological restoration

Severe chronic mucocutaneous candidiasis appears together with progressive cellular immunological defect. To eliminate the latter, the restoration of the immune system with transfusion of immunologically competent allogeneic lymphocytes was introduced [112]. From such a therapy conversion of the candidin skin test to positive, migration inhibition factor (MIF) production by lymphocytes and improvement of the mucocutaneous symptoms may be expected [72a]. However, the effect of the therapy is only transitory: 6–8 months following the transfusion the candidiasis recurs the skin tests become negative again and the MIF production falls to insignificant levels. Administration of the transfer factor of Lawrence (a dialysable extract of peripheral blood leukocytes from a donor sensitive to candidin) was the subsequent step in the therapy. The skin tests turned into positive and MIF was produced to candidin. Repeated injections seem to be necessary in high concentrations and at short intervals [22]. The remission can be prolonged by administering the Lawrence factor preparation in combination with anti-Candida agents (e.g. Amphotericin B) [50a, 196].

FORMS OF CANDIDIDS

Like dermatophytes, Candida species allergize the whole organism. In addition, non-specific factors (light, mechanical irritants, etc.) are known to participate in eliciting candidids. The candidids may be regional localized (Fig. 75-16), remote localized or generalized. Dyshidrosis, eczema, psoriasis-, pityriasis rosea-, prurigo-, strophulus- and urticaria-like mycids may occur in the skin. Generalization following Nystatin therapy of *C. albicans* infection (supposedly caused by a rapid elution of candidal toxin) and intracutaneous injection of candidin have also been published [154a]. Some chronic cases of urticaria may be regarded as mycids, in which gastrointestinal diseases are the primary pathogenetical factors. Holti [83] found the cutaneous test to be positive with *C. albicans* extract in 49 cases out of 270 in chronic urticaria. Szádeczky [216] demonstrated yeasts in the gastric juice of chronic urticarial patients in 57 per cent and in the intestinal juice in 41 per cent. The intracutaneous test with a Candida extract was positive in 40 per cent of these patients.

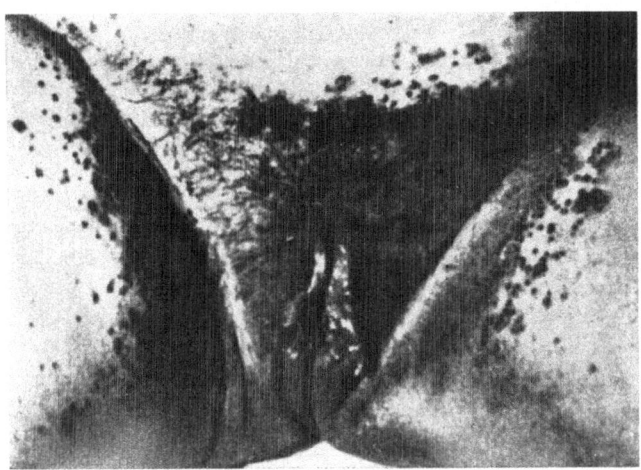

Fig. 75-16. Regional candidid around the primary focus of
a vulvovaginal and genitofemoral candidiasis

The allergic symptoms may involve the internal organs: bronchial asthma, allergic rhinitis, migraine, conjunctivitis, and anaphylactic shock have been observed in experimental animals [39]. Fejér [52e] described the prosthesis disease of mycotic origin. *C. albicans*, hidden under dental prostheses, bridgeworks and badly-fitting crowns may induce eczematoid candidids, mainly of a regional character, on the face, neck and temples. From the immunological point of view a new triad consisting of chronic mucocutaneous candidiasis, myositis and thymoma deserves interest [147]. Myositis is the first manifestation (biopsy shows perivascular interstitial lymphorrhagia). The removed tumour showed numerous small and large lymphocytes as well as larger epithelial-like cells. The fungal infection displayed little spontaneous improvement during the first year after surgery.

MOULD ALLERGY

Among the aetiological components of fungal allergic diseases moulds play an important role in common with dermatophytes and yeasts. Detailed investigations have proved the sensitizing capacity of moulds and the route of invasion of allergens.

Since the investigations of Strom van Leeuven [211] various clinical observations, human and animal experiments, specific skin reactions and serological reactions have corroborated the sensitizing ability of several moulds of the genera Penicillium, Aspergillus, Alternaria, Mucor, Hormodendron, Chladosporium, etc. in inhalant allergy (asthma, etc.) [39, 51a, b, 78, 133, 244]. The often seasonal occurrence of mould-allergic diseases, similarly to pollinosis, is due to the spore content of the air. The spore is the part of fungi with the highest sensitizing capacity (1,000 to 10,000-fold that of the hyphae). Macro- and micro-climatic components play an important role in the propagation of fungi. The spores propagate quickly in dry, windy weather (they may occasionally be demonstrated as high as at 2,000 meters in the atmosphere) but settle down in wet weather [51b, 244]. There are geographic differences in the prevalence of individual moulds, e.g. Alternaria species mainly occur as inhalant allergens in the U.S.A., whereas in Hungary hypersensitivity to Aspergilli and Penicillia is the most frequent [74].

The aetiological role of moulds in skin mycoses has been recognized only recently. They may induce skin mycoses as well as infections of the internal organs [93a, b, c, d, 94, 133, 244]. Moulds may occur as associated pathogens in different processes of the skin, in interdigital and nail mycoses, in eczematous diseases [51b], and in urticaria [200], altering thereby the original character of the process and inducing hypersensitivity.

The following data support the aetiological role of moulds in allergic diseases:

1. Moulds with a proved sensitizing effect in inhalant allergies may be cultivated from the skin processes.
2. The extracts of the same fungi may serve as antigens in serological reactions, induce positive skin tests, and the induced hypersensitivity characterized by immediate reactions can be transferred passively.
3. Different eruptions of a mycid character may be elicited by penicillin, a fungus product, in individuals suffering from penicillin allergy.
4. Secondary diseases due to sensitization heal soon after the elimination of the primary foci.
5. Desensitization with mould antigens may be successful.

Hypersensitivity to penicillin and other antibiotics may occur in mould allergy. According to Ogasawara et al. [157], a lethal anaphylactic shock could be induced in mice with an intravenous injection of penicillin-G 11 days after intracerebral administration of Penicillium chrysogeneum. It is highly probable that the closer the relation of the antigen structure of the mould products participating in the mycotic skin diseases to that of the applied penicillin, the more frequently penicillin allergy occurs. Therefore antibiotics have to be administered to mould-allergic patients with due care. Inhalation of mould spores may also elicit penicillin-allergic symptoms [51b] as has been shown by lethal penicillin shock cases induced in this way.

SKIN TESTS

The antigens of, and consequently, the skin reactions to, moulds are group-specific. Species-specificity occurs rarely. Different commercial extracts produced from different species are available. They are applied in a dilution of 1 : 100. The evaluation of the reaction is hindered by the lack of standardization. A positive skin reaction may often be observed in respiratory diseases [244]. Rajka [181] received positive skin reaction to mould allergens in 25 per cent of patients suffering from atopic dermatitis (prurigo Besnier).

The intracutaneous test does not furnish exact information as to whether in fact there is an infection. Therefore, if applied alone, it has no diagnostic value. The suspected allergen has to be found in great quantities in the patient's environment. Exposure test may be performed on the conjunctiva, on the nasal mucosa or through an inhalative route, the last one being the most adequate [244].

SEROLOGICAL TESTS

In the course of mould infections precipitins appear in the serum. These can be demonstrated by agar gel diffusion methods and by immunoelectrophoresis. The C fixation test yields cross-reactions with other groups of moulds. In children suffering from asthma due to mould allergy the IgE level was found normal [99], although the reagin-type antibodies responsible for the immediate reactions belong in the IgE class. In rabbits immunized with moulds specific IgM and IgG antibodies were found [233a].

Several moulds elicit allergic reactions at an especially high frequency. It seems to be worth while discussing these moulds and the phenomena elicited by them more thoroughly.

ASPERGILLOSIS

Among Aspergilli *A. fumigatus*, a facultative parasite, induces allergic symptoms most frequently. It produces several endotoxins, which elicit a severe tissue damage in animals, which may even be lethal. Manifestation occurs mainly in patients suffering from leukaemia or lymphoma, or in those under permanent corticosteroid, broad-spectrum antibiotic, immunosuppressive or X-ray therapy.

A. fumigatus may cause several types of lesions in the lungs:

1. Aspergilloma
2. Chronic bronchitis (bronchopneumonic form)
3. Bronchial asthma
4. Lesions of the lungs due to fungal septicaemia

Besides, it may elicit sinusitis and/or mycosis of the auditory meatus.

Seeliger [197*d*] has investigated the Aspergillus antibody titre of human sera by the C fixation test and received a positive titre with the *A. fumigatus* antigen only in a single case; in the other cases the titre was very low or negative. Moreover, the C fixation test yields cross-reactions.

Patients allergic to *A. fumigatus* are liable to recurrent pulmonary infections. In a high per cent of these cases precipitins can be demonstrated by means of agar gel diffusion [31, 45, 244]. Both IgE [162*a*] and IgD [137*a*] antibodies against *A. fumigatus* can be detected in sera of patients with bronchopulmonary allergic aspergillosis.

Immunoelectrophoresis yields at least four precipitin lines in pulmonary aspergillosis [39]. Agglutinins could not be demonstrated.

Inhalation of *A. fumigatus* may elicit an immediate urticarial skin reaction which is accompanied by eosinophilia. Pepys et al. [167] observed a simultaneous positive skin test and a positive agar gel precipitation to aspergillus extracts in several cases. In other cases, however, precipitins could not be demonstrated in spite of positive skin reactions.

The indirect immunofluorescent method may be of diagnostic help in clinically doubtful cases [122*a*].

PHYCOMYCOSIS (MUCORMYCOSIS)

Mucoraceae are facultative parasites. The predisposing factors are the same as in aspergillosis. This infection is especially frequent in diabetic acidoses. Subcutaneous, orbital, cerebral, gastrointestinal and pulmonary forms are known. The metabolic disturbance due to diabetes severely damages the phagocytic capacity of leukocytes, and therefore the fungus is able to disseminate by the haematogenous way [39, 133]. Little is known about the immunological relations of this disease. Skin test and a C fixation test with the fungus extract cannot be used for diagnosis. The human organism seems to be highly resistant to mucor infection.

MYCOTIC ECZEMA (ECZEMA MYCOGENES)

Two groups of mycotic eczema are known:

1. Eczematous mycoses
2. Secondary eczematous diseases consequent upon mycotic sensitization.

ECZEMATOUS MYCOSES

Eczematous mycoses develop under the direct effect of fungi. Török [229] used the term mycosis eczematiformis for all mycotic processes that more or less show the polymorphous appearance of eczema. They are characterized by eczematous inflammation first surrounded by a distinct epithelial border which, however, becomes indistinct later on. The eczematous mycoses are characterized by [52*g, i*]:

1. The presence of the pathogenic fungus
2. Clinical manifestations which are not, or hardly, characteristic of the pathogenic agent
3. Positive allergic skin reactions to the adequate antigen in most cases especially in the vicinity of the lesion (the process may still be local)
4. Itching
5. Good response to antimycotic treatment.

This mostly unilateral process occurs especially on the extremities, ano-genital region, on opposed skin surfaces, i.e. in regions where the skin is exposed to physical chemical, and microbial irritation.

Eczematous mycoses may be caused by different types of dermatophytes, moulds and yeasts. Mixed fungal-microbial infections may frequently be found in the background of the disease. Fungal and chemical allergies may also be associated.

SECONDARY ECZEMATOUS DISEASES

The overwhelming majority of mycotic eczemas are dyshidrotic and eczematoid eruptions (Fig. 75-17). The classical form is the sterile, symmetrical, vesicular eczema dyshidroticum. The main factors of the pathogenesis of secondary fungal allergic eczemas are:

1. The sensitizing primary foci
2. Mycotic allergy induced by the primary focus
3. Usually specific, but partly non-specific factors eliciting the disease and determining the localization

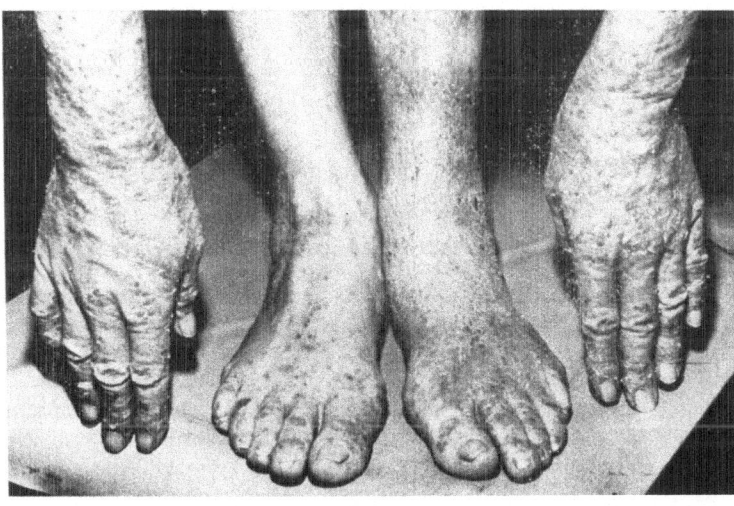

Fig. 75-17. Mycotic eczema. The primary focus is an erosio interdigitalis pedis

4. Sterile eczematoid eruptions

5. Occasional secondary infection of sterile eruptions.

Accordingly, the most important tasks in the clinical diagnostics of mycotic eczemas are as follows:

1. Search for primary foci
2. Establishing the nature of the mycotic allergy (trichophytin, Candida allergy),
3. Revealing the factors eliciting the symptoms
4. Determination of the agent(s) causing infection in the originally sterile eruptions.

The primary foci may be epidermal or situated in internal organs.

(A) *Epidermal foci*:
    1. Interdigital and dyshidrosis-like foot mycosis
    2. Nail mycosis
    3. Mycosis of the female genitals
    4. Perianal mycosis
    5. Balanoposthitis
    6. Mycoses of opposed surfaces and skin folds
    7. Paronychia
    8. Oral candidiasis
    9. Mycosis of the external auditory meatus
   10. Umbilical mycosis
(B) *Foci in internal organs*
    1. Intestinal tract
    2. Tonsils
    3. Bronchi
    4. Lungs

THERAPY OF MYCOTIC ECZEMA

The therapy of mycotic eczema consists in a careful external and sometimes internal antimycotic treatment.

In secondary eczematous diseases complex treatment is needed.

1. Elimination of the primary mycotic focus by local, (occasionally) oral antimycotic treatment. In the therapy of primary foci due to Candida the possible elimination of predisposing factors is very important (treatment of diabetes; discontinuation of corticosteroid or immunosuppressive therapy, etc.).

2. In the acute phase and in cases with severe symptoms of inflammation, a short-lasting corticosteroid, ACTH or antihistamine treatment may be combined with antimycotic treatment.

3. Desensitization with the adequate fungal antigen may be attempted. Before such a therapy the estimation of the degree of hypersensitivity by intracutaneous injection of different dilutions of the allergen seems to be important. Fresh in-

jections should only be given after the previous skin reaction has faded; generally one or two injections are to be administered weekly. If the reaction to the same dilution has shown a declining tendency, the concentration should be increased. A complete desensitization, however, cannot be achieved with the currently available methods. Drugs necessary for overcoming an occasional shock, primarily epinephrine, should always be at hand.

4. Though mycids in themselves are sterile eruptions, their frequent secondary infections may necessitate local—occasionally a general—antiseptic-treatment.

5. The prophylactic hygiene of the regions of the skin which are especially liable to fungal infections (interdigital spaces, opposing skin surfaces, female genitals) is especially important.

IMMUNOLOGY OF DEEP MYCOSES

These may be classified into two clinical groups:

1. *Subcutaneous mycoses* which mainly affect the skin and the subcutaneous tissues (sporotrichosis, chromoblastomycosis, madura mycosis, rhinosporidiosis).

2. *Systemic mycoses* localized to the skin and the internal organs (coccidiomycosis, histoplasmosis, North American blastomycosis, paracoccidiosis, cryptococcosis, actinomycosis).

The fungi causing deep mycoses are, as antigens, less active in inducing the production of protective antibodies; they rather induce severe hypersensitivity.

The same methods may be used for the demonstration of antibodies in these cases as in superficial mycoses. Serological examinations are important mainly for the diagnosis and prognosis but can also be used for epidemiological studies, furthermore, for investigating the taxonomic relations of fungi. The evaluation of the results is hindered by the lack of commercial standard antigens, further, by the frequent cross-reactions between dimorphous fungi. (The term dimorphous fungi is applied to fungi that may alter their shape in the organism and under different conditions of cultivation.)

SUBCUTANEOUS MYCOSES

Sporotrichosis

The aetiological agent is *Sporotrichum (Sporothrix) schenckii*.

The immunology of sporotrichosis has been studied by few investigators only. Circulating antibodies occur in infected experimental animals as well as in patients in variable quantities. The diagnostic value of the sporoagglutination, a serological method frequently used earlier, could not be confirmed by recent investigations. Some authors obtained high-titre (1 : 640) positive results [70, 175] others, however, observed no agglutination or low titres (1 : 10–1 : 20) in verified cases of sporotrichoses [113, 197b].

163

The C fixation test can be used only in diseases of the deep tissues and in disseminated sporotrichosis. McMillen [141] demonstrated the presence of C fixing antibodies in 1 : 2–1 : 16 titres in two-thirds of his patients suffering from cutaneous sporotrichosis, but in the articular and pulmonary forms the reaction was positive in each with a considerable high titre (1 : 16–1 : 256).

According to Seeliger [1976], precipitation is often positive with fungus extract and the positive reaction may persist for a long time after convalescence. Precipitation with fungus extract is positive even if the process is localized, while the positive C fixation test seems to indicate extensive processes. McMillen [141] observed positive agar gel precipitation in the articular and pulmonary forms, and occasionally in the cutaneous form. Roberts and Larsh [188] applied an antigen prepared from the yeast phase of *Sp. schenckii* for the C fixation, precipitation and agglutination tests. The reactions proved to be specific in each of the tested 37 extracutaneous cases of sporotrichosis.

The fluorescent antibody method is mainly suitable for the demonstration of fungi in histological preparations [39, 1976].

Sporotrichin skin test, which is an intracutaneous test, may be carried out with killed vaccines or with the polysaccharide fraction extracted from the fungus. Delayed-type reaction may be observed 24–48 h later in a cutaneous-lymphatic form. Non-infected subjects and those in an early state of infection are negative. The reaction is usually negative in severely disseminated forms as well. The skin test may be positive as early as 5 days after the infection. In endemic regions 24–27 per cent of the population were found to be positive [34d, 39, 242].

The simultaneous occurrence of agglutinins, precipitins and C fixing antibodies is possible. It is probably the skin test which yields the most precise information as regards the nature of the disease. Only the direct examination of histological preparations with labelled antibodies has proved to be more valuable.

Sporotrichids. The 'id' reaction is similar to that observed in trichophytids (lichenoid, pustular, papulonecrotic) [245].

Chromoblastomycosis

The aetiological agents are: *Phialophora verrucosa, Ph. pedrosoi* or *Ph. compacta*. It is easy to diagnose the disease from clinical manifestations and by culturing fungus. Neither the cutaneous test nor the serological reactions (agglutination or C fixation) are suitable for establishing the diagnosis [197]. In patients suffering from chromoblastomycosis Bacquero [11] found the skin test positive with an antigen extracted from *Ph. verrucosa*, but 25 per cent of healthy individuals also displayed positive reactions in endemic regions. These may be explained by a past abortive infection.

Maduromycosis

The aetiological agents are Nocardia, Indiella, Madurella species, *Aspergillus nidulans* and *Monosporium apiospermum*.

Specific antibodies may be demonstrated in the patients' sera by serological reactions (agglutination, C fixation, precipitation) but their production is not regular. The titres decrease with the improvement of the disease. The C fixation test may yield cross-reactions, whereas the precipitation test is more specific. According to Seeliger [197b] the serological reactions have a special diagnostic value in chronic cases.

Rhinosporidiosis

The aetiological agent is *Rhinosporidium seeberi*. Its immunology has not been investigated.

SYSTEMIC MYCOSES

Coccidioidomycosis

The aetiological agent is *Coccidioides immitis*.

Its living and killed arthrospora-mycelium and spherule-endospore forms may be used for immunological tests; for vaccine preparation the spherule-endospore forms are more suitable. Among the serological reactions the qualitative precipitin reaction and the quantitative C fixation test are equally suitable for diagnostic and prognostic purposes.

Precipitins may be demonstrated 2–4 weeks after the infection in 90 per cent of the cases, but they disappear within a short time even if the infection is disseminated. Therefore, they have no prognostic value.

The C fixation test becomes positive only later; 70 per cent of the cases will be positive by the end of the first month, and 90 per cent by the end of the second month. The antibody titre depends on the patient's condition. Its rise above 1 : 16–1 : 32 suggests dissemination, whereas its decrease runs parallel to clinical improvement. A low antibody level can be demonstrated even a few months after recovery under certain circumstances. The precipitins may be found in the IgM fraction, while the C fixing antibodies in the IgG fraction [193]. In coccidial meningitis it is rare to find C fixing antibodies in the serum but their presence can be demonstrated in the cerebrospinal fluid [160]. Pappagianis et al. [161] succeeded in demonstrating antibodies with immunodiffusion in cases which had yielded negative results with both the conventional C fixation test and the tube precipitation method. Though cross-reactions may occur with other dimorphous fungi, the above reactions yield a reliable diagnosis in 90–99 per cent.

Wallraff and Wachs [236] found the anti-IgG globulin labelled with fluorescein-isothiocyanate useful in the diagnosis of coccidioidomycosis.

The antigen used for skin test is an N-containing polysaccharide. The test usually becomes positive 1–3 weeks after the infection, and the positivity may persist for several years. It was found positive in 95–100 per cent of the population in endemic regions. Positivity may indicate prevailing infection or an earlier one. In the early phase of the disease the examination has to be carried out very carefully with a high dilution of the antigen. Cross-reactions with histoplasmin, blastomycin and paracoccidioidin are frequent.

A positive cutaneous test in combination with a negative C fixation test seems to indicate an immune state and is a good basis for prognosis. Negative skin test with an increased C fixation titre, however, suggests dissemination. The delayed hypersensitivity in coccidioidomycosis can be transferred passively with the leukocytes of the patient after a previous treatment with DNase [182]. Lymphocytes of patients with positive skin test results undergo blast transformation *in vitro* [158a]. On the other hand, in patients with negative skin- and lymphocyte transformation tests the initial results of transfer factor therapy are encouraging [208a].

Not only the clinical, but also abortive infections are followed by a persistent immunity.

An immune state could be induced in animal experiments with a vaccine prepared from *C. immitis*. The extract of the spherule-endospore cell wall seems to be the most effective vaccine [119]. No successful vaccination is known in man.

The 'id'-reaction. Three to seven weeks after the subsiding of the early symptoms allergic skin manifestations may be observed in 4 per cent of men and in 10 per cent of women in the form of erythema nodosum and erythema exudativum multiforme, respectively. A progressive, systemic mycosis rarely develops in these patients.

Histoplasmosis

The aetiological agent is *Histoplasma capsulatum*.

As in coccidioidosis, the immune reactions have diagnostic and prognostic value.

The disease is frequently associated with Hodgkin's disease, leukaemia and other systemic fungal processes (e.g. cryptococcosis). Its dissemination is promoted by permanent corticosteroid treatment.

An antigen for serological tests can be prepared from the mycelial and yeast phase of *H. capsulatum*. The antigen obtained from the yeast has proved to be preferable in practice. Campbell [27] and Seeliger [197b] suggest the application of both antigens in serological tests. The antigens may be identified by physico-chemical and immunofluorescent methods [142, 178]. Using various preparations of mycelial culture filtrates, two precipitin lines have been found with the agar gel diffusion method in Histoplasma infections. These were termed H and M bands [81, 142]. The antibodies taking part in the M band may be induced by a positive skin test and may persist for a long time after acute infection. Those taking part in the H band mean an active histoplasmosis, they are not induced by skin test or infections with other dimorphous fungi. The H band may be absent in the early phase of histoplasmosis [133]. Recent experiments have revealed the presence of 7 components in the H and M antigens by means of electrophoresis [47]. Gordon [65] succeeded in demonstrating an Y band, in addition to the H and M bands, by using the yeast phase of the fungus as antigen. The Y band also proved to be specific and indicated active infection.

In the histoplasma serology the frequent cross-reactions with coccidioidomycosis and North American blastomycosis should be taken into consideration. The common polysaccharide antigens of the fungi are responsible for the cross-reactions. It is advisable to perform serial tests in the course of the disease.

Latex or collodion particle agglutination or passive haemagglutination are usually applied. The agglutinins appear and disappear earlier than the C fixing antibodies. The value of the agglutination test resides in establishing an early diagnosis.

The C fixation test becomes positive 2–4 weeks after the infection. The titre runs parallel to the clinical course, increasing significantly during dissemination. Campbell and Hill [28] observed an increasing fixing antibody titre in 7 out of 12 healthy individuals after the application of a histoplasmin skin test. The titre reached 1 : 256. The increased titre persisted for several months. In contrast, Seeliger [197b] could not observe a positive complement fixation or precipitation during 3 years of observation even after 2–4 histoplasmin skin tests.

It is generally admitted that after skin tests the C fixation test can only be evaluated when an antigen of the yeast phase is applied. Conant et al. [34c] observed low-titre C fixing antibodies in 8 per cent of the healthy population in endemic regions. In European patients who have lived in endemic regions even a C fixation titre of 1 : 5 provides some information [197b].

In precipitation tests the precipitins, like agglutinins, appear early, 1–2 weeks after the infection, and disappear within 4–6 weeks. The presence of bands H and Y is of the greatest diagnostic value. The demonstration of precipitins is especially valuable in mild infections, where the C fixation test is usually negative. In such cases the prognosis is good [197b].

The fluorescent antibody method enables the diagnosis of histoplasmosis in histological preparations within 1–2 h. Cross-reactions with dimorphous fungi may occur. To reduce their incidence, sera should be absorbed with B. dermatitidis and C. immitis [39]. Newberry et al. [154] have carried out a lymphocyte transformation test with radioactive thymidine in healthy individuals (with and without histoplasmin positivity) and in patients suffering from acute or chronic histoplasmosis. The thymidin uptake was greater in acute histoplasmosis and in healthy histoplasmin-positive individuals than in chronic forms and in histoplasmin-negative individuals.

For the histoplasmin skin test, histoplasmin is produced from the filtrate of H. capsulatum broth cultures. The antigen is a protein containing polysaccharide; 0.1 ml of the antigen diluted to 1 : 100 should be administered intradermally. The skin test becomes positive earlier than the serological reactions. The positive skin test may indicate an active infection or a past one. The negative skin test excludes histoplasmosis, though Lehan and Furcolow [126] were of the contrary opinion. There may be a cross-reaction with dimorphous fungi, but the reactions induced by the homologous antigen are always stronger than those induced by heterologous ones. As the antibody production is significantly stimulated by the skin test, the serological tests should precede the skin test. In endemic regions, e.g. in the USA, 80 per cent of the population display a positive cutaneous test [34a].

Immunity may be induced in animals with killed cells or cell fractions or with sublethal doses of living cells. This immunity is in no connection with a stimulated phagocytosis of H. capsulatum. Neither the intracellular digestion of the yeast cells nor the intracellular multiplication of Histoplasma seems to be altered [133].

The 'id' reaction may be: erythema nodosum and erythema exudativum multiforme.

North American blastomycosis

The aetiological agent is *Blastomyces dermatitidis*.

This fungus frequently yields cross-reactions with *C. imitis* and *H. capsulatum*. Therefore, a single serological examination is of little diagnostic value. Serial tests carried out with different antigens simultaneously are much more reliable.

The most frequently used serological method is the C fixation test. However, this may be negative in the early phase of the disease and in mild infections. In extended processes high-titre of C fixing antibodies has been found. A negative skin test with a high C fixation titre makes a bad prognosis [204].

Precipitins may be demonstrated transiently in a small quantity. Ball et al. [6] have observed positive agar gel precipitation in 17 out of 300 individuals without blastomycosis. The C fixation test was negative in all of these cases.

The fluorescent antibody method has been used to differentiate the yeast and the mycelial phases of *B. dermatitidis*.

The skin test has not been extensively used because of its divergent results. In blastomycosis the intracutaneous reaction is stronger to histoplasmin than to blastomycin. The difference between the two antigens can also be demonstrated serologically [133]. Among the antigens of *B. dermatitidis* the polysaccharide antigen seems to be the most specific in the skin test. Delayed hypersensitivity to *B. dermatitidis* can be passively transferred with spleen cells [196a].

Paracoccidioidosis

The aetiological agent is *Paracoccidioides brasiliensis*.

The immunological reactions are less useful for diagnostic purposes than for following the course of the disease and judging the results of therapy.

C fixation test can be carried out with a polysaccharide antigen of the yeast form of *P. brasiliensis*. The antibody titre is usually low and may be negative in early cases. The titre is higher in generalized infections. A cross-reaction may occur with histoplasmosis, coccidioidomycosis and North American blastomycosis.

Precipitins are the first to appear upon infection and, after recovery, the first to disappear.

The value of the paracoccidioidin skin test is similar to that of the coccidioidin skin test but the reaction is less intensive. Its positivity may indicate an acute or a subsided infection. The test may be positive in 20–26 per cent in healthy individuals living in endemic regions and in patients suffering from other diseases [39].

Cryptococcosis

The aetiological agent is *Cryptococcus neoformans*.

The disease frequently accompanies Hodgkin's disease, leukaemia, tuberculosis, rheumatic heart disease and hepatic cirrhosis. In the blood of infected patients circulating antibodies are either absent, or only present in low titres, therefore, their demonstration cannot be used for establishing the diagnosis.

The negative serological reactions observed in immunized and infected experimental animals may be explained by the particular characteristics of *C. neoformans* or by an immune paralysis [197]. It is possible that the Cryptococcus is a weak antigen, or the antigen applied in the serological test is inappropriate. The most active antigen is the polysaccharide antigen of the capsule, which is built up of glucose, xylose, mannose, galactose and acid. Evans [49] has differentiated three serotypes of the *C. neoformans* capsule, viz., types A, B and C. Wilson et al. [341] have described a fourth serotype termed type D. Serotype A occurs most frequently (95 per cent) [197d]. The specificity of the capsule antigens is limited; apathogenic Cryptococcus strains may also contain them [197b].

Soluble polysaccharide antigens of the Cryptococcus may be demonstrated in the serum, cerebrospinal fluid and urine of patients (Neill test) [151]. Seeliger [197d, 198] and Goodman et al. [64] recommend the latex particle agglutination technique for this purpose. The reaction is specific and has a diagnostic value.

Opinions vary on the value of the serological examinations. Bannet et al. [15] regard the complement fixation test carried out with the Cryptococcus polysaccharide antigen as relevant. Seeliger [197b], however, failed to detect C fixing antibodies or precipitins in 8 cases of mycologically and histologically verified cryptococcoses.

Decreased lymphocyte transformation in response to *C. neoformans* has been found in human disseminated cryptococcosis [41a]. It has been concluded that the defective function of lymphocytes may reflect increased susceptibility to cryptococcal infection in patients without other known predisposing factor.

The fluorescent antibody method may be used for the demonstration of Cryptococcus in tissues and for serological classification. The reaction is specific, and cross-reactions do not occur. Vogel et al. [234] could demonstrate serum antibodies by the indirect immunofluorescence method in 8 per cent of 339 subjects including healthy individuals and patients suffering from unrelated diseases. The subclinical infection of these patients has been supposed.

Several authors have studied the active and the passive immunization of animals. Gadebusch [61a, b] has observed an anti-Cryptococcus activity in the sera of immunized animals, but failed to demonstrate circulating antibodies. Louria [135] has suggested that the protective antibodies are tissue-bound. Abrahams [1] succeeded in transferring the immunity passively with immune lymphocytes and macrophages to non-immune animals. A significant immunity may be achieved in mice with a sublethal dose of living Cryptococcus, with formalin-treated Cryptococcus or with a purified polysaccharide fraction [1, 61b, 136].

When Cryptococcus cells are mixed with a specific antiserum, the capsule becomes visible, but its diameter does not increase [197b]. This capsule is highly specific and may be used for the serotyping of Cryptococci.

Decapsulated Cryptococcus cells are used as antigen in the skin test. A positive reaction often ensues with this antigen in active infections, though much less frequently in other mycoses [14].

Actinomycosis

The aetiological agents are: *Actinomyces wolff-israeli* and *Actinomyces bovis*. The immunobiological characteristics of this disease are poorly known. Serological tests are not suitable for diagnostic and prognostic purposes, though, circulating antibodies have been demonstrated in experimental animals as well as in man [34b]. The C fixation test does not yield reliable results unless the antigen applied is made from fresh strains. Neuber [153] used aqueous and alcoholic Actinomyces suspensions or extracts as antigen. The patients with a verified actinomycosis yielded positive results in 60–70 per cent. According to Seeliger [197b] the complement fixation test is of greater value than the agglutination test.

Serological reactions may also be used for differentiating *A. wolff-israeli* from *A. bovis*, furthermore for investigating the serological relationship between Actinomyces and Nocardia.

The vaccine treatment widely applied earlier has lost its practical importance since the discovery of antibiotics (first of all, penicillin).

REFERENCES

1. Abrahams, I. and Gilleran, T.: *J. Immunol.* **85**, 629 (1960).
1a. Andersen, P. L. and Stenderup, A.: *Scand. J. infect. Dis.* **6**, 69 (1974).
2a. Aravijszkij, A. N.: *Mycopathologia (Den Haag)* **11**, 143 (1959).
2b. ibid., **16**, 177 (1962).
3. Arzt, L.: *Derm. Wschr.* **75**, 1193 (1922).
4. Arzt, L. and Fuchs, H.: In *Jadassohn's Handbuch der Haut- und Geschlechtskrankheiten.* Vol. XI. Springer, Berlin 1928, p. 607.
4a. Axelsen, N. H., Kirkpatrick, C. H. and Buckley, R. H.: *Clin. exp. Immunol.* **17**, 385 (1974).
5. Ayres, S. and Anderson, N. P.: *Arch. Derm. Syph.* **29**, 536 (1934).
6. Ball, O. G., Lummus, F. L., Sigrest, M. L., Busey, J. F. and Allison, F., jr.: *Amer. J. Hyg.* **72**, 231 (1960).
7. Balogh, É.: *Bőrgyógy. vener. Szle.* **47**, 17 (1971).
8. Balogh, É. and Halmy, K.: *Bőrgyógy. vener. Szle.* **45**, 145 (1969).
9. Balogh, É., Mészáros, Cs. and Halmy, K.: *Bőrgyógy. vener. Szle.* **47**, 58 (1971).
10. Balogh, É., Nagy, E. and Halmy, K.: *Bőrgyógy. vener. Szle.* **45**, 56 (1969).
10a. Balogh, É., Szegedi, Gy., Karmazsin, L., Szabó, G. and Szabolcsi, M.: *Derm. Mschr.* **162**, 100 (1976).
11. Baquero, G. F.: In *Essays on Tropical Dermatology.* Ed. by Simons, R. D. G. and Marschall, J. Excerpta Medica Foundation, Amsterdam 1969, 252.
11a. Basarab, O., How, M. J. and Cruickshank, C. N. D.: *Sabouraudia* **6**, 119 (1968).
12. Bazyka, A. P.: cited by Halmy, K.: *Bőrgyógy. vener. Szle.* **47**, 75 (1971).
13. Bazyka, A. P., Kashkin, P. N. and Siluyanova, N. A.: *Vestn. Derm. Vener.* **40**/5, 46 (1966).
14. Bennett, J. E., Hasenclever, H. F. and Baum, G. L.: *Amer. Rev. resp. Dis.* **91**, 616 (1965).
15. Bennet, J. E., Hasenclever, H. F. and Tynes, B. S.: cited by Louria, D. B.: *New Engl. J. Med.* **277**, 1126 (1967).

15a. Bice, D. E., Lopez, M., Rotschild, H. and Salvaglio, J.: *Int. Arch. Allergy* **47**, 54 (1974).
16. Biquet, J., Havez, R., Tran van Ky, P. and Degaey, R.: *Ann. Inst. Pasteur* **100**, 13 (1961).
17. Biquet, J., Tran van Ky, P. and Andrieu, S.: *Mycopathologia (Den Haag)* **17**, 239 (1962).
18. Bishop, C. T., Blank, F. and Aranisavljevic-Jakovlevic, M.: *Canad. J. Chem.* **40**, 1816 (1962).
19. Bishop, C. Z., Blank, F. and Gardner, P. E.: *Canad. J. Chem.* **38**, 869 (1960).
20. Bishop, C. T., Perry, M. B., Blank, F. and Cooper, F. P.: *Canad. J. Chem.* **43**, 30 (1965).
21. Bläker, F., Fischer, K. and Hellwege, H. H.: *Dtsch.med. Wschr.* **98**, 194 (1973).
22. Bläker, F., Grob, P. J., Hellwege, H. H. and Schulz, K. H.: *Dtsch. med. Wschr.* **98**, 415 (1973).
23a. Bloch, Br.: In *Jadassohn's Handbuch der Haut- und Geschlechtskrankheiten.* Vol. XI. Springer, Berlin 1928, p. 300.
23b. ibid., p. 564.
24. Bloch, Br., Labouchère, A. and Schaaf, F.: *Arch. Derm. Syph. (Berl.)* **148**, 413 (1925).
25. Bolay, G.: *Dermatologica (Basel)* **100**, 288 (1950).
26. Bolgár, E., Fehér, E., Török, H. and Rajka, E.: *Hautarzt*, **11**, 254 (1960).
27. Campbell, C. C.: *Ann. N. Y. Acad. Sci.* **89**, 163 (1960).
28. Campbell, C. C. and Hill, G. B.: *Amer. Rev. resp. Dis.* **90**, 927 (1964).
29. Canales, L., Middlemas III. R. O., Louro, J. M. and Ann South, M.: *Lancet*, **ii**, 567 (1969).
29a. Charpentier, C., Isoard, P. and Fontanges, R.: *Mykosen* **19**, 1 (1976).
30. Chilgren, R. A., Menwissen, H. J., Quie, P. G. and Hong, R.: *Lancet* **ii**, 688 (1967).
31. Coleman, R. and Kaufman, M. L.: *Appl. Microbiol.* **23**, 301 (1972).
32. Collins, J.-P., Grappel, S. F. and Blank, F.: *Dermatologica (Basel)* **146**, 95 (1973).
33. Comaish, J. S., Gibson, B. and Green, C. A.: *J. invest. Derm.* **40**, 139 (1963).
34a. Conant, N. F., Smith, D. T., Baker, R. D., Callaway, J. L. and Martin, D. S,: *Manual of Clinical Mycology.* Saunders, Philadelphia 1955.
34b. ibid., p. 21.
34c. ibid., p. 143.
34d. ibid., p. 180.
35. Cormia, F. E. and Lewis, G. M.: *J. invest. Derm.* **7**, 375 (1946).
36. Cormia, F. E., Lewis, G. M. and Hopper, M. E.: *J. invest. Derm.* **8**, 95 (1947).
37. Crounse, R. G.: *Rev. med. vet. Mycol.* **7**, 187 (1971).
38. Cruickshank, C. N. D., Trotter, M. D. and Wood, R. S.: *J. invest. Derm.* **35**, 219 (1960).
39. Curtis, A. C. and Bocobo, F. C.: In *Dermatologic Allergy.* Ed. by Criep, L. H. Saunders, Philadelphia 1967, p. 428
40. Delamater, E. D. and Benham, R. W.: *J. invest. Derm.* **1**, 451 (1938).
40a. Delanas, G., Vatopoulou, Th., Fotopoulou, A. and Anagnostopoulou, M.: *Acta microbiol. Hellen.* **19**, 246 (1974).
41. Desai, S. C.: In *Essays on Tropical Dermatology.* Ed. by Simons, R. D. G. and Marshall, J. Excerpta Medica Foundation, Amsterdam 1969, p. 226.
41a. Diamond, R. D. and Bennett, J. E.: *J. infect. Dis.* **127**, 694 (1973).
42. Dokudovszky, E. G.: *Veterinariya* **39**, 32 (1962).
43. Dostrovsky, A., Kallner, G., Raubitschek, F. and Sagner, F.: *J. invest. Derm.* **24**, 195 (1955).
44. Drouhet, E.: **35**, *Antonie v. Leeuwenhoek* **35**, Suppl. E-15 (1969).
45. Drouhet, E.: *Arch. roum. Path. exp. Microbiol.* **30**, 65 (1971).
46. Dupperat, B., Lamberton, J. N., Lemonnier, J. V. and Barrade, A.: *Bull. Soc. franç. Derm. Syph.* **63**, 271 (1966).
46a. Eleuterio, M. K., Grappal, C. A. and Blank, F.: *Dermatologica* **147**, 255 (1973).
46b. Elinov, N. P., Kashkina, M. A., Kashkin, A. P. and Iljina, V. P.: *Mykosen* **18**, 407 (1975).
47. Emmons, C. W., Binford, C. H. and Utz, J. P.: *Medical Mycology.* Lea and Febiger, Philadelphia 1970, p. 64.

48. Escande, J. P.: *Presse méd.* **76,** 888 (1968).
49. Ewans, E. E.: *J. Immunol.* **64,** 423 (1950).
50. Fegeler, F.: *Mykosen* **2,** 26 (1958).
50a. Feigin, D., Shackelford, P. G., Eisen, S., Spitter, L. E., Pickering, L. K. and Anderson, D. C.: *Pediatrics* **53,** 63 (1974).
51a. Feinberg, S. M.: *Allergy in Practice.* Year Book Publ., Chicago 1946, p. 356.
51b. ibid., p. 431.
52a. Fejér, E.: *Orv. Hetil.* **91,** 404 (1950).
52b. id., *Bőrgyógy. vener. Szle.* **27,** 48 (1951).
52c. ibid., **27,** 48 (1951).
52d. ibid., **27,** 82 (1951).
52e. ibid., **29,** 13 (1953).
52f. ibid., **31,** 149 (1955).
52g. id., In *Orvosi Mykológia (Medical Mycology).* Ed. by Fejér, E., Oláh, D., Szathmáry, S., Szodoray, L. and Úri, J. (in Hungarian). Akadémiai Kiadó, Budapest 1957, p. 562.
52h. id., *Acta allerg. (Kbh.)* **13,** 427 **(1959)**.
52i. id., In *Allergie und allergische Erkrankungen.* Vol. II. Ed. by E. Rajka, Akadémiai Kiadó, Budapest 1959, p. 551.
52j. id., *Bőrgyógy. vener. Szle.* **37,** 283 (1961).
52k. id., *XIII. Internat. Kongr. Dermat. München. 1967.* Vol. II. Springer, Berlin 1968, p. 867.
52l. id., *Bőrgyógy. vener. Szle.* **47,** 113 (1971).
53. Fischer, E.: *Arch. klin. exp. Derm.* **203,** 270 (1956).
54. Florey, H. W. et al.: *Antibiotics.* Oxford University Press, London 1949, p. 676.
55a. Flórián, E. and Nemeséri, L.: *Magy. Állatorv. Lap.* **15,** 4 (1960).
55b. ibid., **19,** 519 (1964).
56. Flórián, E. and Török, I.: *Derm.-vener. Halad.* **15,** 217 (1971).
57. Folb, P. I. and Trounce J. R.: *Lancet* **ii,** 2112 (1970).
58. Friedrich, E.: *Z. Immun. Forsch. Allergie u. klin. Immunol.* **130,** 373 (1966).
58a. Friedrich, E. and Hollmann, I.: *Mykosen* **18,** 135 (1975).
59. Frisk, A. and Wasserman, J.: *Antonie v. Leeuwenhoek* **35,** Suppl. E-13 (1969).
60. Fukazawa, Y., Shinoda, T. and Tsuchiya, T.: *J. Bact.* **95,** 754 (1968).
61a. Gadebusch, H. H.: *Proc. Soc. exp. Biol. (N. Y.)* **98,** 611 (1958).
61b. id., *J. infect. Dis.* **102,** 219 (1958).
62. Gaudibert, R.: *Rev. franç. Allerg.* **12,** 21 (1972).
63. Geck, P. and Novák, E. K.: *Acta microbiol. Acad. Sci. hung.* **14,** 13 (1967).
64. Goodman, J. S., Kaufman, L. and Koenig, M. G.: *New Engl. J. Med.* **285,** 434 (1971).
65. Gordon, M. A.: cit. by Louria, D. B.: *New Engl. J. Med.* **277,** 1065 (1967).
66. Gordon, M. A., Elliott, J. C. and Hawkins, T. W.: *Sabouraudia* **5,** 323 (1967).
67. Götz, H. and Heitman: cited by *Münch. med. Wschr.* **110,** 2553 (1968).
68a. Götz, H. and Thies, W.: *Derm. Wschr.* **124,** 1193 (1951).
68b. id., *Arch. Derm. Syph. (Berl.)* **194,** 91 (1952).
69. Graffenfried, C. V.: *Derm. Wschr.* **66,** 361 (1918).
70. Grappel, S. F. and Blank, F.: *Dermatologica (Basel)* **145,** 245 (1972).
71. Grappel, S. F., Blank, F. and Bishop, C. T.: *J. Bact.* **93,** 1001 (1967).
72. Greenbaum, S. A.: *Arch. Derm. Syph. (Chic.)* **10,** 279 (1924).
72a. Grob, P. J. and Wuethrich, B.: *J. Obstet. Gynec. Brit. Cwlth.* **81,** 812 (1974).
73. Gróf, P.: *Bőrgyógy. vener. Szle.* **28,** 56 (1952).
74. Hajós, K., Pethő, M. and Pogány, I.: *Orv. Hetil.* **93,** 1025 (1952).
75. Halmy, K.: *Bőrgyógy. vener. Szle.* **47,** 75 (1971).
76. Halmy, K.: *Bőrgyógy. vener. Szle.* **49,** 13 (1973).
77. Halmy, K. and Pintye, I.: *Bőrgyógy. vener. Szle.* **44,** 12 (1968).
77a. Hanifin, J. M., Ray, L. F. and Lobitz, W. C., jr.: *Brit. J. Derm.* **90,** 1 (1974).
78. Hansen, K.: In *Allergie.* Ed. by Berger, W. and Hansen, K. Thieme, Stuttgart 1957, p. 122.
79. Hasenclever, H. F.: In *Jadassohn's Handbuch der Haut- und Geschlechtskrankheiten.* Erg.-Werk. Vol. IV/4. Springer, Berlin 1963, p. 694.
80. Hasenclever, H. F. and Mitchell, W. O.: *J. Bact.* **82,** 574 (1961).

81. Heiner, D. C.: *Pediatrics* **22**, 616 (1958).
82. Holman, J. G.: *Arch. Derm. Syph. (Chic.)* **55**, 512 (1947).
83. Holti, G.: In *Symposion on Candida Infections*. Ed. by Winner, H. I. and Hurley, Rosalinde. Livingstone, Edinburgh 1966, p. 73.
83*a*. Hopfer, R. L., Grappel, S. F. and Blank, F.: *Dermatologica (Basel)* **151**, 135 (1975).
84. Ito, K.: *Mykosen* **1**, 50 (1957).
85. Ito, K. and Kirita, K.: In *Jadassohn's Handbuch der Haut- und Geschlechtskrankheiten*. Erg.-Werk. Vol. IV/3. Springer, Berlin 1962, p. 124.
86. Ito, K., Kuroda, T. and Inoue, T.: *Bull. Pharm. Res. Inst.* **13**, 1 (1957).
87. Ito, K. and Nishitari, N.: *Bull. Pharm. Res. Inst.* **35**, 13 (1961).
88. Ito, Y.: *J. invest. Derm.* **45**, 285 (1965).
89. Ivády, Gy. and Dósa, A.: *Ann. paediat. (Basel)* **189**, 177 (1957).
90. Iwata, K. and Uchida, K.: *Antonie v. Leeuwenhoek* **35**, Suppl. E 39–40 (1969).
91. Jadassohn, J.: *Korresp.-Bl. schweiz. Ärz.* **42**, 24 (1912).
92. Jadassohn, W. and Suter, M.: *Acta allerg. (Kbh.)* **4**, 150 (1951).
93*a*. Janke, S.: *Z. Haut- u. Geschl.-Kr.* **12**, 172 (1952).
93*b*. id., *Derm. Wschr.* **125**, 526 (1952).
93*c*. id., *Hautarzt* **4**, 387 (1953).
93*d*. id.. *Z. Haut- u. Geschl.-Kr.* **14**, 35 (1953).
94. Janke, D. and Roos, G.: *Z. Haut- u. Geschl.-Kr.* **19**, 105 (1955).
95. Janke, R. G.: *Z. Haut- u. Geschl.-Kr.* **15**, 320 (1953).
96. Jelinov, N. P. and Zaikina, N. A.: *Zh. Mikrobiol. (Mosk.)* **30**, 42 (1958).
97. Jillson, O. F., and Hoekelman, R. A.: *Arch. Derm. Syph. (Chic.)* **66**, 738 (1952).
98. Jillson, O. F. and Huppert, M.: *J. invest. Derm.* **12**, 179 (1949).
99. Johansson, S. G. O.: *Proc. Roy. Acad.* **62**, 971 (1969).
99*a*. Jones, H. E., Reinhardt, J. H. and Rinaldi, M. G.: *Arch. Derm. (Chic.)* **110**, 369 (1974).
100. Kabe, J., Aoki, Y., Ishizaki, T., Miyamoto, T., Nakazawa, H. and Tomaru, M.: *Amer. Rev. resp. Dis.* **104**, 348 (1971).
101*a*. Kaden, R.: *Mykosen* **1**, 1 (1957).
101*b*. id., *Arch. klin. exp. Derm.* **211**, 323 (1960).
102. Kaplan, W. and Kaufman, L.: *Sabouraudia* **1**, 137 (1961).
103. Kärcher, K. H.: *Arch. klin. exp. Derm.* **202**, 424 (1956).
104. Kashkin, P. N.: *Medical Mycology* (in Russian). Medgiz, Leningrad 1962, p. 208.
105. Kashkin, P. N., Kokusina, T. M. and Szilujanova, N. A.: *Serological Diagnosis of Mycotic Infections* (in Russian). Medgiz, Leningrad 1959, p. 3.
106. Kashkin, P. N., Krasilnikov, N. N. and Nekasalov, V. Y.: *Mycopathologia (Den Haag)* **14**, 173 (1961).
107. Kaufman, L.: *Mycopathologia (Den Haag)* **26**, 257 (1965).
108. Keeney, E. L. and Huppert, M.: *J. invest. Derm.* **32**, 73 (1959).
109. Kenedy, D.: *Bőrgyógy. Urol. Vener. Szle. Kozmet. (Budapest)* **21**, 59 (1943.
110. Kielstein, P. and Richter, W.: *Arch. exp. Vet. Med.* **24**, 1205 (1970).
111. Kirkpatrick, C. H., Chandler, J. W. and Schmike, R. N.: *Clin. exp. Immunol.* **5**, 375 (1970).
112. Kirkpatrick, C. H., Rich, R. R. and Graw, R. G., jr.: *Clin. exp. Immunol.* **9**, 733 (1961).
113. Kligman, A. M. and Delamater, E. D.: *Ann. Rev. Microbiol.* **4**, 283 (1950).
114*a*. Kogoj, F.: *Arch. Derm. Syph. (Berl.)* **150**, 333 (1926).
114*b*. ibid., **154**, 463 (1938).
115. Korossy, S., Doroszlay, J. and Munkácsi, Á.: *Bőrgyógy. vener. Szle.* **45**, 50 (1969).
116. Korossy, S., Doroszlay, J., Munkácsi, Á., Gombás, Zs. and Dömötör, A.: *Bőrgyógy. vener. Szle.* **47**, 3 (1971).
117. Korossy, S. and Vincze, E.: *Bőrgyógy. vener. Szle.* **45**, 254 (1969).
118. Kozinn, P. J., Taschdjian, C. L., Seelig, M. S., Leona, C. and Teitler, A.: *Sabouraudia* **7**, 98 (1969).
119. Kulaga, V. V.: *Vestn. Derm. Vener. (Mosk.)* **7**, 42 (1966).
120. Kuroda, K.: *Bull. Pharm. Res. Inst.* **15**, 5 (1958).
121. Kuroda, K. and Ohashi, C.: *Bull. Pharm. Res. Inst.* **37**, 4 (1962).
122. Kuroda, T.: In *Jadassohn's Handbuch der Haut- und Geschlechtskrankheiten* Erg.-Werk. Vol. IV/4. Springer, Berlin 1963, p. 712.
122*a*. Kühn, G.: *Derm. Mschr.* **162**, 168 (1976).

123. Kvachevskaya, A.: *Vestn. Derm. Vener.* (*Mosk.*) **38/10**, 44 (1964).
124. Laczkó, L.: In *Asthma, Ekzema.* Ed. by Hajós, K. and Rajka, E. Eggenberger, Budapest 1944, p. 559.
125. Laskownicka, Z., Porebska, A. and Zemburova, K.: *Mycopathologia* (*Den Haag*) **33**, 10 (1967).
126. Lehan, P. H. and Furcolow, M. L.: *J. chron. Dis.* **5**, 489 (1957).
127. Lehner, I.: *Bőrgyógy. Urol. Vener. Szle. Kozmet.* (*Budapest*) **21**, 49 (1943).
128. Lehner, T.: *J. Path. Bact.* **91**, 97 (1966).
129. Lesznyikov, E. P.: *Vestn. Derm. Vener.* (*Mosk.*) **38/11**, 36 (1964)
130. Levine, H. B., Cobb, J. M. and Smith, C. E.: *J. Immunol.* **85**, 218 (1961).
131. Lewis, G. M., Hopper, M. E., Wilson, J. W. and Plunkett O. A.: *An Introduction to Medical Mycology.* Year Book Publishers, Chicago 1958, p. 227.
131a. Lischka, G. and Bonatz, G.: *Z. Hautkr.* **50**, 853 (1975).
131b. Longbottom, J. L., Brighton, W. D., Edge, G. and Pepys, J.: *Clin. Allergy* **6**, 41 (1976).
132. Lorincz, A. L., Priestley, J. O. and Jacob, P. H.: *J. invest. Derm.* **31**, 15 (1958).
133. Louria, D. B.: *New Engl. J. Med.* **277**, 1126 (1967).
134. Louria, D. B. and Brayton, R. G.: *Nature* **20**, 309 (1964).
135. Louria, D. B. and Kaminski, T.: *Sabouraudia* **4**, 80 (1965).
136. Louria, D. B., Kaminski, T. and Finkel, G. J.: *J. exp. Med.* **117**, 509 (1963).
137. Louria, D. B., Smith, J. K., Brayton, R. G. and Marga, B.: *J. infect. Dis.* **125**, 102 (1972).
137a. Luster, M. I., Leslie, G. A. and Bardana, E. J., jr.: *Int. Arch. Allergy* **50**, 212 (1976).
138. Maibach, H. I. and Kligman, A. M.: *Arch. Derm.* (*Chic.*) **85**, 233 (1962).
139. Mariani, G.: *G. ital. Mal. vener.* **64**, 587 (1923).
140. Markert, H. J.: *Münch. med. Wschr.* **68**, 1288 (1921).
141. McMillen, S.: *Abstr. V. Kongr. Soc. Intern. Myc. Paris* 1971, p. 262.
142. McMillen, S. and Devroe, S.: *Amer. Rev. resp. Dis.* **87**, 438 (1963).
143. Melczer, M.: *Orv. Lapja* **4**, 1365 (1948).
144. Meyer, N.: *Amer. J. med. Sci.* **202**, 822 (1941).
145. Miescher, G.: In *Jadassohn's Handbuch der Haut- und Geschlechtskrankheiten.* Vol. XI. Springer, Berlin 1928, p. 378.
146. Miller, H. E., Stewart, R. A. and Kimura, P.: *Arch. Derm. Syph.* (*Chic.*) **44**, 801 (1941).
147. Montes, L. F., Cebullos, R., Cooper, M. D., Bradley, M. N. and Bockman, D. E.: *J. amer. med. Ass.* **222**, 1619 (1972).
148. Müller, H. L.: *Klin. Wschr.* **50**, 809 (1972).
148a. Müller, H. L. and Holtmannspötter, H.: *Mykosen* **18**, 91 (1975).
149. Müller, H. L. and Kranenberg, K.: *Mycopathologia* (*Den Haag*) **38**, 57 (1968).
150. Negroni, R.: *Mycopathologia* (*Den Haag*) **38**, 189 (1969). .
151. Neill, J. M., Sugg, J. Y. and McCauley, D. W.: *Proc. Soc. exp. Biol.* (*N. Y.*) **77**, 775 (1951).
152. Neisser, A.: *Arch. Derm. Syph.* (*Wien*) **60**, 63 (1902).
153. Neuber, E.: *Klin. Wschr.* **19**, 736 (1940).
154. Newberry, W. M., jr., Chandler, J. W., jr., Chin, T. D. Y. and Kirkpatrick, C. H.: *J. Immunol.* **100**, 436 (1968).
155. Newcomer, V. D., Landau, J. W., Lehman, R., Dabrova, N. and Fujiwara, A.: *Arch. Derm.* (*Chic.*) **93**, 149 (1966).
156. Nowakowski, T., Lewandowska, J. and Sielicka, B.: In *Diagnostik und Therapie der Pilzkrankheiten und neuere Erkenntnisse in der Biochemie der pathogenen Pilze.* Ed. by Götz, H. and Rieth, H. Grosse Verlag, Berlin 1970, p. 79.
157. Ogasawara, K., Yamamoto, N. and Kato, N.: *Rev. Allergy* **12**, 464 (1958).
158. Okudaira, M.: In *Essays on Tropical Dermatology.* Ed. by Simons, R. D. G. and Marshall, J. Excerpta Medica Foundation, Amsterdam 1969, p. 226.
158a. Opeitz, G.: *J. infect. Dis.* **132**, 250 (1975).
159. Paldrok, H.: *Arch. klin. exp. Derm.* **227**, 290 (1966).
160. Pappagianis, D.: *Abstr. V. Kongr. Soc. Intern. Myc. Paris* 1971, p. 260.
161. Pappagianis, D., Lindsey, N. J., Smith, C. E. and Salto, M. T.: *Proc. Soc. exp. Biol.* (*N. Y.*) **118**, 118 (1965).

162. Parish, W. E. and Rhodes, E. L.: *Brit. J. Derm.* **79**, 131 (1967).
162a. Patterson, R. and Roberts, M.: *Int. Arch. Allergy* **46**, 150 (1974).
163a. Peck, S. M.: *Klin. Wschr.* **8**, 1357 (1929).
163b. id., *Arch. Derm. Syph. (Chic.)* **22**, 40 (1930).
163c. id., *J. Allergy* **11**, 309 (1940).
163d. id., *Ann. N. Y. Acad. Sci.* **50**, 1362 (1950).
164. Peck, S. M., Bergamini, R., Kelcec, L. C., and Rein, Ch. R.: *J. invest. Derm.* **25**, 301 (1955).
165. Peck, S. M. and Hevitt, W. L.: *Publ. Hlth. Rep. (Wash.)* **60**, 148 (1945).
166. Peck, S. M., Rosenfeld, H. and Glick, A. W.: *Arch. Derm. Syph. (Chic.)* **42, 426** (1940).
167. Pepys, J., Riddel, R. W., Citron, K. M., Clayton, Y. M. and Short, E. I.: In *Jadassohn's Handbuch der Haut- und Geschlechtskrankheiten.* Erg.-Werk. Vol. IV/4. Springer, Berlin, 1963, p. 716.
168. Pepys, J., Riddel, R. W. and Clayton, Y. M.: *Nature* **184**, 1328 (1959).
169. Petrozzi, J. W. and Witkowski, J. A.: *Arch. Derm. (Chic.)* **103, 442** (1971).
170. Plato: Cited by 152.
171. Plötz, C. and Sichert, H.: *Zbl. inn. Med.* **19**, 308 (1964).
172. Pólay, A., Dobozy, A., Hunyadi, J. and Simon, M.: *Bőrgyógy. vener. Szle.* **47**, 141 (1971).
173. Polemann, G.: *Klinik und Therapie der Pilzkrankheiten.* Thieme, Stuttgart 1961, p. 121.
174. Pospišil, L.: *Dermatologica (Basel)* **118**, 65 (1959).
175. Pospišil, L. and Vlašin, Z.: *Dermatologica (Basel)* **120**, 223 (1960).
176. Pöhler, H.: *Derm. Mschr.* **159**, 103 (1973).
176a. ibid., **162**, 104 (1976).
177. Prochacki, H., Cykalewicz, H. and Zielinski, T.: *Mykosen* **14**, 469 (1971).
178. Procknov, J. J., Connely, A. P., jr. and Ray, C. C.: *Arch. Path.* **73**, 313 (1962).
179a. Rajka, E.: *Derm. Wschr.* **76**, 574 (1923).
179b. id., *Bőrgyógy. Urol. Vener. Szle. Kozmet. (Budapest)* **21**, 58 (1943).
179c. id., In *Asthma, Ekzema.* Ed. by Hajós, K. and Rajka, E. Eggenberger, Budapest 1944, p. 45.
179d. id., *Acta derm.-venereol. (Stockh.)* **28**, 585 (1948).
179e. id., *Bőrgyógy. vener. Szle.* **30**, 51 (1954).
180. Rajka, E., Korossy, S. and Gózony, M.: *Dermatologica (Basel)* **107**, 38 (1953).
181. Rajka, G.: *Acta derm.-venerol. (Stockh.)* **43**, Suppl. 54, 11 (1963).
182. Rapaport, F. T., Lawrence, H. S., Millar, J. W., Pappagianis, D. and Smith, C. E.: *J. Immunol.* **84**, 358 (1960).
183. Reiss, F. and Graham, J. B.: *J. invest. Derm.* **7**, 127 (1946).
184. Rimbaud, P., Rioux, J. A. and Bastide, J. M.: *Bull. soc. franç. Derm. Syph.* **67**, 673 (1960).
185. Rimbaud, P., Rioux, J. A., Duntze, F. and Bastide, J. M.: *Bull. Soc. franç. Derm. Syph.* **67**, 689 (1960).
186. Rivalier, E.: In Desaux, A. et al.: *Affection de la Chevelure et du Cuir Chevelue.* Masson, Paris 1953, p. 571.
187. Robbins, W. J., Hervey, A., Davidson, R. W. and Robbins, W. C.: *Bull. Torrey Bot. Club* **72**, 165 (1945).
188. Roberts, G. D. and Larsh, H. W.: *Amer. J. clin. Path.* **56**, 597 (1971).
189. Roth, F. J., Boyd, C. C., Sagami, S. and Blank, H.: *J. invest. Derm.* **35**, 549 (1959).
190. Saeves, I.: *Arch. Derm. Syph. (Wien)* **121**, 161 (1915).
191. Saito, N.: *Jap. J. Derm. Ser. B* **81**, 477 (1971).
192. Saltarelli, C. G.: *Mycopathologia (Den Haag)* **34**, 225 (1968).
193. Sawaki, Y., Huppert, M., Bailey, J. W. and Yagi, Y.: *J. Bact.* **91**, 422 (1966).
194. Schabinski, G.: In *Jadassohn's Handbuch der Haut- und Geschlechtskrankheiten.* Erg.-Werk. Vol. IV/4. Springer, Berlin 1963, p. 694.
195. Schirren, C.: In *Krankheiten durch Schimmelpilze bei Mensch und Tier.* Ed. by Grimmer, H. and Rieth, H. Springer, Berlin 1965, p. 16.
196. Schulkind, M. L., Adler III, W. H., Altemeier III, W. A. and Ayoub, E. M.: *Cell Immun.* **3**, 606 (1972).

196a. Scillian, J. J., Cozard, G. C. and Spencer, H. D.: *Infection Immunity* **10,** 705 (1974).
197a. Seeliger, H. P. R.: *Z. ges. Hyg.* **141,** 110 (1955).
197b. id., In *Jadassohn's Handbuch der Haut- und Geschlechtskrankheiten.* Erg.-Werk. Vol. IV/4. Springer, Berlin 1963, p. 676.
197c. id., *Arch. Hyg. (Berl.)* **151,** 509 (1967).
197d. id., *Mykosen* **12,** 49 (1969).
198. Seeliger, H. P. R. and Christ, P.: *Mykosen* **1,** 88 (1958).
199. Seeliger, H. P. R. and Matheis, H.: *Dtsch. med. Wschr.* **93,** 542 (1968).
199a. Seeliger, H. P. R., Tomšíková, A. and Török, I.: *Mykosen* **18,** 51 (1975).
199b. ibid., **18,** 119 (1975).
199c. ibid., **18,** 149 (1975).
199d. Segal, E., Vardinon, N., Schwartz, J. and Eylan, E.: *Acta allergol.* **30,** 1 (1975).
200. Shelley, W. B. and Florence, R.: *Arch. Derm. Syph. (Chic.)* **83,** 549 (1961).
201. Šikl, D., Masler, K., Bauer, Š., Šandula, J. Tomšiková, A. and Zavázal, V.: *Z. Immun.-Forsch.* **138,** 207 (1969).
202. Sipos, K.: *Derm.-vener. Halad.* **2,** 69 (1955).
203. Sipos, K. and Zlatarov, St.: *Bőrgyógy. vener. Szle.* **31,** 194 (1955).
204. Smith, D. T.: *Ann. intern. Med.* **31,** 463 (1949).
205. Stallybrass, F. C.: *J. Path. Bact.* **87,** 89 (1964).
206. Stanley, V. C., Hurley, R. and Carroll, C. J.: *J. med. Microbiol.* **5,** 313 (1972).
207. Steigleder, G. K.: *Hautarzt* **4,** 35 (1953).
208. Stein, R. O.: *Arch. Derm. Syph. (Berl.)* **132,** 294 (1921).
208a. Stevens, D. A.: *Derm. News* **8**/6, 1 (1975).
209. Stewart-Tull, D. E. S., Timperley, W. R. and Horne, C. H. W.: *Sabouraudia* **5,** 104 (1966).
210. Stikle, D., Kaufman, L., Blumer, S. O. and McLaughlin, D. W.: *Appl. Microbiol.* **23,** 490 (1972)
211. Strom van Leeuwen, W.: *Allergische Krankheiten.* Springer, Berlin 1928, p. 57.
212. Stuka, A. S. and Burell, R.: *J. Bact.* **94,** 914 (1967).
213a. Sulzberger, M. B.: *Arch. Derm. Soph. (Chic.)* **18,** 891 (1928).
213b. id., *J. Immunol.* **27,** 73 (1932).
213c. id., *J. Allergy* **7,** 385 (1936).
213d. id., *Arch. Derm. Syph. (Chic.)* **33,** 374 (1936).
214. Sulzberger, M. B. and Lewis, G. M.: *Arch. Derm. Syph. (Chic.)* **22,** 410 (1930).
215. Summers, D. F., Grollman, A. P. and Hasenclever, H. F.: *J. Immunol.* **92,** 491 (1964).
216. Szádeczky, L. and Heszler, E.: *Bőrgyógy. vener. Szle.* **44,** 257 (1968).
217. Sadokova, E. A. and Kvachevskaya, A. I.: *Zh. Mikrobiol. (Mosk.)* **8,** 147 (1965).
218a. Szodoray, L.: *Bőrgyógy. Urol. Vener. Szle. Kozmet. (Budapest)* **22,** 1 (1944).
218b. id., *Mykosen* **10,** 19 (1967).
218c. id., *Orv. Hetil.* **109,** 617 (1968).
218d. Tagani, H., Watanabe, Sh. and Ofuji: *J. invest. Derm.* **61,** 237 (1973).
218e. Tager, A., Lass, N., Avigad, J. and Beemer, A. M.: *Dermatologica* **147,** 123 (1973).
219. Taschdjian, C. L., Dobkin, G. B., Leona C. and Kozinn, P. J.: *Sabouraudia* **3,** 129 (1964).
220. Taschdjian, C. L., Kozinn, P. J. and Leona, C.: *Sabouraudia* **3,** 312 (1964).
220a. Tausch, I., Böhme, H., Barthelmes, H. and Krolikowski, M.: *Derm. Mschr.* **162,** 143 (1976).
221. Thompson, K. W. I.: *Ing. Clin.* **2,** 156 (1941).
222. Tomomatsu, S.: *Bull. Pharm. Res. Inst.* **35,** 1 (1961).
223. Tomšiková, A. and Novačková, D.: *Z. Immunforsch. Allergie u. klin. Immunol.* **130,** 155 (1966).
223a. id., *Mykosen* **19,** 41 (1976).
224. Tomšiková, A. and Seeliger, H. P. R.: *Mykosen* **12,** 195 (1969).
225. Tomšiková, A., Sikl, D., Masler, L. and Bauer, S.: *Antonie v. Leeuwenhoek* **35,** Suppl. E 5–6 (1969).
226. Török, I.: *Bőrgyógy. vener. Szle.* **46,** 252 (1970).
226a. id., *Bőrgyógy. vener. Szle.* **52,** 38 (1976).
227. Török, I. and Flórián, W.: *Bőrgyógy. vener. Szle.* **49,** 8 (1973).

228. id., *Mykosen* **16**, 29 (1973).
229. Török, L.: In *Asthma, Ekzema*. Ed. by Hajós, K. and Rajka, E. Eggenberger, Budapest 1944, p. 550.
230. Tsuchiya, T., Fukazawa, Y. and Kawakita, S.: *Mycopathologia (Den Haag)* **10**, 191 (1959).
231. Úri, J.: In *Orvosi Mykológia (Medical Mycology)*. Ed. by Fejér, E., Oláh, D., Szathmáry, S., Szodoray, L. and Úri, J. Akadémiai Kiadó, Budapest 1957, p. 898.
232. Úri, J., Juhász, P. and Csobán, G.: *Pharmazie* **10**, 709 (1955).
233a. Vanbreuseghem, R.: In *Precis de Mycologie*. Ed. by Langerson, M. and Vanbreuseghem, R. Masson, Paris 1952, p. 576.
233b. id., In *Orvosi Mykológia (Medical Mycology)*. Ed. by Fejér, E., Oláh, D., Szathmáry, S., Szodoray, L. and Úri, J. Akadémiai Kiadó, Budapest 1957, p. 595.
233c. Vardinon, N., Segal, E., Schwartz, J. and Eylan, E.: *Acta allergol.* **30**, 120 (1975).
234. Vogel, R. A., Sellers, T. F. and Woodward, P.: *J. Amer. med. Ass.* **178**, 921 (1961).
235. Waldbott, G. L. and Ascher, M. S.: *Arch. Derm. Syph. (Chic.)* **36**, 314 (1937).
236. Wallraff, E. B. and Wachs, E. E.: *Amer. J. clin. Path.* **55**, 418 (1971).
236a. Walters, B. A. J., Chick, J. E. D. and Halliday, W. J.: *Int. Arch. Allergy* **46**, 849 (1974).
237. Walzer, R. A. and Einbinder, J.: *J. invest. Derm.* **39**, 165 (1962).
238. Watanabe, S.: *Acta derm.-venerol. (Stockh.)* **53**, 21 (1958).
238a. Wells, R. S., Higgs, J. M., MacDonald, A., Valdimersson, H. and Holt, P. J. L.: *J. med. Genet.* **9**, 302 (1972).
239. Wharton, M. L., Reiss, F. and Wharton, D. R. A.: *J. invest. Derm.* **14**, 291 (1950).
240. Wiedmann, A.: *Zbl. Haut- u. Geschl.-Kr.* **78**, 389 (1952).
241. Wilson, D. E., Bennett, J. E. and Bailey, J. W.: *Proc. Soc. exp. Biol. (N. Y.)* **127**, 820 (1968).
242. Wilson, W. J.: *Clinical and Immunologic Aspects of Fungous Diseases*. Thomas, Springfield 1957, p. 98.
243. Winner, H. I.: cit. by Lehner, T.: *J. Path. Bact.* **91**, 97 (1966).
244. Wirchow, Chr.: *Dtsch. med. Wschr.* **94**, 2508 (1969).
245. Young, C. J., Shackleford, P. O., Lamb, J. H. and Koons, R. C.: *Mycopathologia (Den Haag)* **6**, 235 (1952).
246. Zaslov, L. and Derbes, V. J.: *Derm. int.* **8**, 1 (1969).

CHAPTER 76

IMMUNOALLERGOLOGIC ASPECTS OF GONORRHOEA

by

K. KIRÁLY

Abbreviations used in the text

CF   C fixation
FA   fluorescent antibody
IFA   indirect fluorescent antibody

INTRODUCTION

Gonorrhoea is an inflammatory disease of the mucous membranes, glands and sinuses of the genital organs caused by *N. gonorrhoeae* and transmitted mainly sexually [43]. It may be localized in the rectum and very occasionally in the pharynx. Non-sexual transmission may result in ophthalmia neonatorum, conjunctivitis or, in young girls, vulvovaginitis. Septic complications affecting skin, joints and other internal organs are infrequent.

With the advent of antibiotics and sulphonamides the epidemiologic and clinical pattern of gonorrhoea has radically changed. Formerly a disease of low socio-economic position, it now occurs in both rich and poor. The shorter course of the disease now seen in males and antibiotic treatment have practically eliminated the infection of the posterior urethra, with complications such as prostatic abscesses, epydidimitis and urethral strictures seen in chronic stages of the disease. The natural course of gonorrhoea is unknown; the defence mechanism of the organism has only recently been studied with modern methods of immunology.

The introduction of penicillin resulted in a rapid diminution in the number of cases of gonorrhoea after the Second World War and it was hoped that the disease might be eliminated as a public health problem. This optimistic attitude led to a lessening of interest in certain basic medico-biological aspects of gonorrhoea. Since the mid-fifties a world-wide recrudenscence of the disease has been observed and today gonorrhoea is one of the commonest communicable diseases in the world. Modern society is facing now an endemic situation which cannot be controlled by the treatment schedules and epidemiological methods available no matter how efficient they may be. This review embraces our piecemeal knowledge of the host-parasite interrelationship in gonorrhoea, concentrating on the first strategic goal of up-to-date research, the development of a reliable serological screening method for the detection of asymptomatic carriers.

ANTIGENIC COMPOSITION OF GONOCOCCI

COLONIAL VARIATION

Much of the immunological research undertaken in the past has been hampered by biochemical and morphological changes taking place on subculturing of gonococci on artificial media. Certain morphological [109] and accompanying antigenic changes were noted long ago [20]. S and R colonial variants are mentioned in handbooks [116]. Colonial differentiation between virulent (1 and 2) and non-virulent (3 and 4) types of gonococci, however, was first recognized in 1963 by Kellogg et al. [50]. Types 1 and 2 grow in primary cultures from acute infections, whereas types 3 and 4 arise on subculturing. Association of colonial types 1 and 2 with acute human infection was confirmed in 1967 [96] while types 3 and 4 are held to be non-virulent degenerated gonococci which predominate in laboratory stock strains. The existence of the four different characteristic types of gonococcal colony, their association with virulence [44] and an additional fifth colony variant have been described and analysed [91]. Type 1 was not detectable in old laboratory strains, while a low percentage (0.01−0.1) of type 2 has been found in some laboratory strains of recent origin. Very rarely, the entire population of organisms, cultured from urethral male exudate was colony type 3, when the infection had been of two to three weeks' duration [50]. Jephcott and Reyn [44] found type 1 colonies in one of twenty old laboratory cultures and significant numbers of type 1 and 2 colonies in another old culture.

The varied appearances of the different colonies (when viewed with a stereomicroscope with oblique substage illumination) resulted from the ways in which each type reflected and refracted transmitted light [91]. Type 1 and 2 colonies are small (0.5 and 0.4 mm). They form markedly rough suspensions in saline. The colonies of type 3–5 are larger (1 to 2 mm) and flatter. Type 3 and 5 colonies are of granular appearance with flat edges. Type 4 colonies are non-granular and almost colourless. Types 3 and 4 are easily emulsified and they form smooth suspensions in saline.

It is claimed [48] that the virulence of gonococci of types 1 and 2 can be maintained on artificial media as evidenced by human inoculation: thus the first requirement for rational biochemical work endeavouring to define the antigenic structure of gonococci appears to have been fulfilled. The virulent cell types, if not maintained by selective subculturing, are in *in vitro* cultures quickly overgrown by the avirulent cell type occurring as mutants with an established frequency.

Recently, inter-cellular fibrils (pili) were detected in colony types 1 and 2. They were present only in small numbers, if at all, in the great majority of gonococci in other colony types [45, 98]. This is so far the only visible difference in the ultrastructure between virulent and non-virulent gonococci.

ULTRASTRUCTURE

The ultrastructure of gonococci is similar to other Gram-negative bacteria. The following structures can be recognized in the logarithmic phase of growth: (*i*) a 7.5–8.0 nm thick triple layered wavy membrane, as the outer part of the cell wall. Beneath the membrane a very thin, dense and taut line (the mucopeptide layer) is observed which at intervals is apposed to the inner leaflet of that membrane together with which it constitutes the cell wall. (*ii*) A three-layered cytoplasmic membrane of the same thickness as the wavy part of the cell wall. (*iii*) Inside the cells the nuclear regions appear as light irregular patches within which the electrodense DNS filaments can be seen. (*iv*) Ribosomes are seen as small dark spots. (*v*) Mesosomes appear as intrusions of the cytoplasmic membrane [90, 92]. On negative staining, freeze-cleavage and freeze-etching the outer membrane of the cell wall seems to be composed of round to hexagonal subunits, 8.0 nm in diameter. The membrane is also punctuated by 8.0 nm holes [97a].

Electron-microscopic study of negatively stained specimens revealed that pili (fimbriae) with a diameter of approximately 8.5 nm and a length of up to 4 μm were present on the surface of all type 1 and type 2 gonococci examined and were not seen on any type 3 or 4 gonococci [98]. In the negatively stained preparations, pili radiate from the surface of gonococci, in the freeze-etched preparation they appear to adhere to the surface of microbes [97a]. The lack of pili on the avirulent colony types suggests a possible connection of pili with the pathogenicity of the organism in anchoring it to the urinary epithelium [97b]. In other facultatively pathogenic Neisseria strains, e.g. in *N. catarrhalis*, *N. subflava*, *N. perflava*, short thin filaments (fimbriae) are seen radiating and originating possibly from the outer surface of the wall [118].

Gonococci disposed extracellularly in urethral secretions of patients display many globular and elongated structures around them, which disappear on attachment to the epithelial cell. Gonococci are seized by pseudopods and vacuoles appear in their neighbourhood in the cytoplasm [107a]. Inside the phagosomes of the leukocytes the gonococci may undergo lysis. The lysis in phagosomes is well discernable after antibiotic treatment [80].

ANTIGEN PREPARATIONS

Many Gram-negative bacteria, among them gonococci, contain in their cell walls complex antigens composed of carbohydrate, lipid and a protein or polypeptide-like material. Each of the three components is associated with biological properties. The carbohydrate determines the somatic 'O' antigen specificity, the lipid is implicated in the endotoxic activity and the protein is important for the immunogenic properties. The interest in the deeper layers, consisting of the murein layer and of the cell membrane is limited because the immunity in infectious diseases is mainly related to the more superficial antigens. Systematic, combined electron-microscopic, chemical and immunological approach has only recently been applied to *N. gonorrhoeae*. In the past only a few attempts were made to produce a chemically well-defined antigen from gonococci. Casper [12] isolated a type-specific polysaccharide which gave delayed-type skin reactions in patients with gonorrhoea. This antigen seems now to have been a highly degraded polysaccharide derived from the endotoxin.

Although the study of surface cell wall antigens and serological typing commenced in 1906 [8], the situation even now is not clear and no generally accepted classification of gonococci has been achieved. This is due to the rapid change of the gonococci after isolation from pathogenic material. As gonococci alter their colonial morphology on subculturing, there is an essential change in their antigenic structure, too. Laboratory strains were studied in cross-absorption experiments using agglutination [54, 117], C fixation [89a, b] and immunofluorescence [19f, 23a, 60a]. The existence of at least 8 separate antigens was shown by Wilson [117], four of them were species-specific, the rest were group-specific and were shared by other Neisseria. In subcultures these antigens may disappear, then later reappear again [116]. Recently Hutchinson [42] typed gonococci isolated according to Lancefield's technique into 5 groups. About one-fourth of the strains showed several specificities.

Wilson [117] observed first that freshly isolated gonococci were frequently inagglutinable in immune sera raised by laboratory strains. Later, using immunofluorescent techniques, Deacon [23a] observed that strains freshly isolated from acute cases of gonorrhoea possess an antigen (K) which was preserved by formalin fixation, but destroyed by autoclaving at 120 °C. When grown on artificial media, the K antigen is lost. Since the virulence of meningococci is believed to depend partly upon the antiphagocytic properties of its polysaccharidal capsule, the search for a similar virulence factor in *N. gonorrhoea* was readily at hand. However, Kraus [cited by 33] was unable to demonstrate clear cut capsules by staining methods and failed to isolate polysaccharide antigens from cultures of different colony types of gonococci. It may depend, however, on the culture medium; the gonococcus does produce polysaccharides in a complex medium containing protein hydrolysate [47b]. The labile K antigen has been questioned by other investigators, especially to the stainability of *N. gonorrhoeae* (after subculturing) in the 'delayed' FA test [60a, 79]. Based on recent findings this antigen may be identical with the pili from the surface of the cells in colony type 1 and 2. Buchanan et al. [10] sheared the pili from the surface of gonococci colony type 2. Examined under the electron microscope, the antigen consisted only of pili. In polyacrylamide gel electrophoresis the cleaved preparation has shown a single major peak consisting of proteins with a molecular weight of approximately 24,000. A pilus is a polymer of these protein sub-units with a molecular weight of 20 million as calculated from its dimensions, periodicity and sub-unit size. Immune serum raised in rabbits with purified pili and conjugated with fluorescein isothiocyanate stained the surface of gonococci from colony types 1 and 2 only but not that of several non-pilated strains. The immune serum did not cross-react with other pilated Neisseria strains and seemed to be strictly specific for gonococci. Eighteen pilated gonococcal cultures reacted with the immune serum, i.e. the antigen seems to be representative of different strains of gonococci [11].

The cell membrane antigen of gonococci has hardly been studied. By means of a Ribi cell fractionator Kellogg et al. [52] produced a mixture of protoplasm and cell particulate. The particulate fraction was separated in sucrose solutions resulting in the detection of objects identified as cell walls and 'plasts'. By electron microscopy the latter were shown to consist of spatially oriented granules surrounded by a membrane-like structure only. Cell wall structures were not observed with these 'plasts'. Rabbit anti-cell-wall sera (produced against sonically treated purified cell walls) reacted quantitatively differently with cell walls and 'plasts', but sera from patients with and without gonorrhoea reacted with the cell wall and 'plast' antigen in the same titre.

Disruption of gonococci to obtain 'soluble' or protoplasmic extracts of gonococci has been accomplished by various procedures including ultrasonic disintegration, freeze-thawing, shaking with glass beads and Ribi cell fractionation. The 'soluble' fraction obtained after treatment with the Ribi cell fractionator was also referred to as protoplasm, the 'insoluble' sediment, separated by centrifugation was also referred to as cell wall [71]. The distinction between soluble and insoluble fraction is, however, dubious: precursors of cell wall, capsular material and finely particulate cell wall fragments appear undoubtedly in the so-called protoplasmic fraction. A cell-wall-type antigen and a protoplasmic-type antigen have in fact been separated from virulent gonococci by pressure fractionation and gel filtration techniques [21]. The protoplasmic antigen was soluble, of high molecular weight and was split into five subfractions. The extract and the subfractions were examined by agar gel diffusion with immune sera. The 'same' antigen was produced more rapidly and in a purer form by means of ion-exchange chromatography on DEAE Sephadex A25 [93]. Earlier, in immunodiffusion several protoplasmic antigens have been shown [19f], part of which is shared with meningococci or other Neisseria [19d, e, 61]. Danielsson et al. [21] isolated by gel filtration on a Sephadex G-200 column two fractions of the soluble protoplasmic extract, which reacted with the sera of patients with gonorrhoea both in CF and agar-gel diffusion. Using the protoplasmic antigen Danielsson et al. [22] found that some patients' sera gave a positive reaction only with antigen isolated from their own gonococcal strain, indicating again the importance of strain specificity of protoplasmic antigen.

A polyvalent whole cell antigen was found superior to a monovalent antigen in CF with sera from patients with gonorrhoea. Immunoelectrophoresis experiments with the supernatant from a sonicated whole cell preparation against patients' sera resulted in several precipitation lines. Precipitations were also demonstrated in 14 per cent of blood donors' sera [22].

Another approach was that of Geizer, who used a precipitation technique in an attempt to type laboratory strains [29].

ENDOTOXIN

Endotoxins, generally produced by Gram-negative bacteria, are responsible for harmful effects in many diseases. Recently a review concerning endotoxins was published by Lüderitz, Staub and Westphal [63]. Endotoxins are composed of lipid, carbohydrate and a protein or peptide component.

Killed or living pathogenic and avirulent (laboratory) strains of gonococci are equally toxic: they induce inflammation of the mucous membranes (urethritis, conjunctivitis) or if injected intracutaneously, an inflammatory papule. If a suspension of gonococci is injected into the skin of animals, it will produce inflammation; if it is injected in the peritoneal cavity, necrosis, fever, splenomegaly and degeneration of the parenchymatous organs will ensue; after huge doses the animals even die of shock. The toxic component has been shown to be an endotoxin, which is probably responsible for the most important clinical symptom of gonorrhoea, the acute inflammation. Efforts have been made to isolate and study the endotoxin with the aim of developing a vaccine and a reliable antigen for serological screening of asymptomatic carriers. The toxicity of the isolated preparations can be measured by Shwartzman reaction in rabbits and pathologic changes in chick embryo. The animals develop a haemorrhagic inflammation of the skin at the site of the preparatory intracutaneous injection of endotoxin followed by an eliciting intravenous injection 24 hours later [64b].

The endotoxin is derived from the cell wall [64a] and endotoxin preparations may be used for serotyping of strains [64g]. Possibly two endotoxins are present in gonococci: one in the cell wall and another in the protoplasm. The protoplasmic endotoxin must have a chemical composition different from that in the cell wall because it is soluble in the aqueous phase of phenol extract, but it might be a precursor of the cell wall endotoxin [83]. L forms of gonococci have recently been grown from urethral discharge of males [32] and from the synovial effusion of a patient [41]. This is interesting because of the defective cell walls of L forms when presumably the protoplasmic endotoxin is responsible for the inflammation.

Endotoxin can be extracted from the cells in phenol-water [36], aqueous ether [64d], trichloroacetic acid [5] and alkali [14] and purified by precipitation with acetone. It can also be precipitated from the autolysate of broth cultures with ammonium sulphate and ethanol [114]. The physicochemical, biological and immunological properties of the preparations depend on the method used [64c].

Chanarin [14] extracted two antigen components from the S variant of gonococci by alkaline hydrolysis of the microbes followed by ethanol precipitation. These antigens were probably of polysaccharidal nature. Chanarin suggested that the two antigen components formed a complex antigen on the surface of gonococcus. The first component sensitized red blood cells as shown by a C mediated haemolysis test in the presence of specific immune sera. The second component was detected by its ability to fix complement in the presence of immune serum. Based on the first component, the strains examined could be classified into types 1 and 2. The type 1 antigen was present in meningococci and in a single strain of non-pathogenic Neisseria. The sensitizing component disappeared from the strains after several transfers which resulted in R transformation.

The endotoxin prepared by Tauber and Garson [100] with phenol-water was a lipopolysaccharide with a 22 per cent amino acid content. The amino acids presumably bind the lipids, sugars and amino sugars to a macromolecule [101].

Preparations extracted by other methods all contain protein(s): e.g. the endotoxin extracted with aqueous ether contained nearly 90 per cent protein [64e]. The majority of data regarding the chemical composition of the endotoxin were gained by immunochemical methods using mainly passive haemagglutination technique. The endotoxin is readily absorbed to the surface of formalinized or tanned red blood cells. It was stable at 100 °C for 30 minutes. Immunization of rabbits with erythrocytes sensitized with the endotoxin gave rise to antibodies which could be detected by passive haemagglutination and haemolysis, C fixation, agglutination of gonococci and precipitation reactions [64f]. The antigenic composition of the endotoxin depended upon the method of preparation. In the purified phenol-water extract a single antigenic specificity of polysaccharide nature was present which could be destroyed by periodate oxidation [64b]. The extracts prepared by other methods contained another determinant most likely of polypeptide nature which could be split by pronase digestion [64f]. The polypeptide (b) was a group antigen shared by gonococci and meningococci, but not by other species of Neisseria [64g]. The polysaccharide component (a) had at least 6 different antigenic determinants (a_1-a_6) which were distributed widely among different strains of gonococci. All strains contained however, a factor a_1 and at least one more factor. Part of the polysaccharide antigenic specificity is present in meningococci and non-pathogenic Neisseria [64g]. It was shown recently [65] that endotoxin prepared by phenol-water extraction in comparison with the ether-water extract was predominantly of polysaccharide (a) specificity; the b antigenic determinant was not present in all preparations. The antigenic determinant factors were carried by the polysaccharide molecular complex as in the endotoxins prepared by aqueous ether [66].

Using an indirect haemagglutination technique, Maeland et al. examined the sensitizing effect of saline extracts of gonococci with a view to establishing the relationship between the antigens in these extracts with that in the endotoxin complex. The authors concluded that 'more information is needed' [68].

A toxic lipopolysaccharide was isolated by Nair and Chacko [74] from the amniotic fluid of chicken embryos infected with gonococci by precipitation with ethanol and acetic acid. This antigen had a determinant in common with lipopolysaccharide from meningococci as shown by means of a microprecipitation technique using sera from patients with gonorrhoea and meningococcal meningitis. The lipopolysaccharide prepared from N. catarrhalis did not react with these sera. The antigen was supposed to possess a new determinant which was not present on the surface of laboratory strains [75].

VIRULENCE

The virulence of gonococci has been reviewed by Kellogg and Thayer [51]. Until recently, the experimental production of gonorrhoea in man has been successful only when discharge from patients infected with gonorrhoea was transferred directly to human recipients [38, 70]. Even under these circumstances, not all attempts were successful. Lack of transmissibility by means of discharge or in vitro isolates was ascribed to lack of proper physiologic circumstances, to the presence of immune substances detrimental to the gonococcus, or to the use of avirulent laboratory strains.

In 1963 and 1968 Kellogg et al. [48, 50] inoculated male volunteers intra-urethrally with cells from type 1 colonies of the gonococcus strain F62. Colonial type 1 cells retained their virulence during *in vitro* cultivation for 35 months, or approximately 700 selective laboratory transfers without passage through human tissues. The colonial morphology-virulence relationship was apparently a stable one. The individual patients did not respond to the same infecting strain in a uniform way. The amount and character of exudate varied from negligible and watery to voluminous and purulent. This indicated that the response was more a characteristic of the host than of the strain. The dose of type 1 organism needed to set up infection was about 1.5×10^{10} microbes [119a]. This must be greatly in excess of the infecting dose in naturally acquired infection. The volunteers responded with demonstrable antibody production, which was detected by micro-precipitation and indirect FA techniques, within one to four days post-inoculation. Inoculation with one of the two virulent types resulted in a selection for the alternate virulent type over the original type inoculated as seen by the change in colony types. This change indicates a host-controlled mechanism possibly involving the physicochemical character of the surface of the cells. Those volunteers who received avirulent organisms developed a transient tenderness of inguinal lymph nodes not seen with those who received virulent cells.

The surfaces of avirulent and virulent organisms are different, as indicated by their colony morphology, the increased saline auto-agglutinability and presence of pili on their surface when virulent. The presence of pili (fimbriae) suggests a possible mechanism for attaching to the surface of mucous membranes. This possibility was studied recently by Ward and Watt [107a]. Scrapings of the urethra of male patients with acute gonorrhoea were examined under the electron microscope. Gonococci were attached to the surface of epithelial cells as well as to mucus secreting cells with the membrane of the host cells raised up to surround the base of the organism. Gonococci were deeply embedded within the epithelial cell cytoplasm. This fact excludes a random association of cells and bacteria. No pili could be seen at the magnification used by the authors. Gonococci with pili have a much greater adhesiveness to human fibroblasts than non-pilated mutants of the same strain [31]. Attachment of gonococci to human amnion cells in tissue culture is facilitated as shown by light and electron microscopy if the gonococci bear pili. Pilated colony type 2 gonococci associated with the amnion cells incubated *in vitro* as compared with the non-pilated colony type 4 microorganisms [97b]. A scanning electron-microscopic study of human fallopian tubes maintained in an organ bath during perfusion with pilated gonococci has revealed organisms apparently anchored to the epithelial surface by their pili [107b]. Recently it was reported that the colonial varieties of *N. gonorrhoeae* that are associated with virulence (types 1 and 2) were more resistant to phago-cytosis by rabbit exudating polymorphonuclear leukocytes than colonial types of less virulence, i.e. types 3 and 4. Type 1 gonococci were resistant, and type 4 gonococci susceptible, to phagocytosis by human polymorphonuclear leukocytes. Phagocytosis of both types 1 and 4 gonococci by rabbit and human leukocytes was bactericidal, but rabbit leukocytes were superior to human leukocytes in killing gonococci [102].

Another possible explanation for the enhanced pathogenicity of gonococci to humans might be that man lacks some defence system that is responsible for the destruction of gonococci in immune species. It has been claimed that gonococci survive and even multiply in human leukocytes [95]. This is supported by the everyday observation that in stained smears gonococci inside the leukocytes appear morphologically intact. It was shown, however, in *in vitro* experiments that gonococci were destroyed by leukocytic lysosomes or if engulfed by leukocytes [110]. Less than one per cent of gonococci phagocytosed by guinea pig polymorphs survived after 100 minutes, whereas about twenty per cent of gonococci associated with the human polymorphs were not killed even after three hours. The persisting gonococci were destroyed when the polymorphs were exposed to penicillin, and this indicates that the surviving bacteria lay outside the membrane of the polymorphs. The ultrastructural damage to gonococci in phagosomes of polymorphonuclear leukocytes has been demonstrated using the electron microscope [106]. Both these observations indicate that virulent gonococci are not resistant to destruction by leukocytes of the host. Another explanation must be sought for the high susceptibility of man to gonococcal infection.

Gonococci growing *in vivo* are resistant to killing by serum. A new antigen is present on their surface which confers resistance to natural antibodies and C. In most strains this factor is lost in subculture *in vitro* [108]. This antigen can be sustained in strains grown on media containing prostate extract [111]. Though the virulence of gonococci is not completely elucidated, presumably the presence of pili and an antigenic component present only *in vivo* are decisive factors in this context.

PATHOGENICITY OF GONOCOCCI FOR ANIMALS

N. gonorrhoeae is a human parasite which, under natural circumstances, does not multiply either on the mucous membranes or in the tissues of animals. It provokes temporary inflammation at the site of infection and causes lethal endotoxic shock of the animal in excessive doses. The mechanism which makes the urogenital tract of animals resistant is obscure. Obviously it is not a humoral mechanism. A number of investigators have tried to establish animal infection without success having used guinea pigs treated with methotrexate, neonatally thymectomized mice, and germ-free mice [77]. Recently male chimpanzees have been infected with human urethral discharge containing *N. gonorrhoeae*. A typical gonococcal urethritis developed. The infection was also transferred from chimpanzee to chimpanzee [62]. It was even possible to infect a male chimpanzee with *N. gonorrhoeae* colony types 1 and 2 transferred selectively *in vitro*. The infection was venereally transmitted to the female cagemate. The male showed only a slight urethral discharge and the female remained symptomless [7]. The need remains for a model infection in a small laboratory animal that is more widely available, less expensive and more easy to handle. Mice have been infected intraperitoneally with a mixture of suspension of gonococci and mucin [72], or intracerebrally [26]. Arko [1] used subcutaneous implantation of hollow subcutaneous chambers in the dorsolumbar region of rabbits and guinea pigs with the subsequent infection of these chambers. The fluid in these chambers remained positive for *N. gonorrhoeae* for more than 9 months with a massive gonococcal infiltration of the biopsy specimen of the tissue surrounding the chambers. This artificial model may prove useful in the study of the host-parasite interaction as regards the kinetics of antibody formation. Chorioallantoic membranes of chick embryos have been used to differentiate between virulent and laboratory strains of gonococci. Infection of the chorioallantoic membrane and the chorio-allantoic fluid was produced significantly more often (69 per cent) when cells from type 1 and 2 colonies were inoculated, than when using comparable numbers of cells from type 3 and 4 colonies (11 per cent) [9].

Different techniques for the study of the protective effect of human and animal immune sera have been developed. Gonococci were able to multiply and remained pathogenic after several passages on chick embryos. Non-pathogenic laboratory strains recover virulence after chick embryo passage [104]. Bang [3] claims that cellular changes (focal necrosis of epithelium and leukocytic infiltration) on the chorioallantoic membrane of chick embryo resemble those seen in man more closely than those found in any other animal model. Therefore this technique should fit for the study of virulence and the protective effect of immune sera. Diena et al. [27] developed a tissue culture model using monkey kidney (RE_2) cells. If sera obtained from vaccinated animals and humans contained protective antibodies, the tissue cells were not destroyed by a suspension of gonococci [35].

ANTIBODIES

NATURAL ANTIBODIES

Antibodies which are commonly found in the sera of 'normal' individuals and which are not related to obvious immunization or clinical infection, may be called natural antibodies [57].

Gonococci are killed by the active serum of several animals [116]. The gono-coccidal activity of animal serum is C dependent and can be destroyed by inacti-vation at 56 °C [57]. Active normal human serum is likewise gonococcidal; heat inactivation considerably diminishes its gonococcidal potency [76]. Most people have serum antibodies capable of mediating complement killing of cultured gonococci. By means of the killing effect of both normal and immune human sera, Glynn and Ward [30] were able to divide gonococcal strains into four main types. The antigens involved in the bactericidal reaction seem to be lipopolysaccharides.

Laboratory strains with pili are liable also to the C killing [102]. However, gonococci isolated from gonorrhoeal discharge [108] or those cultivated on media containing prostatic extract [111] did not succumb in the presence of normal or immune serum and C. This seems to suggest that the virulence of gonococci may be related not only to the pili but also to the composition of the bacterial surface.

The immunochemical characterization of these vexing natural antibodies giving false positive results was studied by Cohen [16] who used the indirect fluorescent antibody (IFA) procedure. The natural antibodies of the IgG, IgA and IgM classes react mostly with heat-stable somatic antigens. Immune IgG antibodies were distinguishable from natural IgG antibodies by their ability to recognize heat-labile surface antigens, whereas IgM antibodies from both infected and normal individuals appeared to react with heat-labile antibodies. Immune IgG antibodies were more resistant to heating than were natural antibodies. Their distribution according to immunoglobulin classes varies with the method used [18, 67]. In IFA experiments with monospecific conjugates the natural antibodies seem to belong mostly to the IgG and to a lesser extent to the IgM class of immunoglobulins [16]. Antibodies of the IgG class can even be found in the sera of newborns [18]. In the indirect haemagglutination test using red blood cells sensitized with endotoxin, they seem to belong exclusively to the IgM class, as shown by the inhibition of the agglutination after mercaptoethanol treatment of the sera [67]. The cause of this divergence may be the higher sensitivity of IgM antibodies, as compared with IgG molecules in haemagglutination.

Presumably, natural antibodies are provoked by infections with other Neisseria sharing antigenic components with gonococci. The bactericidal antibodies may be absorbed from normal human sera with various other Neisseria strains [30].

IMMUNOCHEMISTRY OF SPECIFIC ANTIBODY RESPONSE

Though in uncomplicated cases the clinical manifestations of gonorrhoea are largely confined to the mucosal surface of the body, systemic antibody response is often stimulated by the infection. When complications are present a higher percentage of sera are reactive attaining 95 per cent in patients with gonococcal septicaemia [22].

Distribution of antibodies according to immunoglobulin classes during the infection has been studied by the IFA technique with the use of monospecific conjugates [17]. Sequential antibody studies of experimentally infected males have revealed that serum antibodies appear in most instances within 1 to 3 weeks of infection. Antibodies can be found in all Ig classes. In contrast to natural antibodies, those contained in the serum of gonorrhoea patients, except antibodies of the IgA class, react mostly with the thermolabile surface antigen. This difference in preferential antigenic stimulation has clearly been shown when the serum antibody response was examined serially [17] in experimentally infected male volunteers. Nine of the ten patients developed a fourfold increase in reactivity with IgG antibodies to the heat-labile surface antigens. Fewer patients showed increased IgM or IgA reactivity to heat-labile antigens. Heat-stable 'somatic' antigens, in contrast, induced only the production of IgA class antibodies. In the other immunoglobulin classes no increase could be observed. The decline of antibody titre takes place slowly over a period of weeks or months. As shown in another study by mercaptoethanol treatment [67], only one-third of patients with gonorrhoea developed IgG class antibodies against the a and b determinant of aqueous ether endotoxin in the haemagglutination test. With most patient sera the titres of the IgM antibodies were comparable to the titres of normal sera.

Antibodies against gonococci have been demonstrated in vaginal washings [39]. These antibodies belong to the IgA class and they appear promptly after infection and disappear soon after treatment. They seem to show an anamnestic response to a second infection [78]. There is an increase in the number of IgA producing plasma cells in the mucosa of the cervix [15]. Preliminary work has also shown that IgA antibodies are present in urethral secretions of males with gonorrhoea [46]. The bulk of the IgA present was of secretory type. The immune response seems to start locally, since in half of the patients no serum IgA-type antibodies could be found. The secretory IgA system is operative in the local immune response. Interestingly there is no correlation between previous infections and the local IgA level.

CELL-MEDIATED IMMUNE RESPONSE

Cell-mediated immune response seems to play an important role in the natural course of gonorrhoea. The predominance of lymphocytes in the discharge of patients with chronic gonorrhoea, the spontaneous cure of untreated male patients, the lessening of acute urethritis during a complicating epydidimitis, the good therapeutic effect of vaccines given locally to females para-urethrally and into the cervical tissue [53] are all long-forgotten old clinical experiences which may be explained now through terms of cell-mediated immunity. However, studies to pinpoint and analyse the role of cell-mediated immunity in gonorrhoea are extremely scanty. Cellular antibody response as detected by lymphocyte transformation has been shown recently in males with gonorrhoea [55]. A crude sonicated suspension of the F62 virulent colony type 1 gonococci was used as antigen. As the 9–10 days' interval between infection and treatment is too short to evoke delayed hypersensitivity, no significant difference was observed between the controls and the patients with only one infection. A significantly greater degree of transformation occurred in patients with several infections. Possibly cross-reactions between *N. gonorrhoeae* and other Neisseria may account for the high degree of transformation observed in two non-gonorrhoeal subjects. It was stated that females with gonococcal complications did not show a greater degree of transformation than asymptomatic carriers [77].

SEROLOGICAL TESTS FOR THE DETECTION OF GONORRHOEA

As gonococci can be readily cultured, serology is not needed so much as a diagnostic test as for epidemiological screening in the detection of inapparent infection. Asymptomatic females may often harbour gonococci. As reliable diagnosis in women depends on cultures at least from the cervix and rectum, much time and money must be spent when screening low prevalence groups. The present strategy of gonococcal immunological research is to find a simple serological screening procedure sensitive enough to detect a significant percentage of infected females in a population in which the gonorrhoea incidence is suspected to be high. Afterwards the diagnosis might be confirmed by culture. A variety of serological techniques have been used to achieve this objective including CF and IFA tests, passive haemagglutination, radioimmunoassay and several flocculation procedures. Most workers have used relatively crude antigens (intact or sonicated organisms). As *N. gonorrhoeae* shares antigens with other Neisseria species the problem of false positive reactions is one of the most vexing. Because of lack of

190

information on the gonococcal antigens, a serological test applicable to clinical practice has not yet been developed. Recent research is directed, therefore, to finding a chemically and immunologically homogeneous antigen free from the drawbacks of crude suspension of gonococci.

Using the serological techniques mentioned and using crude antigens, detection of asymptomatic female carriers of gonorrhoea has ranged between 65 and 90 per cent. Infected males, who usually come forward early for treatment, show a reactivity of 30 to 60 per cent. Asymptomatic males, however, would be as important a group to detect as the female carriers. False positive reactions have ranged from 1 to 20 per cent with the higher reactivities generally found in those procedures which are the most sensitive for detecting infected individuals.

The results obtained by a given method depend on several factors, e.g. the reproducibility of the antigen preparations, the prevalence of gonorrhoea in the area and the incidence of other infections giving rise to cross-reactions. In addition, limited numbers of sera are often examined. The number of repeated gonorrhoeal infections may also vary from one place to another.

In order not to waste time with a bad preparation or to discard prematurely a good one, the rational testing would be in two steps; first a qualitative and quantitative pilot assay with a set of problem sera from patients well characterized from the clinical and bacteriological points of view, followed in the second step by a field trial with a careful analysis of the discordances. However, most research workers are apt to embark immediately on a study of venereal clientele using carefully selected 'normal' individuals. Therefore the tests (antigens) proposed generally give excellent results in the hands of the inventor but they are hardly reproducible by other investigators. The present review is restricted to the positivity rates found in problem groups (asymptomatic female carriers, patients with other Neisseria infections) and healthy donors.

COMPLEMENT FIXATION (CF) TECHNIQUE
WITH WHOLE CELL SUSPENSION

CF was proposed in 1906 for the laboratory detection of gonorrhoea [73]. The antigen used was a suspension of apathogenic laboratory strains. With the advent of chemo- and antibiotic therapy and more efficient bacteriological techniques, this method has fallen into disuse. A substantial body of knowledge regarding the dynamics of the immune response of the host was gained, however, through systematic study with the CF reaction. These general rules can be transferred also to other tests. The CF test becomes positive in males 2–3 weeks after infection and once positive, it remains so for several months even after successful treatment. If the antigenic stimulus is weak, e.g. the patient was treated successfully with antibiotics in the first few days after the clinical manifestations, the test remains negative. In asymptomatic females less than 35–40 per cent of the patients have shown positive results. To improve the sensitivity of the test, polyvalent antigens have been used at the Statens Serum Institute in Copenhagen [89d]. Recently Danielsson et al. [22] assessed CF by increasing the representativeness of the antigen by using 6 different strains. A doublefold gain in the detection of asymptomatic females was obtained to the detriment of the specificity. In patients with complications (salpingitis, arthritis, epydidimitis) complement fixing antibodies could be demonstrated in as many as 75 to 80 per cent of the cases [69]. This seems now to be the only indication for the use of CF, since gonorrhoeal complications in the females often remain undiscovered. Since antigenic fractions shared with other Neisseria were present in the antigen, false positive results have been fairly frequent especially in patients suffering from various respiratory disorders. In a study from Greenland, where the prevalence of gonorrhoea is very high, it was found that the incidence of positive CF reactions was about three times as high in patients with bronchitis and/or bronchiectasia as in patients from a surgical ward [56]. CF procedures require much time and skillful technicians; other more rapid techniques are therefore used.

THE INDIRECT FLUORESCENT ANTIBODY (IFA) TECHNIQUE

The use of IFA with sera from patients suspected of having gonorrhoea seems to be a rapid and simple procedure for screening. Intact cells of gonococci which are used as antigen, however, display on their surface a mosaic pattern of antigenic determinants in common with other Neisseria and they react also with sera of some healthy donors. Another difficulty is the rapid change in antigenic structure on subculturing which lessens the reproducibility of the results. The method seemed to be successful in detecting antibodies in the sera from patients with gonococcal arthritis [37]. On the other hand, 64 per cent of sera of meningococcus carriers reacted with gonococci and 38 per cent of those defined as 'free of Neisseria' [82]. A new attempt to improve the IFA procedure was made by O'Reilly et al. [79]. An appropriate gonococcus strain with a broad antigenic representation, reacting with a variety of sera from patients with gonorrhoea and which remains reasonably stable on transfer, was selected. Type 1 cells of this strain (No. 9) did not seem to share antigens with other Neisseria as shown by qualitative absorption experiments. In a pilot study [113] 1 : 16 dilution of sera was adopted as the limit of reactivity. Seventy-nine per cent of culture positive females were reactive, and only 2–4 per cent of sera from culture negative patients were non-specifically positive. Further evaluation is, however, needed using problem sera from, e.g. meningococcus carriers, patients with severe bronchitis and bronchiectasia.

While the choice of method is largely based on practical convenience, an appropriate sensitivity and specificity can only be achieved by the development of suitable antigens. It is the search for these which is now occupying most workers. The review of earlier investigations with crude antigens may be found in handbooks [59]. The present paper deals exclusively with the development of new antigens characterized chemically or morphologically.

TESTS PERFORMED WITH ANTIGENIC FRACTIONS OF GONOCOCCI

Ward and Glynn [105] used *lipopolysaccharide antigen* prepared by the phenol-water method from three different strains of gonococci in the passive haemagglutination reaction. The positivity rate varied between 2 and 10 per cent among controls and between 31 and 60 per cent among patients with gonorrhoea depending on the strains used for the preparation of the antigen. Antigen prepared from a laboratory strain of gonococci showed much less specificity and sensitivity than those prepared from two fresh strains. Presumably, false positive reactions were due to cross-reacting antibodies raised against non-pathogenic Neisseria and other organisms. The rate of false positive reactions was especially high (15–63 per cent) with alkali treated lipopolysaccharide in latex agglutination [112]. A possible explanation for this may be that alkali treatment of lipopolysaccharides removes the sugars and O-acetyl groups reducing its antigenic specificity.

A *lipopolysaccharide antigen* prepared from infected chick embryos [74] seems to be sensitive in the micro-precipitation reaction: being positive in male patients 4–6 days after the onset of the discharge [13]. However, its value was not established in females. Gonococci could only be cultured in 20 of 115 women positive with the precipitation test.

The *antigen* (endotoxin?) *prepared by alkali extraction* according to Chanarin [14] was less useful; haemolysing antibodies against sensitized erythrocytes occurred in 55 per cent of sera from blood donors [64a]. In an automated micro-haemagglutination procedure [61] cells sensitized with a similar alkaline extract reacted at low titres with the sera examined. The specificity of this procedure was essentially superior to that of the haemolysis test (6–10 per cent non-specific positives in healthy females) but its sensitivity with sera from gonorrhoeal females was only 49 per cent. If the sera were absorbed with *N. sicca* cells the sensitivity of the test rose to 88 per cent.

Wallace et al. [103] extracted *glycoprotein* from the phenol phase by mixing equal volumes of bacterial cells and 90 per cent phenol. The phenol phase was treated with acetone and the precipitated antigen preparation was dissolved and used in bentonite flocculation test. The test gave a high positivity rate (77 per cent) with the sera of patients with gonorrhoea but the rate was also high (4–21 per cent) in non-venereal patients. The same method was used by Watt, Ward and Glynn [112] who found it unsuitable for discriminating between patient and control sera. An antigen prepared by a similar method was less sensitive in a microprecipitation test: only 54 per cent of sera from women with gonorrhoea were positive but no false positive results were obtained [87].

Buchanan et al. [10] used *pili* labelled with ^{125}I as antigen in quantitative radio-immunoassay. The amount of antigen bound by 79 per cent of sera from patients with gonorrhoea was higher than the highest amount bound by any of the controls. In a later work [11] comprising a far greater and well grouped patient material of a metropolitan venereal disease clinic, they found an antibody level exceeding the highest value seen in a large control group in 50 per cent of males with acute symptomatic and in 33 per cent of males with oligosymptomatic gonococcal urethritis. In asymptomatically infected females the same figure was 89 per cent. Only three (4 per cent) of 75 meningococcus carriers or patients recovered from meningococcal meningitis had higher antibody levels to pili than the highest value in the control group. Antibody to pili appeared 2–3 weeks after infection and returned to normal level one or more months after treatment. Despite the technical difficulties in the performance of the radioimmunoassay, this method seems to be a very promising tool for diagnosing both symptomatic and asymptomatic gonococcal infections.

Using the *purified protoplasmic antigen* of Danielsson et al. [21] Reising et al. [88] found 72 per cent positivity in CF with the sera of infected women; none of the sera of blood donors was reactive. Twelve per cent of presumably non-infected individuals gave, however, positive results with a sediment of the same antigen in a microflocculation test [58]. By means of CF and using the same method for the preparation of the antigen, Watt et al. [112] obtained the same sensitivity, but as high as 12 per cent reactivity in a healthy control group. This discordance may be explained by the fact that although this antigen appeared to be homogeneous by DEAE Sephadex chromatography, it could be split into several bands by polyacrylamide electrophoresis.

Crude protoplasmic antigen: the soluble supernatant of sonicate of gonococci colony type 1 was used in a microflocculation test after adsorption on lecithin-cholesterol particles [86] and in an automated microhaemagglutination procedure [61]. The microflocculation was positive in 5–7 per cent of presumed normal and 79 per cent of gonorrhoeal female sera. The haemagglutination reaction was reactive with 10–19 per cent of presumed non-gonococcal sera and in only 47 per cent of females with a positive cervical culture to gonococci. If the sera were absorbed with sonicates of *N. sicca* and *flava*, the titres were reduced to one twentieth of the original with an essential improvement of specificity (6–12 per cent reactive in healthy female controls) and sensitivity (76 per cent in females with gonorrhoea).* The protoplasmic antigen as described by Martin et al. [71] was used in an automated CF test [81b]. The test was positive in 80 per cent of sera from infected women and 4 per cent of specimens from presumably non-infected persons.

The results as described with tests using protoplasmic antigens were obtained with sera accumulated in the serum bank of the Communicable Disease Center, Atlanta. When a pilot evaluation was performed with these tests using fresh sera from patients attending a venereal disease clinic in a large metropolitan area, antibodies were detected in a lower percentage of sera (39–63 per cent) from patients actually infected and in a high percentage (13–37 per cent) of sera from culturally negative patients. This conspicuous discrepancy may be due to the lack of knowledge concerning the duration of the present and number of past infections. Fresh sera from celibate nuns and virginal college students has shown a low (5 per cent) degree of reactivity [47a] acceptable for screening.

FLUORESCENT ANTIBODY (FA) TECHNIQUE
FOR THE DETECTION OF GONOCOCCI IN SMEARS

Fluorescent antibody (FA) techniques have been increasingly used for the demonstration of various microorganisms. The insensitivity and lack of specificity of the Gram-stained smears promoted investigators to use fluorescent staining for the detection of gonococci. For example, in females an examination of Gram-stained smears of cervical exudate is 30 to 40 per cent less sensitive than the culture method. Furthermore, if a smear is positive, but the culture is negative, the possibility of false positive results should be considered because saprophytic

---

* The minimum   significant titre after absorption was considered to be 1 : 24.

Neisseria are found in about 3–4 per cent of women not infected with gonorrhoea [115]. Overdecolourization while carrying out Gram staining may cause technical errors. Deacon et al. [24] succeeded in demonstrating gonococci with gonococcus immune serum conjugated with fluorescein iso-thiocyanate in smears prepared from specimens taken from male and female patients suspected of having gonorrhoea. This technique took an hour to perform. The processing of specimens was later somewhat modified. It was demonstrated that the gonococci could be identified when smears of secretion were stained (the 'direct' method) but that positive results were significantly less frequent than with culture. When the cotton swabs with secretion were used to inoculate a culture medium (the 'delayed' FA method) the FA technique on the mixed growth gave more positive results than the conventional culture method. Moreover at least 48 to 72 hours were gained if fermentation tests were included among the criteria for identification of gonococci [25]. The 'delayed' FA method came into use in 1961 when Harris et al. [36] established the presence of gonococci in about 20 per cent of female prisoners who had no symptoms of infection. Results on the 'delayed' FA method published since are either in agreement with the first description, or show a pronounced superiority of the method over culture. This is probably due rather to variation in the quality of the medium and in the technique used in culturing than to variability in the FA method itself, which, of course, is dependent on the medium used. The advantage of the delayed FA over conventional culture depends mainly on its independence from contaminating organisms [89c].

The specificity of both methods depends on the gonococcal immune serum which reacts with N. meningitidis and other non-pathogenic Neisseria [19a, 23b, 60d]. Since the genital organs rarely harbour meningococci, this has no practical importance. Cross-reaction with non-pathogenic Neisseria can be eliminated by the dilution of the conjugate [19e]. More disturbing is the staining of certain strains of Staphylococci. With Staph. aureus the Fc piece of immunoglobulins binds non-specifically to one of their surface antigens called protein A [60c] and Staphylococci react even with normal rabbit sera [60a]. It has been eliminated by mixing of the conjugate with unlabelled normal rabbit serum or with rabbit anti-staphylococcal serum (one step inhibition test) [60a], by absorption of the conjugate with strongly fluorescent strains of Staph. aureus [19b] or by mixing the conjugate with rhodamine-B labelled Staphylococcus immune serum [19c]. When this reagent is used both the background and Staphylococci show an orange-red fluorescence. A reliable method of the preparation of a conjugate was recently described [81a]. Rabbits were immunized with fresh isolates of gonococci colonial type 1. After labelling of the globulin fraction with fluorescein isothiocyanate, the conjugate was absorbed with beef bone marrow and a relatively small amount of N. meningitidis group B. Normal rabbit or anti-staphylococcal antiserum was added to inhibit staphylococcal staining. Only well controlled conjugates may be used for the detection of gonococci.

The 'direct' method has also other drawbacks. If only a few gonococci are present in the smear, it has to be examined for a long time before a negative answer can be given. Therefore the positive results are hardly superior to those with Gram staining [60a] and 7 per cent less than those by cultivation [85]. Other drawbacks of the 'direct' method have been eliminated: cross-reaction of the conjugate with non-pathogenic Neisseria is allegedly eliminated by drying the smears at 45 °C [49] and background fluorescence may be counteracted in various ways (staining of the smears with Amido Schwarz or Flazo Orange or Naphthalene Black). Due to its laboriousness and lack of sensitivity, the 'direct' FA method is now used infrequently if reliable culture methods are available.

However, FA staining of smears of exudate from conjunctiva, joint fluids or skin lesions can be used as an adjunct in the diagnosis of these manifestations of gonorrhoea, particularly when commenced or partial therapy may prevent cultural recovery of organisms. As 'direct' FA staining may show non-viable gonococci, it should not be used as a test of cure. Danielsson and Molin [20] reported finding fluorescing organisms in the prostatic secretion of men 2 to 3 weeks after clinically successful treatment of gonorrhoea. Furthermore, instead of the time-consuming fermentation tests, FA staining may be used for the identification of oxidase positive colonies grown on media and giving positive oxidase reaction, since the reactivity of the antigen with the conjugate remains after treatment with either dimethyl-p-phenylene diamine hydrochloride [84] or with tetramethyl-p-phenylenediamine hydrochloride [60b].

INTRACUTANEOUS TEST

The skin test has no value for the diagnosis of gonorrhoea. Killed gonococci injected intracutaneously to healthy persons provoke an inflammatory reaction which reaches its peak after 24 hours. In patients with chronic or complicated gonorrhoea as well as in rabbits immunized with gonococci, the reaction is more violent and lasts longer, indicating the development of an Arthus or delayed-type reaction. The component causing the inflammation is the endotoxin in which the lipid probably acts as the primary irritant. A carbohydrate responsible for the immunological specificity was isolated by Casper [12]. This antigen gave a delayed-type skin reaction only in patients with chronic gonorrhoea. No systematic studies, however, have been undertaken since to isolate an antigen to be used in a diagnostic skin test for gonorrhoea.

IMMUNE PHENOMENA IN GONORRHOEA

IMMUNOLOGICAL BACKGROUND OF CLINICAL SYMPTOMS

Gonococcal infections are usually limited to the mucosal surfaces and more specifically to those of the genitalia, conjunctiva and rectum; however, various other areas of the body may become involved including the mucous membranes of the upper respiratory tract. Synovia of joints, endocardium, capillaries (septicaemia) may be infected by metastatic spreading from primary gonococcal foci of the urogenitary tract. In males, gonococcal infection usually results in an acute symptomatic urethritis, in females infection usually develops an asymptomatic course. Thus, the clinical manifestation of the virulence of gonococci is apparently modified by the interaction with the host's tissues or secretions. The difference in symptomatology between males and females might result from a different virulence potential for female tissues or from a better local antibody response.

The discharge in acute male gonorrhoea is caused by the patchy destruction of the urethral epithelium with accumulation of gonococci in the subepithelial connective tissues with a violent concomitant inflammation. During the 3–5 days' asymptomatic interval that follows upon exposure, gonococci become established on the urethral mucosa. An attachment of gonococci to the epithelial surface precedes the invasion of the deeper tissues. Through the damaged mucosa gonococci may invade the deeper tissues and enter the circulation. They are, however, trapped by the regional lymph nodes and presumably destroyed by 'natural' and acquired antibodies. Intracutaneous injection of gonococci provokes papules or papulo-pustules and abscesses on the site of injection without septicaemia. Complications observed in gonorrhoea (urethral stricture, chronic salpingitis, chronic pelveoperitonitis) with their lengthy duration and formation of abscess cavities and subsequent fibrosis, suggest that cell-mediated hypersensitivity to gonococci may play a role in the development of these processes; their exact immunological background remains, however, unclarified.

GONOCOCCAL SEPTICAEMIA

Gonococcal septicaemia is usually a relatively mild form of metastatic infection. It is a triad of fever, migratory polyarthritis and skin rash. This syndrome occurring with the recrudescence of gonorrhoea is more frequently seen in women than in men (2.3 and 0.4 per cent, respectively, of patients with gonorrhoea) [4] presumably due to a long asymptomatic carrier state and lack of treatment. The fever is generally intermittent and moderate. Arthritis may affect the large and small joints with or without effusion. The patient may have the symptoms of salpingitis.

The skin lesions begin as pinpoint red spots which may be widely scattered but have a preferential localization on the extremities near the joints. Those on the palms and soles tend to remain macular and purpuric, elsewhere they usually evolve through a papular stage to form vesico-pustules with erythematous bases. *N. gonorrhoeac* can be cultured from the blood in about 25 per cent of cases. The clinical diagnosis is based on urogenital gonorrhoea, fever, arthralgia, the typical vesiculo-pustular or haemorrhagic cutaneous lesions plus a response to penicillin therapy. The condition is often misdiagnosed as rheumatic fever, drug eruption, rheumatoid arthritis, systemic lupus erythematosus, etc.

The underlying immunological mechanism of septicaemia remains obscure. This comparatively mild septicaemia cannot be explained by a deficient immune response. Ninety-five per cent of sera of such patients react in CF and there are more precipitation lines using the protoplasmic extract of gonococci in immuno-electrophoresis with these sera than with others [22]. These data speak in favour of an increased immune response.

The histological picture of skin lesions resembles that found in leukocytoclastic angiitis with thrombi, infiltrated blood vessel walls, predominantly with polymorphonuclear neutrophils, a variable admixture of mononuclear cells and minimal to massive haemorrhages. Gonococci are destroyed rapidly and they can be demonstrated by Gram staining only exceptionally. The presence of their debris may be documented, however, by direct FA techniques [4]. The mechanism probably responsible for the production of the skin lesions is the Shwartzman phenomenon. Gonococci arriving in the small blood vessels are phagocytosed by leukocytes or endothelial cells, the endotoxin is released and prepares the site for further bacterial endotoxin arriving via the blood stream and precipitates the Shwartzman reaction. Possibly the vasculitis affects the renal vessels. In a series of female patients where cutaneous lesions were described, 16 per cent were found to have haematuria [40].

The clinical picture, called *keratosis blenorrhagica* has been believed to be gonococcal in origin. Gonococci occasionally have been found in the urethral discharge, and very rarely in the haemorrhagic pustules [99]. This clinical condition is now considered to be a symptom of Reiter's syndrome. In the cases in which gonococci are isolated one cannot exclude a coexistent infection with Chlamydia or the agent responsible for non-gonococcal urethritis. Reports in the literature, however, mention a more severe type of gonococcal septicaemia with a predominant distribution of the skin rash on the palms, soles and fingertips [99].

CARRIER STATE

About 80 per cent of females and 12–15 per cent of males display very mild or no clinical symptoms. Such cases are discovered through screening or contact tracing by cultivation of gonococci. The underlying immunological mechanism is only a matter of speculation. The attachment of gonococci to mucosal epithelial cells and neutralization of the endotoxin are presumably unrelated. Gonococci can adhere and grow on mucosal epithelial cells of these patients without destruction of epithelial cells and invasion of tissues. It has not been examined whether carriers have a high local secretory antibody level which might neutralize the endotoxin of gonococci. As shown by experimental inoculation of male volunteers [6], gonococci grown from asymptomatic female carriers or present in swabs taken from cleaned cervical canal, have the same virulence as those found in symptomatic patients. The consorts of female carriers display the classical symptoms with heavy discharge. For the women, the carrier state is not without danger, either. According to data from the United States, England, Denmark and Sweden, 6–14 per cent of females attending venereal disease clinics or emergency rooms and having positive cultures for gonococci also have pelvic inflammation. Anyway, the carrier state is of paramount epidemiological importance as these persons make up the unknown reservoir of infection. Undoubtedly they contribute greatly to the present epidemic situation.

GONOCOCCAL VACCINE AND IMMUNOPROPHYLAXIS OF GONORRHOEA

Up to the mid-1930s vaccines in combination with instillations were extensively used for the treatment of gonorrhoea. There was, however, little convincing evidence that the vaccines were of any value in the treatment of the acute phase of the disease. With the introduction of sulphonamides and antibiotics, vaccine treatment of gonorrhoea was abandoned.

One effective means of controlling an infectious disease is by active immunization. It is evident that our present methods for controlling gonorrhoea have failed and that the search for an effective vaccine is long overdue. The only possible vaccine until today is a gonococcal autolysate containing three colony type 1 strains prepared by Greenberg et al. [35]. This material has been injected into healthy human volunteers and it stimulated a serum antibody response as shown in a bentonite flocculation test and in a tissue culture neutralization system: 95 per cent of the volunteers who returned after one year still had a measurable antibody level. A small field trial was performed with this vaccine in Inuvik, Canada [34]. The incidence of gonorrhoea within the first three months following the immunization was, however, about the same in the immunized group (30 per cent) as in the controls (24 per cent). It was stressed by the authors that none of the immunized patients who got gonorrhoea developed protecting antibodies as demonstrated in the tissue culture test. The existence of protecting antibodies was considered as a meaningful indicator of immunity [34].

In view of the failures of immunological treatment in the past, the feasibility at all of immunoprophylaxis in gonorrhoea is questionable. The disease itself does not confer immunity in most instances. An impressive number (20–30 per cent) of infections recorded in statistics at present are repeated infections in the same persons [94]. The number of female repeaters is less than that of males, presumably not because of biological but because of behavioural factors. Many persons have been reported to have the disease ten times or more. There are, however, encouraging arguments in favour of the concept that protective immune mechanisms are operating in gonorrhoea. The most convincing is the natural course of the disease. In the vast majority of cases gonorrhoea remains confined to the mucosal surfaces, not giving metastatic complications. It is self-limiting, with spontaneous cure even if no treatment has been given. Though according to clinical experience previous infections do not protect against a new infection, Mahoney et al. [70] in experimental inoculations in male volunteers have, however, found that 43 per cent of volunteers with no previous history of gonorrhoea were infected, but of those with gonorrhoeal antecedents only 24 per cent were infected. This statistically valid difference indicates that an infection leaves a certain degree of protection though its level and mechanism are at present not clear.

Based on the immunological research one can explain the failure of immunoprophylaxis and construct a programme for the elaboration of an effective vaccine.

1. Due to antibiotic treatment and epidemiological measures the duration of the infection is too short to evoke a meaningful immunity. In acute gonorrhoea of males the level of circulating antibodies is too low to be detected by highly sensitive serological methods. The concentration of the local 'secretory' antibodies on the normal mucosa may be even less.

2. 'Wild' strains of gonococci have a heterogeneous antigenic composition and a previous infection does not necessarily provide immunity against other strains. According to the bactericidal pattern of human sera, the endotoxin composition and the surface antigens there may be at least 4 to 8 serological types of gonococci. Recently gonococci have been characterized by means of their bacteriocins, i.e. lethal factors produced by freshly isolated gonococci against other strains [28]. With a set of six indicator (bacteriocin-sensitive) strains 75 isolates gave thirteen reproducible bacteriocinogenic patterns. Though the nature of bacteriocins as

well as their significance regarding the antigenic structure of gonococci is unknown, the phenomenon suggests a higher variability among gonococcal strains.

3. The pathogenicity of gonococci is a complex phenomenon which can hardly be counteracted by a single antibody.

4. The anchorage of gonococci to the epithelial cells is mediated by their pili and the patchy destruction of epithelial cells and inflammation is provoked by the cell wall endotoxin. The carrier state is a clear clinical indication of the dissociation between the ability of gonococci to survive in the human host and that to provoke an acute inflammation.

5. For the immunity an optimal antibody level is needed to counteract all these phases of attachment and invasion of the human urogenital tract by the gonococci.

6. If the problem of immunity against gonorrhoea is looked upon as a complex scientific programme based on our present sketchy knowledge and oriented towards the solutions of these unknowns, the task of producing a vaccine seems not to be hopeless.

ACKNOWLEDGEMENTS

The author expresses his gratitude to Dr. A. Reyn for her kind help, suggestions and criticism; to Prof. A. Glynn, Drs D. Danielsson, B. Diena, D. Kellogg, J. Maeland, R. Willcox and A. Wilkinson for their critical suggestions in the compilation of the manuscript.

REFERENCES

1. Arko, R. J.: *Science* **177**, 1200 (1972).
2. Atkin, E. E.: *Brit. J. exp. Path.* **6**, 235 (1925).
3. Bang, F.: *J. exp. Med.* **74**, 387 (1941).
4. Barr, J. and Danielsson, D.: *Brit. med. J.* **i**, 482 (1971).
5. Boor, A. K. and Miller, C. P.: *J. infect. Dis.* **75**, 47 (1944).
6. Brown, L., Brown, B. C., Walsh, M. J. and Pirkle, C. I.: *J. Amer. med. Ass.* **186**, 153 (1963).
7. Brown, W. J., Lucas, G. T. and Kuhn, U. S. G.: *Brit. J. vener. Dis.* **48**, 177 (1972).
8. Bruck, C.: *Dtsch. med. Wschr.* **32**, 1368 (1906).
9. Buchanan, T. M. and Gotschlich, E. C.: *J. exp. Med.* **137**, 196 (1973).
10. Buchanan, T. M., Swanson, J. and Gotschlich, E. C.: WHO/VDT/RES/GON/73.72.
11. Buchanan, T. M., Swanson, J., Holmes, K. K., Kraus, S. J. and Gotschlich, E. C.: *J. clin. Invest.* **51**, 53 (1972).
12. Casper, W. A.: *Vener. Dis. Inform.* **22**, 119 (1941).
13. Chacko, C. W. and Nair, G. M.: *Brit. J. vener. Dis.* **45**, 33 (1969).
14. Chanarin, J.: *J. Hyg. (Lond.)* **52**, 425 (1954).
15. Chipperfield, E. J. and Evans, B. A.: *Clin. exp. Immunol.* **11**, 219 (1972).
16. Cohen, I. R.: *J. Bact.* **94**, 141 (1967).
17. Cohen, I. R., Kellogg, D. S. and Norins, L. C.: *Brit. J. vener. Dis.* **45**, 325 (1969).
18. Cohen, I. R. and Norins, L. C.: *J. clin. Invest.* **47**, 1053 (1968).
19a. Danielsson, D.: *Acta derm.-venereol. (Stockh.)* **43**, 451 (1963).
19b. ibid., **45**, 61 (1965).
19c. ibid., **45**, 74 (1965).
19d. id., *Acta path. microbiol. scand.* **64**, 243 (1965).
19e. ibid., **64**, 267 (1965).
19f. id., *The Demonstration of N. gonorrhoea with the Aid of Fluorescent Antibodies.* Acta Universitatis Upsaliensis, No. 24 (1965).

20. Danielsson, D., and Molin, L.: *Acta derm.-venereol. (Stockh.)* **51**, 73 (1971).
21. Danielsson, D., Schmale, J. D., Peacock, W. L. and Thayer, J. D.: *J. Bact.* **97**, 1012 (1969).
22. Danielsson, D., Thyresson, N., Falk, Y. and Barr, J.: *Acta derm.-venereol. (Stockh.)* **52**, 467 (1972).
23a. Deacon, W. E.: *Bull. Wld Hlth Org* **24**, 349 (1961).
23b. id., In *Proceedings of the XII. Intern. Congress of Dermatology, September 1972, Washington D. C.* Vol. 2. Excerpta Medica Foundation, Amsterdam, 1963, p. 921.
24. Deacon, W. E., Peacock, W. L., Freeman, E. M. and Harris, A.: *Proc. Soc. exp. Biol. (N. Y.)* **101**, 322 (1959).
25. Deacon, W. E., Peacock, W. L., Freeman, E. M., Harris, A. and Bunch, W. L.: *Publ. Hlth. Rep. (Wash.)* **75**, 125 (1960).
26. Diena, B. B.: Personal communication (1972).
27. Diena, B. B., Wallace, R., Kenny, P. and Greenberg, L.: *Canad. J. Microb.* **17**, 13 (1971).
28. Flynn, J. and McEntegart, M. G.: *J. clin. Path.* **25**, 60 (1972).
29. Geizer, E.: *An Attempt at Serotyping N. gonorrhoeae.* WHO/VDT/RES/GON/71.59.
30. Glynn, A. A. and Ward, M. E.: *Infection and Immunity* **2**, 162 (1970).
31. Glynn, A. A. and Watt, P. J.: *Annual report to WHO for 1972.*
32. Gnarpe, H., Wallin, J. and Forsgren, A.: *Brit. J. vener. Dis.* **48**, 496 (1972).
33. Gottschlich, E. C.: *Immunochemical composition of gonococci.* Paper delivered at the Annual Meeting of the Amer. Soc. Microbiol. Philadelphia, 1972.
34. Greenberg, L., Diena, B. B., Ashton, F. A., Wallace, R., Kenny, C. P., Znamirowski, R. and Ferrari, H.: *Gonococcal Vaccine Studies in Inuvik.* WHO/VDT/RES/GON/72.68.
35. Greenberg, L., Diena, B. B., Kenny, P. and Znamirowsky, R.: *Bull. Wld Hlth Org.* **45**, 531 (1971).
36. Harris, A., Deacon, W. E., Tiedemann, J. and Peacock, W. E., jr.: *Publ. Hlth. Rep.* **76**, 93 (1961).
37. Hess, E. V., Hunter, D. K. and Ziff, M.: *J. Amer. med. Ass.* **191**, 531 (1965).
38. Hill, J.: *Amer. J. Syph.* **27**, 733 (1943).
39. Hirschberg, N.: *Hlth. Lab. Science* **7**, 84 (1970).
40. Holmes, K. K., Counts, G. W. and Beaty, H. N.: *Ann. intern. Med.* **74**, 979 (1971).
41. Holmes, K. K., Gutman, L. T., Belding, M. E. and Turck, M.: *New Engl. J. Med.* **284**, 318 (1971).
42. Hutchinson, R. I.: *Brit. med. J.* iii, 107 (1970).
43. Jadassohn, J. (Ed.): In *Handbuch der Haut- und Geschlechtskrankheiten.* Vol. XX/1. Springer, Berlin 1934, p. 34.
44. Jephcott, A. E. and Reyn, A.: *Acta path. microbiol. scand.* **79**, 609 (1971).
45. Jephcott, A. E., Reyn, A. and Birch-Anderson, A.: *Acta path. microbiol. scand.* Sect. B **79**, 437 (1971).
46. Kearns, D. H., O'Reilly, R. J., Lee, L. and Welch, R. G.: *J. infect. Dis.* **127**, 99 (1973).
47a. Kellogg, D. S.: *HSMHA Hlth. Rep.* **88**, 13 (1973).
47b. id., Personal communication (1973).
48. Kellogg, D. S., Cohen, I. R., Norins, L. C., Schroeter, A. L. and Reising, G.: *J. Bacteriol.* **96**, 596 (1968).
49. Kellogg, D. S. and Deacon, W. E.: *Proc. Soc. exp. Biol. (N. Y.)* **115**, 963 (1964).
50. Kellogg, D. S., Peacock, W. L., Deacon, W. E., Brown, L. and Pirkle, C. L.: *J. Bacteriol.* **85**, 1274 (1963).
51. Kellogg, D. S. and Thayer, J. D.: *Ann. Rev. Med.* **20**, 323 (1969).
52. Kellogg, D. S., Turner, E. M., Callaway, C., Lee, L. and Martin, J. E.: *Infect. Immun.* **3**, 624 (1971).
53. Király, K.: Unpublished observations (1972).
54. Kovács, E.: Personal communication (1972).
55. Kraus, S. J., Perkins, G. H. and Geller, R. C.: *Infection and Immunity* **2**, 655 (1970).
56. Krebs-Lange, P., Reyn, A., Bentzon, M. W. and Lind, I.: *Ugeskr. Laeg.* **128**, 409 (1966).

57. Landy, M. and Weidanz, W. P.: In *Bacterial Endotoxins*. Ed. by Landy, M. and Brause, N. Inst. of Microbiol. Rutgers University Press, New Brunswick 1963, p. 275.
58. Lee, L. and Schmale, J. D.: *Infection and Immunity* **1**, 207 (1970).
59. Leinbrock, A.: In *Jadassohn's Handbuch der Haut- und Geschlechtskrankheiten*. *Ergänzungswerk*. Ed. by Schuermann, H. and Leinbrock, A. Vol. VI/1. Springer, Berlin 1964, p. 1.
60a. Lind, I.: *Acta path. microbiol. scand.* **70**, 613 (1967).
60b. ibid., **76**, 279 (1969).
60c. ibid., **80**, 281 (1972).
60d. id., In *Proceedings of the Northern Dermatological Society 1952, Lund*. Hakon Ohlsons Biktryckeri, Lund 1963, p. 53.
61. Logan, L. C., Cox, P. M. and Norins, L. C.: *Appl. Microbiol.* **20**, 907 (1970).
62. Lucas, C. T., Chandler, F., Martin, J. E. and Schmale, J. D.: *J. Amer. med. Ass.* **216**, 1612 (1971).
63. Lüderitz, O., Staub, A. M. and Westphal, O.: *Bact. Rev.* **30**, 192 (1966).
64a. Maeland, J. A.: *Acta. path. microbiol. scand.* **67**, 102 (1966).
64b. ibid., **69**, 145 (1967).
64c. ibid., **73**, 413 (1968).
64d. ibid., **76**, 475 (1969).
64e. ibid., **76**, 484 (1969).
64f. ibid., **77**, 495 (1969).
64g. ibid., **77**, 505 (1969).
65. Maeland, J. A. and Kristoffersen, T.: *Acta path. microbiol. scand.* **79**, 226 (1971).
66. Maeland, J. A., Kristoffersen, T. and Hofstad, T.: *Acta path. microbiol. scand.* **79**, 233 (1971).
67. Maeland, J. A. and Larsen, B.: *Brit. J. vener. Dis.* **47**, 269 (1971).
68. Maeland, J. A., Wesenberg, F. and Tönder, O.: *Brit. J. vener. Dis.* **49**, 256 (1973).
69. Magnusson, B. and Kjellander, J.: *Brit. J. vener. Dis.* **41**, 127 (1965).
70. Mahoney, J. F., van Slyke, C. J. Cutler, C. J. and Blum, H. L.: *Amer. J. Syph.* **30**, 1 (1946).
71. Martin, J. E., Peacock, W. L., Reising, G., Kellogg, D. S., Ribi, E. and Thayer, J. D.: *J. Bact.* **97**, 1009 (1969).
72. Miller, C. P.: *Amer. J. Syph.* **28**, 620 (1944).
73. Müller, R. and Oppenheim, M.: *Wien. klin. Wschr.* **19**, 894 (1906).
74. Nair, G. M. and Chacko, C. W.: *Ann. Ind. Acad. Med. Sci.* **2**, 35 (1966).
75. id., *Ind. J. Derm. Vener.* **33**, 53 (1967).
76. Norgaard, O.: *Acta derm.-venereol. (Stockh.)* **29**, 421 (1949).
77. Norins, L. C., and Miller, J. N.: In *Progress in Immunology*. Ed. by Anos, B. Academic Press. New York 1971, p. 1193.
78. O'Reilly, R. J., Lee, L., Welch, B. G., Peacock, W. and Schmale, J.: Paper delivered at the *120th Annual AMA Convention*, (1971).
79. O'Reilly, R. J., Welch, B. G. and Kellogg, D. S.: *J. infect. Dis.* **127**, 77 (1973).
80. Ovcinnikov, N. M. and Delektroskij, V. V.: *Brit. J. vener. Dis.* **47**, 419 (1971).
81a. Peacock, W. L.: *Publ. Hlth. Rep.* **85**, 733 (1970).
81b. id., *HSMHA Hlth. Rep.* **86**, 706 (1971).
82. Peacock, W. L., Martin, J. E., Thayer, J. and Schroeter, A. L.: In *Antimicrobial Agents and Chemotherapy*. Ann Arbor 1964, p. 649.
83. Peacock, W. L. and Schmale, J. D.: *Nature (Lond.)* **221**, 760 (1969).
84. Peacock, W. L., Welch, G., Martin, E., and Thayer, J. D.: *Publ. Hlth. Rep.* *(Wash.)* **83**, 337 (1968).
85. Price, E. V.: Paper delivered at the *14th Annual Symposium on Recent Advances in the Study of Venereal Diseases, Houston*. 1964.
86. Reising, G.: *Appl. Microbiol.* **21**, 852 (1971).
87. Reising, G. and Kellogg. D. S.: *Proc. Soc. exp. Biol. (N. Y.)* **120**, 660 (1965).
88. Reising, G., Schmale, J. D., Danielsson, D. G. and Thayer, J. D.: *Appl. Microbiol.* **18**, 337 (1969).
89a. Reyn, A.: *Acta path. microbiol. scand.* **26**, 234 (1949).
89b. ibid., **26**, 252 (1949).
89c. id., *Bull. Wld Hlth Org.* **40**, 245 (1969).

89d. id., Personal communication (1972).
90. Reyn, A., Birch-Andersen, A. and Berger, U.: *Acta path. microbiol scand.* **78,** 375 (1970).
91. Reyn, A., Jephcott, A. E. and Ravn, H.: *Acta path. microbiol. scand.* **79,** 435 (1971).
92. Reyn, A., Murray, R. G. E. and Birch-Andersen, A.: WHO/VDT/RES/GON.1 (1963).
93. Schmale, J. D., Danielsson, D. G., Smith, J. F., Lee, L. and Peacock, W. L.: *J. Bact.* **99,** 469 (1969).
94. Siboulet, A., Niel, G., Egger, L. Majewasky, E. and Busquet, P. Y.: *Les infections urogenitales gonococciques ; étude clinique, thérapeutique et épidemiologique.* Rapport Annual à l'OMS pour 1972.
95. Smith, H.: *Bact. Rev.* **32,** 164 (1968).
96. Sparling, P. F. and Yobs, A. R.: *J. Bact.* **93,** 513 (1967).
97a. Swanson, J.: *J. exp. Med.* **136,** 1258 (1972).
97b. ibid., **137,** 571 (1973).
98. Swanson, J., Kraus S. J. and Gottschlich, E. C.: *J. exp. Med.* **134,** 886 (1971).
99. Tappeiner, J. and Wodniansky, P.: In *Jadassohn's Handbuch det Haut- und Geschlechtskrankheiten Ergänzungswerk.* Ed. by Schuermann, H. and Leinbrock, A. Vol. VI/1. Springer, Berlin 1964, p. 283.
100. Tauber, H. and Garson, W.: *J. biol. Chem.* **234,** 1391 (1959).
101. Tauber, H. and Russel, R.: *Bull Wld Hlth. Org.* **24,** 385 (1961).
102. Thongthai, C. and Sawyer, W. D.: *Infection and Immunity,* **7,** 373 (1973).
103. Wallace, R., Diena, B. B., Yugi, H. and Greenberg, L.: *Canad. J. Microbiol.* **16,** 655 (1970).
104. Walsh, M. J., Brown, B. C., Brown, L. and Pirkle, C. I.: *J. Bact.* **86,** 478 (1963).
105. Ward, M. E. and Glynn, A. A.: *J. clin. Pathol.* **25,** 56 (1972).
106. Ward, M. E., Glynn, A. A. and Watt, P. J.: *Brit. J. exp. Pathol.* **53,** 289 (1972).
107a. Ward, M. E. and Watt, P. J.: *J. infect. Dis.* **126,** 601 (1972).
107b. id., *Brit. med. J.* i, 485 (1973).
108. Ward, M. E., Watt, P. J. and Glynn, A. A.: *Nature (Lond.)* **227,** 382 (1970).
109. Wassermann, A.: *Z. Hyg. Infekt.-Kr.* **27,** 298 (1898).
110. Watt, P. J.: *J. med. Microbiol.* **3,** 501 (1970).
111. Watt, P. J., Glynn, A. A. and Ward, M. E.: *Nature (Lond.)* **236,** 186 (1972).
112. Watt, P. J., Ward, M. E. and Glynn, A. A.: *Brit. J. vener. Dis.* **47,** 448 (1971).
113. Welch, R. G. and G'Reilly, R. J.: *J. infect. Dis.* **127,** 69 (1973).
114. Werch, S. C.: WHO/VDT/RES/GON/5 — 27 April 1964.
115. Wilkinson, A. E.: *Brit. J. vener. Dis.* **28,** 24 (1952).
116. Wilson, G. S. and Miles, A. A.: *Topley and Wilson's Principles of Bacteriology and Immunity.* Ed. by Wilson, G. S. and Miles, A. A. 5th ed., Vol. I. Arnold, London, 1964, p. 678.
117. Wilson, J. F.: *J. path. Bact.* **72,** 111 (1954).
118. Wistreich, G. A. and Baker, R. F.: *J. gen. Microbiol.* **65,** 167 (1971).
119a. World Health Organization: *Meeting in Neisseria Research.* First Report WHO/VDT/RES/GON/8.65.
119b. id., WHO/VD/MEN/1.65.

CHAPTER 77

IMMUNOALLERGOLOGIC ASPECTS OF CHANCROID

by

K. KIRÁLY

INTRODUCTION

Chancroid is an acute, localized, auto-inoculable, sexually transmitted disease caused by *Haemophilus ducrey* and characterized clinically by painful necrotic ulcerations at the site of the infection. The ulcers generally heal spontaneously, sometimes, however, they erode deeply into the tissues. The genital lesions frequently are accompanied by an inflammatory swelling and suppuration of the regional lymph nodes. After the introduction of sulphonamides and antibiotics the disease had practically disappeared from developed countries. In the rest of the world, especially in tropical countries, it is still endemic. There is a close association between chancroid, poverty and poor standards of hygiene. Under abnormal conditions, such as war, chancroid tends to increase. In white American troops in Korea chancroid was fourteen times as common as syphilis [1]. Like many other venereal diseases, chancroid is a disease of towns.

ANTIGENIC STRUCTURE

H. ducrey is a small, Gram-negative, non-motile, non-spore-forming, aerobic bacillus which requires, for primary isolation, enriched media containing blood or its derivates. In contrast with other species in the *Haemophilus* group, *H. ducrey* needs only the heat stable X factor which was shown to behave like haematin while other species of the group require another growth factor called V as well, replaceable by either coenzyme I or coenzyme II.

The antigenic structure of *H. ducrey* was hardly studied by modern biochemical methods. Suspensions of the microbe grown on blood agar are readily agglutinable by antisera. By this method no antigenic difference could be shown between different isolates. As cultivated strains are non-pathogenic, the antigenic structure

205

undergoes modifications not clarified yet on artificial media. Pathogenicity is studied by intradermal inoculation to rabbits or humans. Rabbit lesions appear to be self-limiting and have shown little or no evidence of tissue invasion. In humans infection can be produced by surface scarification, and tissue invasion is obvious. The infective process in humans and rabbits does not appear to be identical. Cultures showing loss of virulence may regain their original pathogenic properties by passage through fresh blood clots. Stock cultures, however, do not regain their virulence and may be cultivated only in inactivated blood.

A thermostable acid-soluble polysaccharide can be prepared from the culture of the organism, which may be precipitated with sera of chancroid patients and evokes a delayed-type reaction if injected intradermally. Nomura [2] isolated an antigenic mixture composed of polysaccharides and proteins. Measured by the intracutaneous test the mixture appeared to be the most potent antigen. As judged by the fever seen in patients treated with *H. ducrey* vaccines, the existence of a thermostable endotoxin may be presumed.

DIAGNOSTIC TESTS

COMPLEMENT FIXATION TECHNIQUE

Complement fixing antibodies are demonstrable in the sera of the patients with lymphadenopathy. The antibodies persist long after the patient's recovery. The diagnostic value of the antigens depends on the media used for cultivation.

At present the test is not used for diagnostic purposes and no antigen is available.

INTRACUTANEOUS TEST

Two antigens are used: sterilized bubo pus or killed bacterial vaccine (Ito-Reenstierna test). The latter is more suitable for standardization and gives earlier and more clear-cut reactions. Antigens prepared from organisms cultivated in a medium containing rabbit serum instead of whole blood has the advantage of being free of rabbit cell debris. It was not warranted, however, that presence of red cell debris would affect the value of antigens for human use. 0.1 ml of the vaccine is injected intracutaneously. A reaction is positive if an induration of 7 mm diameter appears 48 h afterwards. The reaction becomes positive from 8 to 25 days after the appearance of the ulcer, the average being 12 to 14 days. Hence, when the result is negative, the test should be repeated. The reaction probably remains positive throughout the whole life. A positive reaction permits a diagnosis of present or past infection. The test is of value in mass use in assessing the prevalence of chancroid in the community. A negative reaction may be obtained in the presence of a small and localized lesion. With lymph node involvement the test is invariably positive. False positive reactions are observed in diverse conditions (asthma, moniliasis, trichophytic infections, lymphogranuloma venereum, syphilis) and in an African milieu even in a considerable number of normal population [4]. This co-reaction, however, is not as clear-cut and on repetition is usually negative. This diagnostic method is now generally considered as obsolete and production of the commercial vaccines has ceased.

Auto-inoculation of a drop of pus from the ulcer is a justifiable procedure in dubious cases, regarded as the most certain method of diagnosis. Material obtained from the lesion is rubbed into a scarified area on the thigh. Two or three days later tiny vesicopustules appear at the site of inoculation, which break down to give a typical ulceration. The bacterium can be demonstrated more readily in the auto-inoculated lesion. This method has largely fallen into disuse and is seldom used today.

Detection of *H. ducrey* in smears, in culture from the ulcer or from the bubo pus are overweighing skin tests. The patients receive nowadays adequate treatment prior to their positivation.

IMMUNOLOGICAL MECHANISM OF CLINICAL SYMPTOMS

H. ducrey penetrates the broken epidermis. The tissue necrosis may be caused by the endotoxin. As shown by the auto-inoculation test, the infection takes, after exposure, almost always. The variation in the incubation (1 to 5 days) may be due to a difference of the virulence of the infectious agent. This suggests a lack of natural immunity. The ulcer continues growing for 2 to 3 weeks until immune mechanisms become activated. Consequently, the diameter of the ulcer rarely exceeds 2 to 3 cm. The organisms spread in the intercellular space of the corium and along the lymphatic vessels. They spare the subcutaneous fat, and the fibrous tissue of the corpus cavernosum of the penis and of the vagina. The bubo is a painful absceding lymphadenitis caused by the microbes trapped in the lymph nodes. Involvement of the pelvic lymph nodes has not been described. Bacterial debris getting into the blood vessels may provoke erythema nodosum or multiforme-like vasculitis.

There are clinical varieties of chancroid which show a different clinical course. The serpiginous type spreads by extension from the original genital lesions to the groin or thigh. The ulcerations are shallow but show no tendency to heal. This form of chancroid may persist for months or years. The phagedenic type is a rapidly destructive form of the disease. It is caused by a super-added fuso-spirochaetal infection and may produce considerable tissue destruction.

NATURAL COURSE OF THE DISEASE

The disease is a self-limiting one. The primary ulceration may heal gradually within 4 to 6 weeks. Inguinal adenitis may be minimal in approximately one half of the cases. This suggests the involvement of immune mechanisms in the disease. This could be promoted by vaccine, which, with the advent of antibiotics, became obsolete. The mechanism of the spontaneous cure is not clear. Auto-infection is possible in patients positive in complement fixation test. Repeated infections observed earlier suggest that the disease does not provoke a total immunity. Some evidence has been presented which purports to show that there are carriers of Ducrey's bacillus [3]. It may well be that some prostitutes remain carriers of the organism long after chancroidal lesions have healed.

REFERENCES

1. Asin, J.: *Amer. J. Syph.* **36,** 483 (1952).
2. Nomura, Y.: *Jap. J. Derm.* **61,** 181 and 189 (1951) rev. *Zbl. Haut- u. Geschl. Kr.* **81,** 379 (1952).
3. Saelhof, C. C.: *J. Urol.* **13,** 485 (1925).
4. Willcox, R. R.: *Amer. J. Syph.* **36,** 284 (1952).

CHAPTER 78

IMMUNOALLERGOLOGIC ASPECTS OF LYMPHOGRANULOMA VENEREUM

by

K. KIRÁLY

CLINICAL DEFINITION AND AETIOLOGY

Lymphogranuloma venereum (LGV) is a venereally transmitted disease of man, caused by a chlamydial agent and characterized by a small fleeting primary lesion followed by the development of a usually suppurative regional adenitis.

The clinical course of the disease varies, with the outcome ranging from spontaneous remission to chronicity. In the classical clinical course three consecutive stages might be distinguished:

1. Within a few days after exposure, vesicles develop on the genitalia that subsequently burst, leaving a painless, shallow, greyish ulcer.

2. The regional lymph nodes in the groins in males, and the intrapelvic and perianal lymph nodes draining the vagina and rectal regions in females, enlarge. Lymphadenopathy may be accompanied by systemic manifestations. The lymphadenitis may resolve spontaneously or, in many instances, with suppuration.

3. The obstruction of lymphatic vessels causes an elephantiasis of external genitalia or anus. A proliferative proctitis results, which may lead to rectal stricture with vaginorectal, perirectal and/or perianal fistulas (anogenital syndrome).

As with chlamydial infections in general, there are, however, two types of infection: an acute one with symptoms and readily proven by microbiologic evidence, or a chronic infection with maintenance of agents in the host but with less evidence of active infection. The diagnosis may be proved by the Frei test and/or the complement fixation test.

The pathogenic mechanism may be based on two major direct effects of infection on cells—cytocidal, or functional impairment of phagocytic cells. Obviously these may act together, and immune mechanisms may also be involved in the disease pathogenesis.

Bergey's *Manual of Determinative Bacteriology* (1948) describes the chlamydial agent found generally in patients with LGV as a well-determined microorganism with the name *Miyagawanella lymphogranulomatis*, showing the following characteristics: sensitivity to sulphonamides and virulence for mice when inoculated by the intracerebral and intranasal routes, but not by the intraperitoneal route. This description is, however, valid only for Chlamydia LGV strains from a closed population group. Recently isolations have been made from clinical LGV with the characteristics of the avian Chlamydia strain (sulpha resistant, highly virulent for mice and non-productive of glycogen) [18, 19]. Trachoma inclusion conjunctivitis (TRIC) agent (non-virulent for mice by the intracerebral route) has been isolated from seamen returning from South-East Asia [17, 19].

Because of this variety of properties within Chlamydiae causing the disease, the term LGV might more appropriately be reserved for clinical disease rather than to describe a particular agent: microorganism isolated from LGV patients present a spectrum of qualities within the Chlamydia group. Sometimes even the clinical symptoms are a combination of diseases caused by chlamydial agents: patients may exhibit the symptoms of Reiter's disease complicated by suppurative inguinal lymphadenopathy [20].

GENERAL CHARACTERISTICS OF CHLAMYDIAE

ANTIGENIC STRUCTURE

Chlamydiae comprise a large number of antigenically related, culturally, morphologically and tinctorially similar microorganisms. Their form is spherical. The infectious form has a diameter of 300 nm. They are obligate, intracellular parasites, which multiply in the cytoplasm of the host cell and form cytoplasmic inclusions consisting of micro-colonies of the agent. A unique characteristic differentiating Chlamydiae from other microorganisms is their growth cycle. After infecting the host cell they go through a complicated development cycle. The infecting organisms transform into large homogeneous bodies—up to 1,000 nm in diameter—which multiply by division and differentiate into small infectious units. The large forms are either not infectious, or their infectivity is very low. The growth cycle explains the impossibility of obtaining homogeneous, reproducible and well-characterized antigenic preparations.

Two different types of antigens — group- and species-specific — are presently known. The group-specific antigen is the major antigenic component. It is heat-stable and shared by all chlamydial agents. It may be detected throughout the growth cycle and is located in the cell wall structure. It can be extracted from partially purified suspensions with desoxycholate, acid, alkali, diethyl ether, acetone, phenol, urea or water. It is not known whether the same antigenic components are present in commercially available antigens prepared by different methods. Their chemical structure is not established. The extracts contain protein and lipopolysaccharide. Group-specific antigens are detected by means of complement fixation, radioimmunoassay, haemagglutination inhibition and intracutaneous tests. The haemagglutinin is a lecithin–nucleoprotein complex. It agglutinates the erythrocytes of mice and hamsters.

Species-specific antigens may be identified by the reaction between untreated chlamydial suspensions and hyperimmune serum, from which group-specific antibodies have been absorbed with boiled antigen. At present techniques for preparing purified isolate-specific antigens are not available. Species-specific antigens may be obtained from sonically disrupted and potassium periodate or lecithinase-treated Chlamydia cells, where the group-specific antigen(s) have been destroyed. The antigens responsible for infectivity are also species-specific. In many Chlamydia strains, labile species-specific toxins, causing the toxic death of mice, are present. Both are associated with the surface structure of chlamydial agents. Species-specific antigens are detected by neutralizing antibodies and immunofluorescence. The microimmunofluorescent method for typing Chlamydia isolates has proved very reliable [23]. By this test LGV isolates can be readily distinguished from TRIC agents and they have been divided into three serotypes, the majority belonging to LGV Type II [22]. The human Chlamydia strains studied may, up to the present, be divided into twelve subgroups. The antigenic specification does not give any clue to the understanding of the different clinical pictures caused by chlamydial agents.

The toxin is located within the elementary bodies: it is species-specific, and its effect is neutralized by corresponding antisera. The toxic effect can be suppressed by treatment with formalin or by keeping it at a temperature of 37 °C. Toxin combined with the sera of LGV patients fixes complement [7].

ANIMAL PATHOGENICITY

The Chlamydia cell has no active mechanism of penetration into the host cell. To gain entrance it must depend on the phagocytic activity of the host. It is taken up in a phagosome and the developmental cycle takes place there. How the Chlamydia cell avoids the release or action of lysosomal enzymes is not known.

Monkeys and mice show the strongest susceptibility to the infection. The monkey was the first animal to be infected by intracerebral inoculation. The infected monkeys died of meningo-encephalitis. Intraperitoneal infection gives rise to peritonitis, while preputial or urethral inoculation causes chronic lymphadenitis. The monkey is the most suitable model of human infection. The mouse is susceptible to intracerebral and intranasal infection, but is not sensitive to intraperitoneal, subcutaneous and intravenous infection. Meningo-encephalitis ensues if a simultaneous cerebral injury is occasioned by the injection of saline, which was the first method used for the demonstration and isolation of the causative agent of LGV. It seems now, however, that LGV agents are not necessarily virulent for mice. Therefore a major criterion for differentiating between LGV and TRIC agents has been lost. Rats, guinea pigs, dogs and cats are less susceptible and birds are resistant to Chlamydia LGV.

CULTIVATION

All the known Chlamydia strains infect, and multiply in, the entodermal cells of the yolk sack of six- to eight-day-old developing chicken embryos. This method is used for isolation from clinical material and for pathogenicity tests for examining antibiotic and sulphonamide sensitivity. Depending on size and the rate of development of the infecting inoculum, the chicken embryos die between 3 and 14 days after infection. Chicken embryos can be infected also by chorioallantoic inoculation. Chlamydial infection induces small, opaque, pock-like lesions, due to the hyperplasia of ectodermal cells. This method of propagation has been widely used for immunologic studies, since it gives rich harvests of Chlamydial agents which can be conveniently purified.

Chlamydial agents can be adapted and propagated in tissue cultures, though the tissue culture system currently in use is not suitable for producing large yields of Chlamydiae. Irradiated McCoy cell monolayers are, however, more sensitive than yolk sac inoculation, particularly if elementary bodies present in the clinical specimen have been centrifuged on to it [5]. Subgroup A Chlamydia strains (TRIC agent, most LGV agents, etc.) develop as an iodine-staining inclusion.

It must be kept in mind, however, that cytological detection and agent isolation methods of diagnosing LGV infection are relatively insensitive.

ANTIBODIES

NATURAL ANTIBODIES

The sera of healthy individuals contain substances which are destroyed at 60 °C [21].

PROTECTIVE ANTIBODIES

Antisera obtained from chickens inhibit the killing effect of Chlamydia LGV on chick embryos, but do not ensure immunity against other chlamydial agents, despite cross-reaction in complement fixation [8]. If a challenge strain maintained in the yolk sac is incubated with the serum of a patient infected 12–17 days previously, it fails to kill mice even by intracerebral inoculation. These neutralizing antibodies have been stated to be species-specific. However, no important immunological difference between LGV and TRIC agents could be seen by means of the neutralization test: sera strongly protective against Chlamydia LGV were also highly protective against TRIC agents [15].

COMPLEMENT FIXING ANTIBODIES

These antibodies react with the thermostable group-specific antigenic component. Absorption of patients' sera with boiled LGV antigen removes the group antibodies and the remaining activity is specific for LGV [14].

212

DIAGNOSTIC TESTS

COMPLEMENT FIXATION

The antigen generally used is prepared from the yolk sac of Chlamydia LGV infected chick embryos. The antigenic component involved is a group-specific extract. Other chlamydial agents — causing enzootic abortion of ewes [2] and meningopneumonitis as well as 6 B C psittacosis isolate [20] — may also be used. Extracts of non-infected chick embryos serve as controls. Dilution 1 : 40 are regarded as positive. With lower dilutions the complement is fixed even after inflammations of the upper respiratory tract, or in eye diseases caused by TRIC agents [3].

Positive reactions are observed after Chlamydia-induced pneumonia, in 25 per cent of patients with cat scratch disease, and sometimes, without clinical symptoms, in patients with urethral discharge, in promiscuous persons and in about 20 per cent of drug addicts [1]. It is not known if a latent infection is the cause of positive reactions.

The reaction may be positive as early as one week after the infection, reaching its highest titre after several weeks. A rising titre is more suggestive of the disease than a single positive finding. Reactivity remains for several years after recovery [4]. Serological tests are, however, rather insensitive. As in Chlamydia infections generally, they become positive too late. Serological testing may be used more profitably to study reactor rates in the population, as an indication of overall Chlamydia exposure. On the other hand, Frei's test seems to be more sensitive: it gives positive results when complement fixation fails [9].

False positive results may be caused by the presence of antibodies in guinea pig serum used as a source of complement [21]. Due to its lipid composition, yolk sac extract (infected or non-infected) reacts with the sera of patients with syphilis and with chronic biologically false positive reactors for syphilis. The reactivity runs parallel to that of the VDRL test. The antibodies can be removed by absorption of sera with Kahn's antigen [10].

INTRACUTANEOUS (FREI'S) TEST

This simple test is extremely useful to clear the aetiology of bubo, of the anogenital syndrome, and to screen asymptomatic carriers.

Types of antigen used:

1. Lygranum (Chlamydia LGV infected chicken embryo yolk sac extract); stored at 4 °C, it remains active for 3–4 months. 0.1–0.2 ml of the antigen is injected i.c. into one forearm and, as a control, 0.1 ml yolk sac extract into the other forearm.

2. Antigens prepared from the brains of mice and monkeys infected with Chlamydia LGV were used earlier. They frequently gave false positive results.

3. Pus aspirated from unbroken abscesses of LGV patients is inactivated at 60 °C for three hours. The suspension is controlled by injecting healthy individuals and it is diluted until it gives no reaction in them. The antigen can be

stored for 12–18 months at 4 °C. False positive reactions are observed with pus contaminated with bacteria. This test, though described in manuals, is of historical interest only.

4. Inverted Frei test: heat inactivated pus aspired from a suspected LGV bubo is given to a known sufferer of the condition. This method may be used to prove the diagnosis when a negative Frei test is obtained in a case of suppurative bubo.

In positive reactions, erythematous papules of more than 6 mm diameter, surrounded by a hyperaemic area, are seen after 48 or 72 hours, and remain for 7 days. Controls show no reaction, only a slight erythema without infiltration may appear at the site of injection. If Lygranum is used, the size of the hyperaemic area caused by the antigen exceeds that caused by the control. Histologically, the infiltrate consists of neutrophils and lymphocytes followed by the appearance of epitheloid cells [13, 14].

The time elapsing between infection and a positive skin test is variable: it is usually, but not always, positive by the time of the appearance of the bubo (i.e. 5–8 weeks after infection). Once delayed-type hypersensitivity has developed, it will not show reversal in spite of intensive and successful treatment.

Opinions regarding the specificity of the test are equivocal. The antigen is thermostable and common to other Chlamydia. Consequently, the skin test is positive in cases of Chlamydia pneumonia; on the other hand, psittacosis antigen may elicit positive reactions in patients with LGV [16]. Reyman [16], performing the test in 95 healthy persons, observed only a single case of reactivity. However, Lygranum gives positive reactions in 18 to 50 per cent of promiscuous females and patients with venereal diseases without any symptoms of LGV. It is not clear whether this indicates symptomless infection, a carrier state or earlier infection with other Chlamydiae.

The agent of another suppurative lymphadenitis, cat scratch disease, shows no cross-reaction with Chlamydiae in the skin test: pus aspired from bubo of these patients (Reilly's antigen) remains non-reactive if injected into the skin of LGV patients, as Frei's reaction is negative in patients with cat scratch disease [11].

MICROIMMUNOFLUORESCENCE TEST

With Chlamydiae there is a particular need for typing systems, e.g. the distinction between the TRIC agent and the LGV agent in the laboratory has, until recently, depended on the rather irregular patterns of pathogenicity of the two agents to animals. Hence, the labelling of an isolate as LGV rather than as TRIC has been made primarily on its clinical origin. With the aid of microimmunofluorescence, it is possible to distinguish between the two agents and to identify serotypes of Chlamydiae for the preparation of the intracutaneous test.

IMMUNOALLERGOLOGIC PHENOMENA IN THE COURSE OF INFECTION

An infectious immunity develops during the disease: patients are immune to the intracutaneous inoculation of the agent; a papule develops on the injection site without involvement of the regional lymph nodes. Superinfection immunity is preserved even in the phase of esthiomène [7]. How early it is established is not known. The prolonged course of the disease and the frequency of exacerbations suggest that immunity is not complete. Relapse, with enlargement of lymph nodes and a rise of LGV complement fixation titre, may be observed, even several years after infection in patients previously symptomless. The relapse indicates a frail balance between persisting Chlamydia and the host organism.

There are certain facts indicating that the disease does not always follow the classical clinical course. Sometimes just a slight enlargement of lymph nodes and leukorrhoea are the only symptoms in promiscuous females named as contacts and it has not been possible to isolate chlamydial agents [7, 15]. On the other hand, an asymptomatic carrier state seems highly probable. A frequent positivity of complement fixation and Frei's test (or both) among venereal disease patients [9], homosexuals [6], and promiscuous females without any clinical symptoms, speaks in favour of the existence of such a state. The natural course of the disease, i.e. how many subclinical cases and how many chronic cases exist, has not been established.

LGV in developed countries is regarded as a rare disease, which is imported only from tropical countries. However, local outbreaks have been described without any overseas contact, indicating that Chlamydia LGV is present in the population even in industrialized countries [15]. Suppurative inguinal adenitis is often seen by doctors in tropical countries and considered as tropical or climatic bubo. On clinical grounds LGV may be suspected. Due to many other causes of suppurative lymphadenitis in these countries (tuberculosis, syphilis, pyogenic infections, leishmaniasis, etc.), it is difficult to form any accurate estimate of its prevalence.

Cross-immunity between Chlamydiae has hardly ever been examined. Infected animals after cure, or immunized with a heat-inactivated agent, are claimed to be resistant only to challenge with the original agent. However, a cross-immunity between TRIC and LGV agents could be demonstrated [24]. No generally accepted vaccine for LGV infection is available.

Allergic symptoms appear such as erythema multiforme, scarlatiniform or morbilliform exanthema, urticaria, papular, vesicular, bullous, pustular or ecthyma-like lesions, with predilection for surfaces exposed to sunlight [12]. Erythema nodosum may follow the performance of Frei's test or intravenous administration of pus obtained from an abscess [7]. Whether arthritis and iritis, sometimes accompanying LGV, is caused directly by Chlamydia agents or antigen–antibody interaction, remains to be determined.

REFERENCES

1. Cherubin, C. E. and Millian, S. J.: *Ann. intern. Med.* **69,** 739 (1968).
2. Dane, D. S.: *Med. J. Austr.* **1,** 382 (1955).
3. Dömök, I.: In *Lymphogranuloma venereum.* Ed. by Bakács, T. and Farkas, K. Medicina, Budapest 1965, p. 397.
4. Goldberg, J. and Banov, L.: *Brit. J. vener. Dis.* **32,** 37 (1956).
5. Gordon, F. B., Harper, I. A., Quan, A. L., Treharne, J. D., Dwyer, R. S. C., and Gerland, I. A.: *J. infect. Dis.* **120,** 451 (1969).
6. Greaves, A. B.: *Bull. Wld Hlth Org.* **29,** 797 (1963).
7. Hellerström, S.: In *Handbuch der Haut- und Geschlechtskrankheiten.* Erg. Werk. Vol. VI/2. Part B. Ed. by Jadassohn, J. Springer, Berlin 1962, p. 426.
8. Hilleman, M. R.: *J. infect. Dis.* **76,** 96 (1945).
9. King, A. J., Barwell, C. F. and Catterall, R. D.: *Brit. J. vener. Dis.* **32,** 209 (1956).
10. Lassus, A., Johanson, E. A., Sonck, C. E., and Aho, K.: *Brit. J. vener. Dis.,* **47,** 169 (1971).
11. Lèques, B., Verdaguer, S., Vergnas, J. and Régnier, M.: *Bull. Soc. franç. Derm. Syph.* **76,** 256 (1969).
12. Melczer, N.: In *Handbuch der Haut- und Geschlechtskrankheiten.* Erg. Werk. Vol. VI/2. Part B. Ed. by Jadassohn, J. Springer, Berlin 1962, p. 496.
13. id., *Lymphogranuloma inguinale.* Eggenberg, Budapest 1942.
14. Meyer, K. F.: In *Viral and Rickettsial Infections on Man.* Ed. by Rivers, Th. and Horsfall, F. L. Lippincott, Philadelphia 1959, p. 716.
15. Philip, R. N., Hill, D. A., Greaves, A. B., Gordon, F. B., Quan, A. L., Gerloff, R. K. and Thomas, L. A.: *Brit. J. vener. Dis.* **47,** 114 (1971).
16. Reymann, F.: *Acta derm.-venereol.* (*Stockh.*) **31,** 257 (1951).
17. Salim, A. R.: *J. trop. Med. Hyg.* **72,** 134 (1969).
18. Schachter, J.: *J. Ophthalmol.* **63,** 1049 (1967).
19. Schachter, J. and Meyer, K. F.: *J. Bact.* **99,** 636 (1969).
20. Schachter, J., Smith, D. E., Dawson, C. R., Anderson, W. R., Doller, J. J., Hoke, A. W., Smartt, W. H. and Meyer, K. F.: *J. infect. Dis.* **120,** 372 (1969).
21. Terzin, A. L.: *J. Hyg.* (*Camb.*), **62,** 179 (1964).
22. Trehrane, J. D., Davey, S. J., Groy, S. J. and Jones, B. R.: *Brit. J. vener. Dis.* **48,** 18 (1972).
23. Wang, San-pir, and Grayston, J. T.: *Amer. J. Ophthal.* **70,** 367 (1970).
24. Werner, G. H.: *C. R. Acad. Sci.* **261,** 2410 (1965).

CHAPTER 79

IMMUNOALLERGIC MANIFESTATIONS OF HUMAN PROTOZOAN AND HELMINTH DISEASES

by

M. JANKÓ and GY. BÁNKI

INTRODUCTION

The protozoan and helminth parasites of animals have a complex molecular structure and enzymatic activity and, consequently, also a complex life function. They have a well defined life cycle in which the developmental stages follow in a strict sequence. The stages may, however, differ in respect of preference for host tissues, organs or cells and further in antigenic properties [321].

For instance, living parasites elicit an immune response by virtue of their surface and/or exoantigens, among others the ES (excretion–secretion) antigens. The latter may, apart from other substances, contain invasive and/or nutritive enzymes or enzyme inhibitors. Acetylcholinesterase, recently identified as a component of the ES antigen in a number of nematodes [206, 243, 253], influences the intestinal functions of the hosts, acting as a biochemical holdfast [205] and, additionally, as an inducer of specific antibodies.

Anti-parasitic immunity is probably associated with the production of protective antigen at a particular stage of the life cycle of the parasite. The antigen itself has generally not been identified, but the stage responsible for it has become known with several parasites, above all with helminths. The protective antigen is in all probability an ES antigen, maybe the exsheathing fluid itself [274, 275]. The first anti-parasitic vaccine, employed by veterinarians for the prevention of lung worm disease in calves, was elaborated on the basis of the foregoing observations [130]. Vaccination is carried out by oral administration of irradiation attenuated third stage larvae. If the exposure is adequate, the larvae deteriorate in the host after undergoing a single moult, and produce a satisfactory degree of protective immunity.

Intestinal immuno-expulsion of the parasites is another protective mechanism: the primary parasite population is expelled by the defense reaction and the host becomes resistant to reinfection.

Immuno-expulsion can essentially be regarded as a three-step process [158]. In the first step, the parasites are damaged by the antibodies, being thereby rendered susceptible to further untoward influences. The next step requires the presence of functionally intact, sensitized T-lymphocytes and finally the process is accomplished by probably not sensitized myeloid cells.

The interaction of the two cell types probably elicit a prostaglandin response which is also presumed to play a role in the process.

However, parasite infection is rarely as immunogenic as to confer lasting protection. The intermediate developmental stages may establish themselves in the host for long periods without eliciting a reaction. Their activation or deterioration may nevertheless evoke a strong response.

One interesting theory offered for the explanation of the absence of reaction is the molecular mimicry of the parasites which serves to mislead the immune recognition mechanism of the host [39, 58, 271]. It seems also fairly certain that some parasites are capable of adaptation to an immune host [134].

As to allergic manifestations in protozoan infections, these are as a rule of the delayed hypersensitivity type, immediate hypersensitivity phenomena being rare in such conditions. For instance, the periventricular lesions developing in neonatal toxoplasmosis probably correspond to an Arthus-type reaction [99d].

In contrast, immediate-type reactions are frequent in helminth infections,

218

although delayed hypersensitivity often plays a decisive role in the pathogenesis of the disease and the related immunological events. Egg-granulomatosis for example, which is a fundamental lesion in schistosomiasis, arises in consequence of a cell-mediated immune response.

Helminths cannot only induce a homologous immediate-type response, but they can also potentiate the reagin response elicited by heterologous antigens or haptens [131, 211]. This effect probably develops through the stimulation of carrier-specific helper T cells [164]. Thus the helminths, apart from being capable of eliciting certain allergic diseases in themselves, may also aggravate the course of such processes as co-factors.

Apparently, however, the level of the IgE production elicited or potentiated by the parasites parallels the severity of the clinical manifestation only in primary infections, whereas in recurrences the systemic hypersensitivity symptoms gradually become milder and a certain protective immunity develops in the pathological sense although the IgE antibody level continues to rise [88a, 220a].

Infections with metazoan parasites have been reported to potentiate or depress the humoral response to heterologous antigens. A number of other metazoan parasites have been reported to stimulate cellular immunity [194a]. Further there is a difference between the humoral and cellular immune response as based on the bioanatomial characteristics (tropism, localization) of the parasitosis [39a].

The mode and intensity of host-parasite relationship may vary even in case of infection with one and the same parasite species.

A characteristic clinical-pathological example is presented by leishmaniasis. While disseminated, cutaneous leishmaniasis or Kala-Azar is characterized by the absence of cell-mediated immunity, lupoid leishmaniasis is regarded as exaggeration of cell-mediated immunity [302].

A relationship between the immune system and parasitic infection is shown, e.g. in malaria. In experimental malaria, antibody response to sheep erythrocytes or protein antigen but not to hapten was markedly reduced. Allograft rejection and contact hypersensivity were not impaired either [88]. Apparently, this infection did not affect the functions of T cells. At the same time, observations on mouse lymphoma [135] and Burkitt's lymphoma in African children [152] seem to affirm the suppressive effect of malaria on tumour immunity.

Latent strongyloidosis may develop into a lethal endogenous auto-infection in patients under immunosuppressive treatment, showing that the life cycle of the parasite becomes altered by immune response.

The complications associated with several important parasitic infections are suggestive of immune complex or autoimmune disease.

The great advances in immunobiology and related disciplines have stimulated new approaches to the problem on cellular, subcellular or even molecular levels. Nevertheless, answers are still lacking to most questions raised in the field of immunopathology of parasitic diseases and there certainly are still further questions which have not even been asked.

GIARDIASIS

The parasite *Giardia lamblia* is cosmopolitan and infects children more frequently than adults.

It has a flagellated vegetative form and an oval cyst form. Its localization is in the small intestine.

G. lamblia infects exclusively humans. Its vegetative form passed with the stool, but above all its cyst form, are transmitted either by direct contact or by contaminated food or water.

On ingestion by the host, *G. lamblia* parasites adhere by help of their sucker plates to the small intestinal epithelium, which results in mechanical interference with the absorption of digested food, while toxic metabolic products of the parasite may sensitize the host organism. Thus, a local inflammatory eosinophilic cell reaction develops, which inhibits the absorption of chiefly the fat and the lipid-soluble vitamins A, D and K. It was shown experimentally in both humans and animals that *G. lamblia* not only adheres to, but also invades the mucosal tissue of the small intestine.

Symptoms in the early stage of giardiasis are predominantly intestinal, ranging from mild to acute acid diarrhoea (even steatorrhoea).

Chronic giardiasis, often affecting children for periods of 2–3 years, may cause growth retardation, gastrointestinal symptoms, anaemia or rachitis concomitant upon metabolic disorders. Adults show, apart from enteric symptoms, signs of gall bladder and liver involvement. Occasionally urticaria or asthma develop as an allergic response to *G. lamblia* [202].

An antigen recently prepared from *Lamblia intestinalis* culture gave an agar precipitation reaction with rabbit immune serum and antibodies were detected in human serum by immunofluorescence technique [212]. The IgG, IgA and IgM levels of infected individuals were normal [193].

Cysts copiously passed with the faeces are easily identified on microscopic examination.

Metronidazole and quinacrine derivatives have been employed as effective chemotherapeutics against giardiasis.

TRICHOMONIASIS

Among the various Trichomonas infections urogenital trichomoniasis, caused by *Trichomonas vaginalis*, is the most important in view of its pathological and public health significance all over the world [113, 114, 141, 291a]. The protozoan is found in the urogenital tract of men and women. *T. vaginalis* exists exclusively in tropozoite form, as a rule in an extracellular localization. It deteriorates rapidly outside the host, whence its transmission occurs chiefly by sexual intercourse, the male acting as the vector, the female as reservoir. The degree of the lesions relates to the lytic and agglutinating activity of the serum and to the associated bacterium flora as well [231, 290]. In the invaded area degeneration of epithelial cells occurs, followed by inflammation with leukocytic infiltration. It was shown in infection experiments that leukocytes play an important part in the pathogenesis of trichomoniasis. The deteriorated leukocytes give rise to tissue destruction, and serve at the same time as nutriment for the parasites. Several investigators observed that tissue lysis, oedema, hypersensitivity and the development of the immune mechanism are closely interrelated with the metabolic products of the parasite. Certain atypical cell changes, arising in the advanced stage of trichomoniasis, can scarcely be differentiated from cancer cells.

The acute stage of trichomoniasis is accompanied by burning and itching and the production of abundant discharge in the affected region. The disease takes a sub-acute course becoming chronic after a shorter or longer time. The parasite, ascending to the higher regions of the urogenital tract, gives rise to colpitis, urethritis, prostatitis and/or cystitis [15].

Hormonal changes, involving oestrogens, progesterone and gonadotropin, may activate latent trichomoniasis. Hormonal influence, manifested by exaggerated symptoms, chiefly comes into display during pregnancy or the menstrual cycle.

Immunological studies aimed at strain differentiation revealed dissimilar antigenic patterns in *T. vaginalis* [110, 144, 167]. Several hundred strains surveyed by a team were found to belong to four antigenic types (TLR, TN, TRT and TR) [291b, c, 292]. Studies on local vaginal and general immune responses [156, 157, 201b] have suggested that protective antibodies against *T. vaginalis* and *T. foetus* are, in fact, produced in trichomoniasis, but their activity is unrelated to the type of antigen used for challenge and to the titre obtained in the serological diagnostic test.

Agglutination tests for the serological diagnosis of trichomoniasis had initially been performed with an antigen prepared from *T. foetus* [160]. Later, using *T. vaginalis* antigen, it was found that the test, although it is a suitable tool for diagnostic and epidemiological surveys is not conclusive enough for the evaluation of therapeutic results, owing to the persistence of a gradually decreasing antibody level for several months [201a].

Haemagglutination tests performed in the early post-infection stage of urogenital trichomoniasis showed that *T. tenax* and *T. hominis* may cross-react at low titres and that antibodies may also be present in sera of non-infected individuals [110, 183]. This finding was confirmed later and haemagglutination has become the most reliable diagnostic approach to chronic trichomoniasis. Reports on the serological diagnosis of trichomoniasis have chiefly been based on the C fixation test [55, 126, 166]. The antigen should be prepared from several types of Trichomonas strains, to ensure a greater reliability. For the fluorescent antibody technique, formol-treated *T. vaginalis* obtained from an axenic culture has been used as antigen [169]. Cutaneous tests applied for the demonstration of delayed hypersensitivity in urogenital trichomoniasis have not been suitable for routine work, owing to discrepancy between their results and the microscopic findings [5]. Recent investigations have shown that the results of the cutaneous test are related to the antigen employed — heterologous antigens give better results — and to the time of infection [2, 125, 293]. Negative findings may also be due to the anergic state of the subject examined.

Therapy with metronidazole and tinidazole has been successful.

LEISHMANIASIS

CUTANEOUS LEISHMANIASIS

The disease produced by *Leishmania tropica* is endemic in areas of the Near East, the Caucasus, in Sudan and Nigeria.

The parasite is transmitted by sandflies of the genus Phlebotomus and the dog and wild rodents act as reservoirs. Man to man transmission can also occur by direct contact.

An itching papule develops at the site of the insect bite, surrounded by infiltrating epitheloid and lymphoid cells, the macrophages harbouring many parasites. Later dilatation of the capillaries and tissue lysis give rise to ulceration. Secondary bacterial infections are frequent.

Two types of cutaneous leishmaniasis are known, one being the dry or urban type caused by *L. tropica minor* and characterized by late chronic ulceration, and the other the moist or rural type due to *L. tropica major*, in which early acute ulceration occurs.

In dry cutaneous leishmaniasis, a long latency (6–18 months) is followed by the development of dry, rough-surfaced papules at the inoculation site; later on these undergo ulceration and heal by cicatrization.

Moist cutaneous leishmaniasis becomes clinically manifest after a shorter latency (4–6 weeks). Multiple nodules are formed around the crater-like ulcer arising in place of the papules. Healing by fibrosis usually takes about six months.

MUCOCUTANEOUS LEISHMANIASIS OR ESPUNDIA

The disease produced by *Leishmania brasiliensis* is endemic in Mexico and South America in the region between latitudes 21 degrees North, and 25 degrees South.

It is transmitted by Phlebotomus species, domestic and wild dogs and wild rodents acting as reservoirs.

At the site bitten by the insect, infiltrating lymphocytes and macrophages appear in the subcutis and submucosa. In the verrucose form, a tuberculoid inflammatory process develops.

The disease has three types, each being caused by a different strain. (*i*) In the Mexican type, the ulcers appear in the auricular region. Chronic, new and healing ulcers may be present simultaneously with few parasites. (*ii*) The Uta, or papulous type is characterized by ulcers packed with parasites in the early stage. Infrequently espundia-like mucosal lesions also develop. The ulcers heal spontaneously in most cases, leaving a pigment-free scar tissue. (*iii*) Classical mucocutaneous espundia is a disseminated cutaneous leishmaniasis with mucosal lesions. The latter are initially limited to the nasal and labial areas, but later they may spread to other parts. The inflammatory process destroys the surrounding tissues, and may therefore cause deformity of the nose, while the laryngeal processes may give rise to constriction of the airways.

The histological findings, spontaneous healing of the cutaneous changes and variations in the severity of the clinical course unequivocally indicate the involvement of acquired immunity. The degree of the latter, however, depends on the condition of the host, and on the virulence of the parasite as well [108]. Cutaneous leishmaniasis may be caused by two different Leishmania strains [254], and two different explanations have been offered concerning immune response to the causative agents. According to certain investigators, the strains differ antigenically, as judged from the marked resistance to challenge with the homologous parasite strain and partial or complete cross-resistance to the heterologous parasites in animal expriments [4, 142]. Against this, other workers — apart from confirming cross-protection by moist against dry leishmaniasis — were able to demonstrate cross-protection between the two strains in infection experiments [17]. Allergic skin tests with antigen prepared from Leishmanias have been positive in cutaneous leishmaniasis, except in its diffuse form which is due to the anergic state of the host. Delayed hypersensitivity is transmissible passively by lymphoid cells [30,197].

Patients recovered from L. tropica and L. brasiliensis infections become infected once more only very rarely. This observation stimulated the development of a vaccine.

The serological reactions are usually negative in all forms of cutaneous leishmaniasis showing the absence of notable antibody production. A low level of antibodies has recently been demonstrated by immunofluorescent technique in the serum of an experimentally infected subject [234]. At present the Leishmania (Montenegro) cutaneous test is an immunodiagnostic method offering some help.

For chemotherapy chiefly antimony preparations, pyrimethamin and amphotericin B are used, the latter having, however, a toxic side-effect.

VISCERAL LEISHMANIASIS OR KALA-AZAR

Kala-Azar is an infection with *Leishmania donovani* occurring in India, in central China, in northern and central Africa and in South America. It is endemic in certain parts of these regions. Transmission occurs by sandflies of the genus Phlebotomus. The dog serves as the main mammalian reservoir.

In the human or animal bodies the parasite occurs in the form of small round or oval intracellular bodies. In vectors it develops flagella and the leptomonad form is transmitted to the new host with the insect bite.

The parasite then passess to lymph nodes and visceral organs via blood and lymph circulation. The cutaneous lesions arising at the inoculation site are surrounded by a zone of hyperpigmentation. Many centrally aggregated parasites are seen on microscopic examination of the lesion and some also appear in the enlarged lymph nodes. The liver and spleen are markedly enlarged. Reticuloendothelial hyperlasia of the splenic pulp is found on histological examination. Many Leishmania organisms are seen inside mononuclear phagocytic cells. In the liver, hyperplasia of the Kupffer cells, mononuclear cells containing phagocytosed parasites and eosinophilic cells are found.

The symptoms appearing a few weeks after the insect bite are not characteristic. Usually there is general malaise and subfebrility. A febrile course, associated with enlargement of the spleen and liver, as well as of lymph nodes, follows after several months of latency. The parasites multiply in the meantime and stress, undernourishment and intercurrent disease aggravate the symptoms of Kala-Azar. The skin becomes dry and yellowish-grey, and dysentery-like symptoms bring about emaciation and anaemia. Patients recovering from Kala-Azar develop an immunity against the disease.

Experimental observations and epidemiological surveys have unequivocally shown that resistance to Leishmania infection is influenced by several factors.

Comparative studies on the incidence of visceral leishmaniasis in various age groups have suggested that it is associated with the strain of the protozoan rather than with the age of the host. In India, the classical form of Kala-Azar is more frequent in adults than in children. It does not occur in dogs, whereas in the Mediterranean region, the disease is more common in children and also affects dogs and wild animals. Another markedly virulent strain is responsible for the Sudanese Kala-Azar, which again is predominant in the adults and does not spread to dogs. This form is characterized by cutaneous lesions and resistance to antimony therapy. Studies on sex distribution have shown a greater frequency among males, owing probably to more frequent exposure. In animal experiments, females appeared to be more resistant than males to visceral leishmaniasis [84]. In mice, deprivation of protein and pyridoxine caused lowering of both natural and acquired resistance [3]. *In vitro* and *in vivo* studies on the effect of environmental temperature on parasite multiplication showed that it is enhanced at 25–28 °C and inhibited at 36 °C [101, 322].

The development of active immunity in leishmaniasis is indicated by the occurrence of asymptomatic and atypical cases, by the frequent spontaneous recoveries and rarity of recurrences. Studies on the development of resistance and incidence of reinfection have affirmed the cross-immunity of different Leishmania strains [180, 277]. In humans, inoculation with *L. adleri* rendered the subjects immune to *L. donovani* infection [276]. In animals even premunition can be established [107, 213].

The cellular reactions are not characteristic in visceral leishmaniasis. After the infection, the predominant host cells are macrophages and plasma cells [287]. Recently protection against *L. donovani* infection could be transmitted with lymphoid cells from immunized animals to non-immune recipients [189].

Leishmania infection is followed by the appearance of humoral antibodies. Antigens for antibody demonstration can be prepared from both homologous and heterologous strains, but the former are more reliable because the specificity of serological reactions is usually low in leishmaniasis.

C fixation and indirect haemagglutination tests have long been employed for the serological diagnosis of Kala-Azar [7, 30, 162]. Recently the latex test, agar gel test and fluorescent antibody technique have been preferred [72a, 228], being more specific than either C fixation or haemagglutination.

Antimony and diamine preparations proved to be effective chemotherapeutics against visceral leishmaniasis.

TRYPANOSOMIASIS

AFRICAN TRYPANOSOMIASIS (SLEEPING SICKNESS)

Trypanosoma gambiense is responsible for sleeping sickness in West Africa, whereas *T. rhodesiense* in Eastern and Central Africa. The protozoan parasites are found in the blood and can easily be recognized by the elongated shape of their body equipped with a single motile flagellum and also by their characteristic movement. The parasite is transmitted by various species of Glossina flies. *T. gambiense* causes disease almost exclusively in humans and the course is mostly chronic, whereas *T. rhodesiense,* whose reservoir are rodents, attacks both humans and ungulates and the infection usually takes an acute course.

Vectors engorging on infected humans or animals gain access to the agent in the blood of the host and convey it to other hosts after about 20 days of their life cycle. The bite of these flies is not painful. As the two trypanosome species scarcely differ from one another in morphology and life cycle, the changes caused by them cannot be grossly differentiated from one another in most of the cases. In the early stage of trypanosomiasis, the reticuloendothelial system and the heart are affected while in the advanced stage a chronic meningoencephalitis develops. Histologically proliferation of the plasma cells and a marked fibrosis are found in the enlarged lymph nodes. Infection by *T. rhodesiense* causes dilatation and hypertrophy of the heart. Microscopically lymphocytes, plasma cells and histiocytes are seen in the epicardium and myocardium. The brain parenchyma shows oedema and petechiae, and plasma cells and histiocytes are found in it on microscopic examination.

Clinically the first signs are the appearance of a painful, inflamed papule at the site of inoculation and regional lymphadenitis. After 1–2 weeks fever and chills appear at the time of trypanosomal invasion of the blood. A generalized lymphadenitis develops and lymph nodes become characteristically enlarged in the posterior cervial region. Cutaneous rashes, erythema and oedema are also frequent.

T. gambiense infections involve the central nervous system in the advanced stage. The patient becomes depressed and lethargic: death usually occurs due to an intercurrent illness. The disease may last as long as 2–6 years. Apart from the chronic form symptomless carriership may also occur; such hosts harbour the trypanosomes in lymph nodes and cerebrospinal fluid.

T. rhodesiense infections take an acute course. Pancarditis and serous inflammation develop and the patient usually dies before the central nervous symptoms can develop. The course usually takes no longer than a year.

Human serum has a certain trypanocidal effect which is lost on heat inactivation for 30 min at 62–64 °C. The serum level of the trypanocidal factor depends on age—being higher in adults than in newborn—and on liver function [187, 240, 295]. It is associated with the β and γ fractions of serum globulin. In animal experiments, susceptibility to infection by trypanosomes was found to have increased after splenectomy and blocking of the reticuloendothelial system [66].

It has been shown that experimental animals can be rendered resistant to trypanosome infection by pretreatment with spirochetes or bacterial endotoxin

[78, 268]. A protective hyperimmune state could, however, only be provoked in animals born in endemic areas and exposed to infection early in postnatal life.

Antibodies formed in response to trypanosome infection are demonstrable by serological methods. The C fixation test becomes positive 7–15 days after infection [64, 215]. The C fixing antibody titre falls or becomes nil in the advanced stage when the nervous system becomes involved. C fixing antibodies also disappear in response to treatment. Opinions differ as regards the value of the agglutination test; some authors regard it as species-specific, others as strain-specific [87b, 273].

Indirect haemagglutination with an appropriate antigen is a sensitive and reliable test in all protozoiases, including trypanosomiasis [82]. Precipitation test is used for antigen analysis rather than for diagnostic purposes [260, 317]. The fluorescent antibody test cannot be applied in trypanosomiasis, because it very often cross-reacts with antibodies to malaria [251].

Immunization experiments against trypanosomiasis have been conducted for more than 50 years, above all with trypanosomes recovered from the blood because the forms developing in the vector failed to show any immunogenic effect [87a, c]. Experimental immunization of mice was successful [139].

Arsenic and antimony preparations have been used for the therapy of trypanosomiasis. Chemotherapeutics are applied for prophylactic purposes.

SOUTH AMERICAN TRYPANOSOMIASIS (CHAGAS' DISEASE)

Chagas' disease produced by *Trypanosoma cruzi* occurs in almost all countries of South America. It is transmitted by various Rhodnius and Triatoma blood-sucking bug species.

Vectors biting infected humans, monkeys, dogs or cats engorge the parasite with the blood and the metacyclic trypanosomes are passed in the faeces 8–10 days or more after initial infection. Infection of the host takes place through the skin, into which the bug rubs the excretion and with it the parasites at a subsequent bite. The spread of the disease is closely related with the housing conditions and the multiplication of the vectors, whence in those areas where the vectors are indigenous and social conditions are poor, single houses may become endemic focuses. Transmission can also occur by the transplacentar route or with blood transfusion.

The acute stage of Chagas' disease is characterized by inflammatory and degenerative changes. Lymphocyte and plasma cell infiltration, as well as macrophages packed with parasites appear in various organs.

At a later stage, cardiac hypertrophy and — microscopically — lympho- and plasmacytic infiltration and myocardial cellular hypertrophy are found. Megaoesophagus, megacolon and destruction of neurons may also occur.

An inflammatory granuloma (chagoma) develops in Chagas' disease at the site of inoculation. Bites are predominantly found on the face, a unilateral oedematous swelling being characteristic.

The disease may be symptomless, with or without transition to chronic course, but an acute form may also develop, above all in children. Swelling of the pre-auricular lymph nodes in the acute stage is followed by ascending fever in the night, and an often lethal myocarditis may set in.

If the disease runs a chronic course, dyspnoea, oedema and thoracic pain appear owing to heart failure. The patients usually die within six months to one year, but a protracted course of five years is not infrequent. If the thyroid gland is also involved, symptoms of myxoedema develop, and affection of the central nervous system may cause regional paralysis and tremor.

On transplacental transmission *T. cruzi* causes a condition reminiscent of acquired Chagas' disease in the newborn infant.

The relationship between infection and host resistance has been extensively studied. Chagas soon realized that young people are more severely affected than older ones [44]. An increase of the parasite population was found during pregnancy in mice experimentally infected with *T. cruzi* [35, 79, 170]. The role of endocrine factors were also examined. Activation of latent trypanosomiasis was observed in monkeys treated [262], whereas ACTH showed an opposite effect in dogs [237]. The earlier view that hypothyroidism predisposes for *T. cruzi* infection could not be substantiated experimentally. Susceptibility becomes lowered in hosts on high protein diets. Restriction of pantothenate, pyridoxine and vitamin A in the diet was found first to increase, later to decrease the resistance of the host [319]. Studies on the relationship between parasitaemia and temperature in mice showed an increasing tendency of the former below 37 °C [14, 301].

Many aspects of natural resistance and cell-mediated and humoral immunity to Chagas' disease are still unclear. In animal experiments, humoral antibodies appeared earlier after the infection than the cell-mediated immune response [304]. The phagocytic activity of macrophages, supported by the action of non-lytic or opsonin-like factors, is a very important element of protection against the parasite [223, 224].

Demonstration of antibodies as well as isolation and identification of the parasite are very difficult in all stages of Chagas' disease except the acute period. The C fixation test has since long been widely employed for serological diagnosis. Standardization of antigen and technique was proposed by the Pan American Health Organization in 1966 [11, 95, 178, 289]. The test procedures elaborated by various teams are sufficiently specific for use in epidemiological surveys.

Indirect haemagglutination test has the advantage over C fixation that it detects the antibody sooner after infection [195] also at high dilution (above 1 : 1,000), and cross-reactions with antibodies to malaria, amoebiasis, tuberculosis and syphilis do not yield false positive results.

The fluorescent antibody test has also been gaining ground in the immunological diagnosis of trypanosomiasis. It is more specific and sensitive than the C fixation and haemagglutination in the acute stage of the disease [12]. The determination of the IgM fraction is of diagnostic value in the acute and connatal forms of Chagas' disease [86]. Immunization experiments in mice have yielded promising results [163].

No effective chemotherapeutic has yet been found, although recently good results have been obtained with nitrofurazone [16, 31].

AMOEBIASIS

The cosmopolitan protozoan *Entamoeba histolytica* usually causes a mild disease in the moderate climatic zone, but extraintestinal amoebiasis and amoebic dysentery are frequent in subtropical and tropical regions.

E. histolytica is an intestinal parasite. It has two forms: the trophozoite, which is responsible for the pathogenic effect, and the inactive cyst, which is surrounded by a resistant wall.

The source of *E. histolytica* infection is the infected individual. As trophozoites deteriorate rapidly when passed to the exterior, the more resistant cyst form plays the major role in the spread of the protozoan. It is transmitted primarily by direct contact (hand to mouth), but indirect transmission by contaminated water, soiled vegetable and fruit as well as flies also frequently occurs.

The cysts are swallowed and being resistant to the action of digestive juices, pass uninjured into the ileocoecal segment of the intestine, where they find an optimum milieu for the excystation of the trophozoites. The excysted stages are passed into the large intestine and some of them may even reach the appendix. In part of the cases they establish themselves in the intestinal lumen, in part they penetrate the intestinal wall by means of their proteolytic enzyme. Apart from the virulence of the parasite population, penetration is greatly influenced by the general condition, immunological status and feeding habits of the host, by climatic conditions, by the local resistance of the intestinal wall and by the bacterial flora of the intestines. The amoebas establishing themselves in the intestinal wall invade the tissues, thereby causing ulceration, often in association with a secondary bacterial infection. The parasites in the ulcerated areas may erode the blood vessels and pass into various organs via the blood stream.

An inflammatory response arises in the invaded tissues, which later progresses to necrosis. The inflamed area around the necrotic lesions is invaded by eosinophilic cells, lymphocytes, degenerated cells and amoebas.

E. histolytica infection may elicit a wide variety of conditions, ranging from symptomless carriership to severe, often lethal complications. Extra-intestinal processes may also supervene. The acute stage of amoebiasis is marked by severe dysenteric symptoms, such as haemorrhagic and/or mucous diarrhoea, high fever and acute abdominal pain. Tissue invasion may give rise to hepatitis or metastatic ulceration in the liver, brain or lungs. The outcome of the disease may be fatal, but spontaneous recovery may also occur. In mild forms, the coecal and sigmoid ulcers are either less numerous or less extensive so that no intestinal symptoms besides the diarrhoea occur.

After the acute clinical symptoms subside, transition to the chronic stage may occur. Chronic amoebiasis is characterized by gastrointestinal symptoms, colitis and nervous symptoms: focal hepatitis or hepatosis may also develop.

Activation of chronic amoebiasis may occur at any time, giving rise to reappearance of the acute clinical form. As acute and chronic processes may alternate, transition of intestinal to extra-intestinal form is always possible.

Frequent reappearance of the condition may cause a circumscribed thickening of the intestinal wall. In such cases the elements of inflammatory granuloma become predominant in the proliferating connective tissue. This condition may produce the clinical signs of a colon tumour.

Cutaneous amoebiasis is rare, occurring mainly in the perianal region, but ulceration due to fistula formation may take place in any cutaneous region. In some cases amoebiasis is accompanied by allergic skin phenomena, such as eosinophilic erythrodermia, or Quincke's angioedema.

The symptom-free state of a considerable number of infected individuals suggests the presence of some kind of immunity to parasite, which, however, could not be proved so far.

In related studies on animals, experimental evidence was presented of the dissimilar susceptibility of guinea pigs and hamsters [170].

Relatively little attention has been paid to the study of acquired immunity in humans [258]. In dogs once acquired immunity was established, reinfection could only be produced in very few animals [285].

The specific antibodies formed in the host in response to amoeba infection may be utilized for the diagnosis. Indirect haemagglutination was found to be the most specific diagnostic test [72b, 104, 161, 176, 188, 278, 288], especially in patients with liver abscess; it is less reliable in the detection of cases with intestinal involvement. The initially high haemagglutination titre falls markedly within one year. The gel-diffusion test has also been widely employed, because apart from its diagnostic use, it is also suitable for studying the structure of the E. histolytica antigen [18, 173, 309]. The percentage of positive reactions is greater in tissue amoebiasis than in the intestinal form. The C fixation test has largely been superseded by the above reactions. Recently the presence of an amoeba immobilizing factor has been demonstrated in the sera of infected patients, which passes the placental barrier and can therefore be utilized for the detection of incipient infections in infants born in endemic areas, if the maternal serum is tested parallelly [25, 60]. The immunofluorescent technique has also been widely employed lately. It should, however, always be borne in mind that only the high antibody titres can be regarded as specific [85a, b, 132, 288].

As to allergic manifestations, a regular hypersensitivity reaction cannot be expected on the basis of either clinical picture or histological lesions. Studies with skin test have shown that in amoebiasis, delayed-type reactions are mostly restricted to the stage of tissue invasion and even then are of short duration. The cutaneous test, being much less sensitive than the serological reactions, should be employed for epidemiological studies with due criticism [174]. In amoebiasis, like in other parasitic diseases, there is a rise of certain immunoglobulins in the serum. Certain authors observed a significant rise of IgA and IgM levels in the early stage of tissue invasion by E. histolytica [175], while others found an elevated IgG level in the intestinal form and rise of IgE in both forms of amoebiasis [60]. It is expected that counter-immunoelectrophoresis, a rapid and simple technique, will contribute to the immunological diagnosis of invasive amoebiasis [179].

Comparison of the results of serological and faecal examinations has indicated that the microscopical examination of faeces is indispensable for the reliable diagnostic evaluation of amoebiasis [105].

For therapy of amoebiasis emetin and its derivatives, halogenated quinolines, organic arsenicals and metronidazol are applied; antibiotics are used as indirect amoebicidals against supervening bacterial agents.

MALARIA

Malaria is transmitted by anopheline mosquitoes. It is endemic in the region between latitudes 40 degrees North and 30 degrees South.

Plasmodium vivax is responsible for tertian malaria: *Pl. ovale*, which resembles *Pl. vivax* morphologically, also causes tertian malaria. Quartan malaria is caused by *Pl. malariae* and the estivo-autumnal form by *Pl. falciparum*.

The parasite passes part of its life cycle in the mosquito (sporogony) and part in the blood of man (schizogony). The microgametes taken into mosquito hosts feeding on infected humans fertilize the macrogametes and the sporozoites thus formed are inoculated with the mosquito bite into man. The sporozoites soon disappear from the blood of the human host, establishing themselves in various organs, above all in the RES cells of the liver, spleen and bone marrow, further in the brain, where they develop into trophozoites. These invade red blood cells where merozoites develop by asexual division. The mature merozoites swarm out of the red cells and from some of them gametocytes (sexual plasmodial cells) are formed capable of initiating the sexual cycle when reaching the stomach of the mosquito host.

The pathological changes associated with malaria can only be understood if both the life cycle of the parasite and human immune response are taken into account. The merozoites leaving the red blood cells act as foreign bodies and at the same time cause the release of toxic substances by the disrupted erythrocytes. Merozoite release takes place at regular intervals, the length of which is characteristic for each Plasmodium species, and the process is accompanied by high fever. Accordingly, recurrent attacks of fever are the most characteristic symptom of malaria. The severity of the febrile course depends primarily on the resistance and immune response of the host. No complete immunity or protection develops against malaria, but a certain degree of resistance is acquired in the course of the recurrent infections. The acquired resistance is species- and strain-specific and is broken by massive infections, while recurrent mild infections may strengthen it. Patients with acquired resistance show milder symptoms and shorter febrile paroxysms.

In vertebrates malaria infection confers a low grade acquired immunity upon the host. The role of natural immunity is negligible. Resistance may be absolute, phase-linked or incomplete, depending on various factors, above all on the function of the lymphoid tissues and macrophages. Splenectomized experimental animals lose immunity, developing severe malaria on experimental infection [109, 226, 316]. Certain observations suggest that the liver may play a more important role in the maintenance of immunity than the spleen [89]. The role of genetic factors has been suggested by the observation that a high percentage of Europeans died in malaria in certain parts of Africa while the native population usually remained free from infection [313]. Natural immunity to *P. vivax* infection has been demonstrated in West African Negroes [320]. Recent findings on genetic abnormalities associated with natural resistance to *P. falciparum* have attracted attention to sickle cell anaemia in which the abnormal haemoglobin inhibits multiplication of the Plasmodium and to glucose-6-phosphatase enzymopathy. The influence of p-aminobenzoic acid has been pointed out by several investigators [47, 171, 318a] in connection with milk diets.

Age also plays a role in natural immunity: all human malaria agents except *P.falciparum* cause a more pronounced parasitaemia in young than in older persons.

Antibodies formed in the course of malaria may be utilized in the diagnosis. Acquired immunity is transmitted by antibodies through the placenta and later with mother's milk [33]. Protective antibody studies with *in vitro* cultivated Plasmodia require a careful checking *in vivo*. According to experimental observations, protective immunity may be of different degrees [264], being low if the disease takes a rapid, fatal course, full-value if a complete recovery takes place, and premunition only if the condition becomes chronic. The serum immunoglobulin level has been found to be higher in malaria [34]. IgM antibodies were demonstrated throughout the course of parasitaemia; their level kept rising until the appearance of IgG antibodies. A very high IgM level is demonstrable in adults by immunodiffusion [244]. Recently increasing importance has been attached to IgE in acute malaria [218].

Cell-mediated immune response to malaria is also believed to play a certain protective role [221, 318*b*].

In immunization experiments with attenuated strains or irradiated parasites a diminution of parasitaemia and prolongation of the survival of experimental animals have been observed.

For the serological diagnosis of malaria various tests have been applied. C fixing antibodies are demonstrable shortly after the onset of parasitaemia and persist in the blood several months after the elimination of the parasites from circulation. In the indirect haemagglutination test, the antibodies react with the homologous antigen at higher titres than with the heterologous (group-specific) antigen [279]. The gel diffusion test is suitable for serial examinations [184]. The stained slides can be used for comparative examinations later in the course of the disease. The immunofluorescent antibody test which is suitable for identification of the immunoglobulin classes has recently become widely used for diagnostic purposes [49, 299].

Chemotherapeutics used in malaria (*i*) must not be toxic for the patient; (*ii*) should kill all asexual forms of the parasite immediately and thereby relieve clinical symptoms; (*iii*) should act on exoerythrocytic forms and prevent relapses; (*iv*) should kill the gametocytes preventing thereby the infection of mosquitoes, i.e. vector transmission. Curative and prophylactic treatment are equally important. Acute malaria is usually treated with chloroquine diphosphate or sulphate, or amodiaquine dihydrochloride. In infections due to *Pl. vivax*, *Pl. malariae* or *P. ovale*, complementary medication with primaquine phosphate is required to destroy the exoerythrocytic forms. Both chloroquine and amodiaquine may be replaced with quinacrine hydrochloride, quinine sulphate or quinine dihydrochloride. Malaria caused by drug-resistant strains should be treated with sulphorthominidine, either alone or in combination with pyrimethamine, or simply with quinine. Chloroquine diphosphate or sulphate and pyrimethamin have been most widely used for prophylaxis. Apart from drug treatment, protection against mosquito bite is an important element of prevention in endemic areas.

TERTIAN MALARIA

The incubation period of tertian malaria is 8–31 days, but it may be longer in the temperate, climatic zones. Prodromal symptoms preceding the febrile paroxysms are headache, nausea, muscle soreness and enteric troubles. Recurrent infections fail to produce prodromal symptoms. The first stage of the disease is characterized by attacks of chills, followed by a stage of high fever lasting 6–8 h; during the third, sweating, stage the patient abruptly breaks out into a profuse perspiration and temperature drops to normal. The paroxysms last 8–12 h and recur on alternate days. Ten to twelve attacks are followed by a spontaneous recovery due to immunity developed in the meantime. Relapses of malaria depend on the Plasmodium strain involved and on the general condition of the patient. Tertian malaria may persist as long as three years.

Tertian malaria caused by *Pl. ovale* is manifested after an incubation period of 11–16 days. The clinical course is in every respect similar to vivax malaria except that it is somewhat milder.

QUARTAN MALARIA

The incubation period is 28–37 days. The paroxysms occur at intervals of 72 h. The rise of temperature is less abrupt and its fall is more rapid than in tertian malaria. The disease may reappear after a period as long as 30–40 years following the first infection and spontaneous recovery is rare.

ESTIVO-AUTUMNAL MALARIA

Synonyms: Tropical, malignant tertian malaria. The incubation period is 7–27 days and paroxysms occur every 36 to 48 h. This type of malaria is the most severe of all, because the afebrile intervals separating the febrile attacks are extremely short and the multiplying parasites may obstruct the capillary vessels of the visceral organs. Cerebral, septicaemic and intestinal involvement may occur depending on the localization of the parasite.

TOXOPLASMOSIS

Although the incidence of the causative agent *Toxoplasma gondii* is high, affirmed cases of human toxoplasmosis are relatively rare.

The life cycle of *T. gondii* includes sexual and asexual stages. Sexual development occurs exclusively in the final host, the cat, while asexual forms may be found in all the intermediate hosts including man, various animals and the cat itself [98, 122].

Since the parasite may occur in practically all animal species, the sources of infection for man are unlimited. Infection can take place by alimentary, aerogenic and transplacental routes.

According to experimental observations the pathological effect of Toxoplasma depends on the presence of the so-called Jettmar factor, on age—being more frequent in young people—and on the hormone levels of the host (oestrogen and cortisone promote the process) [99*b*, 127*a*, 136, 168, 286]. The virulence of the strain is another decisive factor [24, 248].

After infection the Toxoplasma tachyzoites multiply rapidly in the lymph nodes and may be carried to various organs via the blood and lymphatic circulation. The parasites have the greatest affirmity to the central nervous system and RES cells. Antibody production begins 5–6 days after infection; the Toxoplasmas form clusters and become encysted. The protozoa enclosed by the cyst, the bradyzoites, are sheltered from the action of antibodies. Rupture of the cyst wall may occur under the influence of cytostatic chemotherapy, corticosteroid treatment or gravidity, and the trophozoites released may give rise to a new generation and to reappearance of the pathological symptoms [99c, 305].

In the lymph nodes and involved organs the parasites cause an inflammatory cellular reaction with infiltration by mononuclear cells, macrophages and, infrequently, also by neutrophils; this is followed by the development of necrotic foci. Encysted Toxoplasmas may persist in skeletal muscles, myocardium, brain, etc. which are often only detected at post mortem examination.

The greater part of Toxoplasma infections are either symptomless or take an inconspicuous clinical course. Severe symptoms only occur in a small percentage of the cases, frequently assuming a non-characteristic form.

Toxoplasmosis may either develop as an intrauterine disease (congenital toxoplasmosis) or postnatally (acquired toxoplasmosis). Intrauterine toxoplasmosis may show the so-called classical triad of symptoms, namely chorioretinitis, hydrocephalus and intracerebral calcification [71], or it may be generalized with purpura, hepatitis and splenomegaly. The central nervous system and the eyes are frequently involved but these symptoms may appear as late as several months or years after birth [50].

In the course of acquired toxoplasmosis acute, subacute, chronic and relapse stages can be distinguished. These cannot sharply delimited because the principal symptoms of toxoplasmosis may occur at any stage.

The acute stage is generally characterized by an influenza-like, polysymptomatic condition with fever, fatigue and muscle soreness. Subsequently either of the following forms may develop: (i) febrile (exanthematous); (ii) neural (meningoencephalitis); (iii) pulmonary (interstitial pneumonia); (iv) hepatic; (v) myocardial. The cases of glomerulonephritis associated with acute toxoplasmosis indicate that T. gondii should be included in the group of agents which can give rise to immune complex disease [82a].

Subacute toxoplasmosis is most frequently manifested as lymphadenitis, affecting chiefly young women. Usually the cervical, sub-occipital and axillary lymph nodes, less often the inguinal and mesenteric lymph nodes are involved. Differentiation of toxoplasmal lymphadenopathy from similar conditions due to other agents is only possible by histological examination and serological tests. Toxoplasma infection may also cause myocarditis, encephalitis, or chorioretinitis, depending on the localization of the parasites.

Chronic toxoplasmosis is characterized by predominantly ophthalmic symptoms. Cysts in the retina become ruptured as a result of immunosuppressive action and the released trophozoites cause the characteristic toxoplasmal lesions in and around the macula. Congenital toxoplasmosis causes more severe ocular symptoms than the acquired form and it is also characterized by the simultaneous presence of healed and active processes. Granulomatous anterior uveitis may also occur; it is probably related to hypersensitivity [203].

Relapses in chronic toxoplasmosis have been extensively studied experimentally in different kinds of animals. Spontaneous occurrence of parasitaemia was demonstrated in mouse, rabbit and rat [128, 232, 314]. In pregnant parasitaemic animals the foetus also becomes infected [117].

Toxoplasma infection during pregnancy is important because the intrauterine damage of the foetus may result in abortion, premature delivery, and/or congenital toxoplasmosis. Opinions vary concerning the intrauterine damage in chronic toxoplasmosis and the therapy of Toxoplasma infection during pregnancy [8, 23, 65, 140, 220, 241].

As the symptoms of toxoplasmosis are not specific, the disease can mostly be diagnosed by laboratory methods.

Investigations into humoral immunity to toxoplasmosis have partly been concerned with the effect of antibodies on the parasites, partly with the diagnostic utilization of antibody assays. The effect of antibody on Toxoplasmas has also been studied electron microscopically [150, 265, 282, 296]. It was found that the antibodies first penetrate, then destroy the trophozoites. Antibodies are, however, ineffective against cysts because they cannot penetrate the homogeneous wall formed around the parasites.

In the cell-mediated immune reactions an important role has been attributed to the cells of the lymphoid-macrophage system (LMS) [83a, b, 216]. In mice, Toxoplasma infection stimulates phagocytic activity.

Sensitization of the host by Toxoplasma infection is demonstrable by the intracutaneous allergic test.

The Sabin–Feldman dye test which is a method for demonstration of antibodies has proved to be of great practical value in the diagnosis of toxoplasmosis. It is specific and a high-titre positivity is obtained shortly after the infection.

The C fixation reaction has also been widely employed; it is specific and reliable if pure Toxoplasma antigen, free from other cells, is used. The C fixing antibodies disappear earlier after the infection than the antibodies demonstrable with the dye test. C fixing antibody titres above 1 : 10 and Sabin–Feldman reactions above 1 : 1,000 are indicative of active toxoplasmosis. Low-titre reactions are not conclusive.

Standardization of the reagents is an essential requirement for both C fixation and indirect haemagglutination tests.

Diagnosis of toxoplasmosis by fluorescent antibody test has become more frequent lately, because the test procedure is rapid, sensitive and the reaction is specific [97, 101a]. It can also be employed for determination of the serum protein level, like in other infectious diseases, and the presence of certain γ-globulin fractions may furnish information on the infection: IgM rises in acute processes, whereas the IgG in chronic ones [297]. IgM and IgG levels may be sensitive indicators of therapeutic effect in acquired toxoplasmosis, and are probably even more important in the diagnosis of the congenital form [8, 233]. IgM antibodies are not transmitted to either foetus or newborn, appearing only if the latter is capable of an active response.

Toxoplasma infection induces a delayed-type hypersensitivity in the host. The intracutaneous test, which is suitable for routine diagnostic application, becomes positive within a few weeks after infection and this response persists for a long period, occasionally even for a lifetime [99a, 137].

Both humoral antibodies and cellular factors play an important role in immunity to toxoplasmosis but do not, unfortunately, confer a notable protection upon the host [198, 283].

As to the control of toxoplasmosis, prevention by vaccination would be the method of choice, but efforts along this line are still in the experimental phase [259].

Ideal chemotherapeutics against toxoplasmosis also remain to be found. Sulphonamide-pyrimethamine and spiramycin kill the tachyzoites, but have no effect on cysts.

SCHISTOSOMIASIS (BILHARZIASIS)

The disease can be caused by three species of blood flukes, *Schistosoma mansoni* and *S. japonicum* being the causative agents of intestinal schistosomiasis, *S. haematobium* of vesical schistosomiasis.

In the warm climatic zone, the number of persons exposed to infection has been estimated to be 350 million, that of infected persons 120 million. In Latin America *S. mansoni*, in Africa and South-West Asia *S. mansoni* and *S. haematobium*, in the Far East *S. japonicum* have been identified as causative agents.

The adult sexual stages live in the mesenteric and portal veins and in the venous plexuses of the urinary bladder. The eggs penetrate the perivascular tissues and the lumen of the respective organs by enzymatic action and are evacuated with faeces or urine. Ciliated miracidia hatch from the eggs coming in contact with fresh water. The miracidia develop to cercariae in snails acting as intermediate hosts. Man becomes infected on contact with water into which cercariae have been discharged by snails. The cercariae penetrate the skin or mucous membrane of humans and the schistosomules reach the lungs and then the liver of the host via the blood stream, where they develop to adults and copulate. Oviposition begins on reaching the final residence, the mesenteric and vesicular venules.

The pathological phenomena are elicited by migration of the subsequent developmental stages (cercariae, schistosomules, adult worms, eggs) in tissues and blood, by toxic and antigenic secretions and excretions of living parasites and somatic substances of deteriorating ones.

Schistosomiasis may have three clinical forms: (*i*) cercarial dermatitis (swimmer's itch), (*ii*) acute or toxaemic schistosomiasis (Katayama's disease) and (*iii*) chronic fibroobstructive schistosomiasis.

Swimmer's itch is manifested by the appearance of itching, papular skin lesions at the site of penetration of the parasites. Primary infection may take place without provoking a cutaneous reaction, but oedematous and erythematous large exanthems will appear on repeated exposure. Histological study of the skin lesions and passive transfer experiments have shown that both humoral and cell-mediated immune mechanisms are involved in cutaneous reactions to cercariae [48].

The main causative agents of swimmer's itch are cercariae of Schistosoma species parasitic in birds and rodents rather than in man.

Acute, toxaemic schistosomiasis is relatively rare, but severe and sometimes lethal. It is usually elicited by a massive primary infection, above all by *S. japonicum*.

The symptoms appear 16–60 days after infection, corresponding to the time of the schistosomules' migration and the beginning of oviposition. The main symptoms are recurrent fever, abdominal pain, diarrhoea, lymphadenopathy, hepato-splenomegaly, marked eosinophilia and general toxic signs.

The pathomechanism of acute schistosomiasis is practically unknown. While formerly the toxaemia hypothesis had generally been accepted, information emerging from newer findings suggests that the condition is essentially a specific kind of immune complex disease [176a, 221a, 311a]. The antibody level is low over the migration period of schistosomules but it rises rapidly at the beginning of oviposition under the influence of the massive antigenic stimulus, and as antigen is continuously present in excess, soluble antigen–antibody complexes are formed.

The immunological theory of schistosomiasis seems to be substantiated by the serum-sickness-like characteristics of the disease and by the development of glomerulonephritis in S. mansoni infections as well [15]. Immune lesions, viz. subendothelial or subepithelial depositions of γ-globulin in the glomerules were also found in monkeys infected with S. mansoni [32].

Chronic fibroobstructive schistosomiasis lasts for several years or decades, causing irreversible lesions. The lesions caused by adult parasites become manifest in the chronic stage. The blood flukes metabolize host substances, ingest erythrocytes and release substances and a haematin-like pigment. Parasites deteriorating spontaneously or killed by chemotherapeutics may also elicit pathological reactions either through release of somatic substances or mechanically, being carried by the blood stream as emboli.

The damage caused by the above factors is, however, negligible compared with the effects of eggs. The greater part of eggs deposited by S. haematobium in veins of the urinary bladder and S. mansoni and S. japonicum in those of the small and large intestines, migrate in the right direction towards elimination with urine or faeces, but a still substantial part of eggs escape excretion, being either trapped in the tissues of bladder or intestinal wall, or carried to the liver, lungs or other organs by the blood stream.

Eggs in the tissues soon become surrounded by an inflammatory granuloma called pseudotubercle. The tissue reaction may reach a size one hundred times larger than the egg itself. The granuloma progresses to necrosis and ulceration, or heals by scar formation.

Depending on the organ or organ system involved, the disease has also been termed urinary, intestino-hepato-lienal, cardio-pulmonary or ectopic granulomatous schistosomiasis.

The principal mechanism is practically the same in all the above forms. Infiltration of the parenchyma by eggs induces a tissue reaction which in turn affects the local blood supply. Granulomatous lesions of the vascular system lead to occlusion and hyaline thrombus formation which further interfere with both the local and regional blood supply.

The fibro-obstructive lesions arise as a result of the above damages. Thus, apart from the decay of the intestinal or bladder wall, hepato-splenomegaly, portal hypertension, probably even liver cirrhosis, ascites, oesophageal varix formation with or without an associated pulmonary hypertension may develop.

In mice, Symmers fibrosis of the liver can be elicited by infection with only a few cercariae [68]. Periportal fibrosis, portal hepatitis and septal fibrosis are sequels to primary granulomatous endophlebitis arising in the portal system.

Thus fluke eggs and granulomatous reaction to them play a fundamental role in the pathogenesis of chronic schistosomiasis. The eggs secrete an antigenic substance through ultra-microscopic pores in the egg shell. The secretion is of glycoprotein nature, having a molecular weight above 100,000 daltons [28].

Histological study of the granulomas and experiments with living eggs or isolated soluble egg antigen (SEA) have unequivocally shown that granuloma formation is a manifestation of SEA-induced delayed hypersensitivity, i.e. a cell-mediated immunological phenomenon.

Presensitized mice showed accelerated formation of larger-sized granulomas on intravenous challenge with eggs [312].

Histologically the central mass of the egg granuloma contains epitheloid cells and giant cells surrounded by a zone of fibroblasts and by an external zone of mononuclear cells, with a few eosinophils between them. The lesion is similar to the granulomas formed in tuberculosis, leprosy, sarcoidosis or berylliosis [116]. Passive transfer of hypersensitivity was only possible by lymph node or spleen cells, or by a transfer factor obtained from leukocytes [320a]. Studies by lymphocyte transformation and macrophage inhibition tests as well as investigations relating the eosinophil stimulation promoter have been conclusive of the presence of cell-mediated immunity [311b]. The antigen excreted by schistosoma elicited MIF production at a concentration as low as 10 μg/ml [21].

The bentonite granuloma appears to be an excellent model for the study of infectious and foreign body granulomas [27]. Untreated bentonite particles or those coated with heterologous antigen elicit a foreign body reaction, whereas particles coated with homologous antigen (Schistosoma, Mycobacterium, Histoplasma, etc.) induce the formation of large granulomas resembling those found in hypersensitivity reactions. Specific hypersensitivity is transferable to syngeneic recipients by immunologically active lymphoid cells.

Although the above considerations are unequivocally indicative of the pathological significance of the granulomatous reaction, no hasty conclusion as to the need for immunosuppression should be drawn. It has, namely, been found that in mice depleted of thymus dependent lymphocytes even more severe lesions developed; focal hepatitis with severe destruction of the parenchyma and liquefactive necrosis of the intestinal mucosa developed followed by toxaemia, septicaemia with high mortality [96].

The different stages of the parasite represent various antigenic stimuli to the host. In mice, 27 antigenic fractions could be demonstrated 6–7 weeks after infection with *S. mansoni* [103]. Some fractions were identified as proteolytic enzymes, capable of inducing immediate hypersensitivity in nanogramme amounts [263], others were unknown antigens inducing the production of 'lethal antibodies' to schistosomules. Among the latter C dependent lethal antibodies as well as antibodies activating protective cell systems were found [51]. As shown by *in vitro* studies, humoral antibodies, the C system and cooperation of normal leukocytes are fundamental elements of the protective mechanism against schistosomules [61].

Attempts to provide protection against the infection have either been based on cercariae attenuated by X-ray irradiation [115], or on cercarial antigens, e.g. the granular fraction prepared from the pre-acetabular gland of the cercariae, which contains the secretion inoculated into the dermis at infection [37]. Such experiments have as yet been only of theoretical importance.

Apart from egg demonstration, which is still an indispensable diagnostic tool, various immunological methods have been employed for the diagnosis of schistosomiasis.

The intracutaneous test becomes positive 4–8 weeks after exposure to cercariae. Its efficiency varies between 74 and 95 per cent. The immediate-type reaction is more sensitive; the positive response may persist for several years even in face of successful therapy, but false positivity is also frequent. The delayed-type reaction is more specific, but less persistent [320a].

C fixation with Chaffee-type antigen [43] may be valuable in early diagnosis, because positive reactions can be obtained from the third week after infection, i.e. prior to the beginning of oviposition.

The circumoval precipitin test [208a] can be used for evaluation of the activity of the process and the efficacy of chemotherapy, because it turns negative about eight months after the deterioration of eggs in the tissues.

Immunofluorescent antibody test performed, e.g. on cryostatic sections of adult schistosomes, appears to be suitable for evaluation of the degree of oviposition [294].

In the *Cercarienhüllenreaktion* (CHR) [307] positivity is shown by swelling and shedding of cuticular membrane of living cercariae incubated in immune serum. The sensitivity of the reaction is restricted.

As to the chemotherapy of schistosomiasis, at present hycanthon can be regarded as the drug of choice.

LARVAL CESTODES

CYSTICERCOSIS

Cysticercosis produced by *Cysticercus cellulosae*, the larval stage of *Taenia solium* is widespread in certain South American countries, but a sporadic occurrence has been noted is all regions where *Taenia solium* is indigenous.

Man is the definitive host of the tapeworm *Taenia solium*, the detached proglottids of which contain a great many eggs. The intermediate host is the pig, which becomes infected by ingestion of eggs containing the hexacanth embryo or oncosphere. The latter—being freed from the egg by the physical and chemical stimuli of the gastric and intestinal juice—penetrates the intestinal wall. Being carried into the tissues by the blood stream, it develops into the cystic larval stage, the cysticercus. When infected pork is eaten, cysticerci in man develop into adult tapeworms.

Man may also act as an accidental intermediate host if he swallows the eggs of *T. solium* and the embryos develop into cysticerci in tissues of the human body. The condition known as cysticercosis is infection with this larval stage of *Taenia solium*. Infection of subjects harbouring the tapeworm can also take place by endogenous or exogenous autoinfection. In the former case, eggs are passed into the stomach by regurgitation and then are returned to the small intestine, where they become activated and invade the tissues. In humans, the sites of predilection in which cysticerci develop are in order of frequency the subcutaneous connective tissue, muscles, brain, meninges, liver and lungs.

The full development of cysticerci takes about 9–12 weeks. The fully-grown stage is a 5–8 mm long bladder, containing clear, yellowish fluid and scolex. A special degenerated form is *Cysticercus racemosus*; this may be 4–6 cm in diameter and carries processes; it is often found in the brain or meninges.

The oncosphere invades the intestinal wall by help of the secretions of its penetration gland [267]. This process may elicit haemorrhage and cellular reaction in case of heavy infection. The oncopheres presumably lodge in the lymphatic pathways [269].

Fully grown cyticerci are often found in tissues without indication of any reaction. The majority of authors hold the view that a strong tissue reaction is only elicited by degenerating or dead cysts [181]. The elements of the cell reaction are polymorphonuclear cells, less often eosinophils, epitheloid cells, lymphocytes, plasma cells, macrophages and giant cells; the infiltrate formed by them later becomes fibrotic and finally it may calcify.

The symptoms are mild in most cases. The invasion by oncospheres may be accompanied by fever, and allergic or toxic phenomena. Cutaneous or muscle cysticercosis may give rise to a palpable swelling, periodic pain and calcification. Glaucoma, or an inflammatory reaction may develop in the eye; in case of nervous involvement, meningitis, focal symptoms, increased tension in the brain or hydrocephalus may appear. Radiological abnormalities and eosinophilia, pleocytosis, rise of protein and fall of glucose content of the cerebrospinal fluid may also be present.

The lack of reaction around mature cysticerci is an intriguing problem. In animal experiments, a protective immunity could be elicited with *Cysticercus pisiformis* oncospheres or developing larvae cultured for a maximum of 15 days, whereas live, fully-grown cysticerci had no such effect [106]. Condensation of collagen and infiltrating lymphocytes, macrophages and neutrophiles were also found around young, developing larvae of *Cysticercus bovis* [266]. Irradiation-attenuated *Taenia saginata* oncospheres conferred a firm protection against challenge in cattle [73].

Investigations along similar lines have indicated that active immunogenic substances are chiefly produced by pre-encystment stages, whereas in post-encystment stages either the enzymic activity of the parasite becomes altered, or the cyst wall layers produced by the host and the parasite successfully separate the two organisms in an immunological sense. A third alternative explanation is that the encysted parasite escapes immune recognition by the host.

On death of the cysts, structure-bound somatic substances of the parasite are presumably also acting on the host as antigenic stimuli.

There are indications that even fully-grown cysts may be killed in a host following exposure to homologous antigenic stimuli [148]. Other pathological conditions, e.g. tuberculosis, may probably also activate the latent parasitosis as has been observed in a fatal case of generalized cysticercosis [91].

For the immunological diagnosis of cysticercosis, most authors have preferred the immunofluorescent test. Sections of *T. solium* or *T. saginata* embryos or worms may be used as antigen. The reaction being group-specific, positive results may be obtained in tapeworm infection, echinococcosis, coenurosis and in other types of cysticercosis as well [36, 59, 247].

Effective chemotherapeutics against cysticercosis remain to be found. The evaluation of experimental therapy with mebendazole, metrigonate and other preparations would be premature.

The disease has two forms depending on the causative tapeworm species. Hydatid disease is produced by *Echinococcus hydatidosus*, the larval stage of the cosmopolitan *E. granulosus*. The dog is the definitive host and sheep, hogs, cattle and man are intermediate hosts. *Echinococcus alveolaris*, the larval stage of *E. multi-locularis*, is responsible for the alveolar hydatid disease. The fox and cat are the definitive hosts and microtine rodents act as intermediate hosts. This second type occurs focally in certain regions of Europe and the Arctic zone.

Humans become infected by eggs evacuated in the faeces of the definitive host. Human echinococcosis is in many respects similar to cysticercosis. In this case, too, man is acting as an accidental intermediate host. Oncospheres hatched from eggs in the small intestine are capable of invading the tissues, but unlike cysticerci, most embryos are retained in the liver, the rest in the lungs, developing to larvae in these organs. Oncospheres gaining access to the arterial blood stream may be carried to any organ or tissues, such as muscles, kidney, bones, brain, etc.

The cystic larval form of *E. granulosus* contains abundant fluid and it is sharply demarcated against its surroundings, whereas that of *E. multilocularis* is a solid, tumour-like body, closely associated with the surrounding tissues, owing to infiltrative growth. The inner structure is alveolar and necrosis of the central part is frequently found in stages lodging in man.

The fertile cysts contain many invaginated protoscolices, which infect the carnivorous definitive hosts when ingested. The hydatid cyst is filled with a transparent or slightly opalescent, colourless fluid of antigenic nature, whereas the alveolar hydatid cyst contains proliferating vesicles filled with a gelatinous mass and surrounded by a fibrous stroma. The protoscolices released on disruption of the hydatid cyst may give rise to secondary cysts. The alveolar hydatid cysts found in humans are generally infertile, no scolices being formed in them.

Oncospheres establishing themselves in tissues may become encapsulated by infiltrating mononuclear and eosinophilic cells and, as a result, may die.

The developing larval stages become surrounded by three reactive layers, (*i*) an inner coat composed of mononuclear cells and eosinophils, (*ii*) an intermediate layer of fibroblastic granulomatous tissue and (*iii*) an outer fibroblast layer [315]. Finally, the host surrounds the parasite with an adventitial protective capsule.

The clinical symptoms are usually due to the following effects of the parasite [133]: mechanical compression, infection, secondary pulmonary complications, toxic-allergic phenomena, rupture, concomitant anaphylactic events, obliteration of bile duct and deterioration of the cyst.

The diagnostic criteria of alveolar hydatid disease are regular or nodular hepatomegaly with or without obstructive jaundice, eosinophilia, high alkaline phosphatase level and hyperproteinaemia with hypergammaglobulinaemia. Laparoscopy and liver biopsy are indispensable for diagnostic evaluation [229].

Both immediate and delayed hypersensitivity related to larval echinococcosis can be detected by cutaneous test. The IgE level was above 700 IU/ml, on average 1,670 IU/ml, in more than half of the cases studied [40, 67*a*]. Reaginic response can also be employed as a diagnostic test in hydatid disease [9]. The PCA test performed on albino guinea pigs showed positive reaction with 94.4 per cent of sera.

Positive inhibition was found in the leukocyte migration test, performed on a few occassions to affirm the presence of delayed hypersensitivity [40].

It is, nevertheless, still unclear which are the factors of the host-parasite relationship with which these mechanisms might be linked. The problem of common antigenic factors also needs consideration. Human serum protein components [154], P blood group substance [270] as well as other host-specific or Forsmann antigens have been found inside the echinococcus cyst. It is not known whether these phenomena, also observed with other helminths can be interpreted as signs of the adaptive effort of the parasite to obviate imminent destruction by immune response of the host.

C fixation and haemagglutination tests can now be regarded as classical serodiagnostic procedures. The efficiency of the C fixation test has been estimated to be about 60–70 per cent [1, 80]. The sensitivity and specificity of the haemagglutination test seem to be more favourable being about 90 per cent [80, 280].

The Casoni skin test although sensitive, often produces reactions which are biologically not specific [80].

Diagnosis should always be based on several tests. Good results have been obtained combining the Casoni test with determination of the eosinophil count and ESR, and with latex agglutination [81].

The diagnostic value of immunofluorescent antibody test, which has recently been employed for detection of hydatid disease [245], cannot be judged until further experience becomes available.

Chemotherapeutic approach to human echinococcosis remains to be found. In sheep, promising results have been obtained by immunization [74]. Animals immunized actively or passively with hydatid antigen + vitamin B_{12} as adjuvant, or hydatid antigen + immune γ-globulin, showed abnormal thickening of the adventitia, calcification of the cyst wall and degeneration of the germinal layer.

DIRECT INFECTION INTESTINAL NEMATODES WITH TRANSITORY LARVAL TISSUE STAGE

ASCARIASIS (ROUNDWORM INFECTION)

Ascariasis is produced by the roundworm *Ascaris lumbricoides*. On oral infection with eggs, the larvae hatch in the small intestine, penetrate the mucous membrane and are carried to the lungs via the lymph or blood stream. They break out of the pulmonary capillaries into the bronchial tree, ascend the trachea and migrate up to the glottis and enter the digestive tract again. They reach their final residence in the small intestine, where the larvae develop to sexually mature adult worms.

In the course of migration the larvae may be retained by various tissue barriers and may be killed there by the cellular reaction. Such barriers are the intestinal mucosa or submucosa, the lymph nodes, and—for larvae finding their way into the portal circulation—the liver and finally the lungs. The trapped larvae become surrounded by infiltrating eosinophils and histiocytes.

The tissue reaction is stronger on reinfection so that fibrinoid necrosis and epitheloid and giant cell granuloma occasionally even a haemorrhage may develop around the dead larva.

The symptoms appearing 5–7 days after infection are fever, disorders of respiration and pulmonary circulation and, probably, an itching cutaneous rash. Among the many supervening conditions ileus, obstruction of the choledochus or pancreatic duct and intestinal perforation constitute the greatest risks.

The pathogenic effect of the adult roundworms is much more complex. These synthesize many biologically active substances. A very potent allergen, capable of eliciting a positive P–K reaction already in $10^{-8}-10^{-9}$ μg amounts, was isolated from adult stages [121]. Ethiopian children with ascariasis showed a 25-fold increase of the IgE level over normal controls [138]. Hypersensitivity reactions are aggravated by ascariasis, as shown by application of the Bordet phenomenon [284]. In guinea pigs infected with eggs of Ascaris the lethality of anaphylactoid reaction elicited by intraperitoneal administration of *E. coli* was significantly greater than in controls. At the same time, the activity of certain resistance factors becomes lowered in ascariasis. Rats infected with eggs of *A. suum* showed a threefold decrease of the complement titre, twofold decrease of lysozyme and 10 to 15 per cent reduction of the phagocyte index [225].

Various immunogenic enzymes have been demonstrated in roundworm extracts, e.g. malonic acid dehydrogenase [235] and aldolase [192], as well as anti-enzymes, among others an anti-tryptic fraction, which also strongly reduced the activity of leukocytic proteinase [151].

The polysaccharides of ascarids not only act as specific antigens, but also exert a powerful stimulating action on haematopoiesis [208b]. Extracts of Ascaris were found to contain a human A_2 isoagglutinogen-like substance, which presumably plays a role in the hypersensitivity mechanism [208c].

The mechanism of the granulomatous reaction induced by the larvae is still unclear. It is, nevertheless, certain that circulating humoral antibodies have a deleterious effect on the larvae [52]. Antigen-stimulated peripheral leukocytes showed immunoadherence to larvae sensitized with antibodies [196]. This phenomenon was C independent. The information emerging from both *in vivo* [149] and *in vitro* studies [323] suggests the fundamental role of cell-mediated immunity. A positive correlation was found between infection, the degree of leukergy and the result of migration inhibition test made with splenic cells.

Several tests have been tried to be applied for the serological diagnosis of ascariasis [53, 147, 153a] most of these, however, still cannot be used for routine purposes because of frequent non-specific and cross-reactions.

Levamisole and mebendazole proved to be highly active chemotherapeutics against ascariasis.

HOOKWORM DISEASE
(ANCYLOSTOMIASIS, NECATORIASIS)

This clinical syndrome is caused by infection with two closely related parasite species. *Ancylostoma duodenale* and *Necator americanus*.

Hookworm infections are especially prevalent in warm and moist climates necatoriasis being predominant in American countries and ancylostomiasis in the respective regions of other continents.

The larvae hatching from eggs passed in the faeces develop into infective, filariform larvae; these penetrate the skin or mucosa of the host, reach the lungs via the blood stream and, breaking through the alveolar walls, ascend to the glottis, are swallowed and pass into the upper third of the small intestine. The penetrating larvae produce itching, erythematous, papular lesions on the skin which are called ground itch. Tissue reaction to larval migration is usually milder than the granulomatous lesion caused by ascarid larvae.

Extensive lesions are chiefly found in the jejunum, where the adult worms are attached to the mucosa by means of their strong buccal cavity and feed on tissue fluids, mucosal fragments and blood.

The lesions are predominantly intestinal degenerative phenomena developing under the influence of local mechanical and toxic irritation which gives rise to haemorrhage, necrosis and, finally, to fibrosis. Loss of blood and lymph means loss of iron, protein and electrolytes as well, and consequent iron deficiency anaemia, hypoproteinaemia and electrolyte imbalance are particularly deleterious in undernourished populations.

Apart from a few observations on rise of IgE [38, 165], IgM, IgG and IgA antibody levels [182], little is known about the immunological background of hookworm disease in humans.

Experimental observations have chiefly been available on *Ancylostoma caninum* infection in dogs. Promising results have been obtained by vaccination of dogs with irradiated filariform larvae secured from a sterile culture [191].

Cryostatic sections of *A. caninum* can be utilized for the serological diagnosis of human infections using the immunofluorescent antibody technique [233].

Recently successful maintenance and transfer of *N. americanus* in gold hamsters has been reported [207, 261] creating new possibilities for *in vivo* studies.

The life span of the larva may be excessively prolonged, which accounts for the extremely long latency period of hookworm disease in some cases. Retarded development—as has been proved for trichostrongylid larvae—is due to factors affecting the infective larval stages outside the host, such as cold, lack of moisture, etc. Such larvae persist in a dormant state after infection. Living L_3-stage larvae were isolated from guinea pigs 29 months after infection with *A. caninum* [281], and in a human self-induced *A. duodenale* infection, eosinophilia developed eight months after infection, the eggs appearing in the faeces another month later [257].

Various chemotherapeutics have been used against hookworm disease, of which mebendazole, thiabendazole, pyrantel and bitoscanate appear to be the most satisfactory.

STRONGYLOIDIASIS

The life cycle of the causative agent *Strongyloides stercoralis*, is particular. The non-infective rhabditiform larvae hatch in the intestinal tract of the host and after being passed in the faeces may develop into infective filariform larvae in two ways either directly by metamorphosis or indirectly through a generation of free-living adult worms, the rhabditiform larval progeny of which become transformed to filariform larvae. A third type of development is auto-infection. In this case, rhabditoid larvae become transformed into filariform larvae inside the host.

Strongyloidiasis is endemic chiefly in subtropical moist regions, but outbreaks may also occur in groups of humans living under poor hygienic conditions (e.g. mental homes).

Infection takes place through cutaneous penetration and larval migration follows the same paths as in hookworm disease. The helminths typically inhabit the crypts of the doudenal and upper jejunal mucosa.

Percutaneous penetration elicits an itching macular or — on repeated exposure — papular exanthem, similar to the ground itch caused by ancylostomatid larvae. The pulmonary changes are more severe than in ancylostomiasis, their degree depend on the intensity of infection. Larval migration frequently produces Löffler's syndrome or a severe, haemorrhagic bronchopneumonia. This stage is characterized by marked eosinophilia which may occasionally reach 70–90 per cent. The intestinal symptoms are those of catarrhal, oedematous or ulcerative enteritis, depending on the severity of infection.

Strongyloidiosis presents certain remarkable features in respect of the host-parasite relationship. Unlike animal hosts of related species of Strongyloides, no protective response to *S. stercoralis* is observed in the human host [77]. This may account for the practically unlimited persistence of infection if no therapeutic measures are taken. At a recent survey of farmers who had been POWs during World War II, infection was still demonstrable in 10 per cent by faecal examination, and in as many as 40 per cent when the serum IgE level was also checked [185].

It appears that the immune state of the host also influences the mode of larval development in addition to genetic properties of the parasite strain and its adaptability to nutritional and climatic-environmental conditions. Recent findings in strongyloidiasis of pigs strongly suggest that larval development is always direct in the initial stage and a switch to the indirect mode must be connected with the development of host immunity [303].

Many fatal cases of strongyloidosis have been reported, in which death was due either to an acute abdomen, to haemorrhagic enteropathy, or to other reasons. In every case extensive filariform larval invasion was found in various organs, indicating auto-infection. Histologically, absence of eosinophils was often observed, suggesting an anergic state of the host. A common characteristic of the patients succumbed to strongyloidiasis was that they either had been under immuno-suppressive treatment [10, 227, 230] or suffered from some disease affecting the immune apparatus [214, 238]. It follows that suppression of the immune system may promote the development of the dangerous hyper-infective form of strongyloidiasis.

As to the serological diagnosis of the disease, the immunofluorescent antibody test seems to be the method of choice. In regions, however, where filariasis is endemic previous absorption of the test serum with filaria antigen is necessary to avoid cross-reactions [57].

Of the various chemotherapeutics tested, thiabendazole seems to be the most efficient preparation acting apparently not only on intestinal stages, but also on those lodged in different tissues.

DIRECT INFECTION NEMATODES WITH LONG-LASTING LARVAL TISSUE STAGES

TRICHINELLOSIS (TRICHINOSIS)

The causative agent is *Trichinella spiralis*. The disease is cosmopolitan in distribution. Relatively high incidence has been found in the United States and in certain European countries.

The adult parasites inhabit the duodenum and jejunum, are viviparous and begin to produce larvae as early as the fifth day after infection. Larval migration takes place via the lymph and blood stream. The young larvae pass from the pulmonary to systemic circulation and are widely distributed to all tissues but can only establish themselves in skeletal muscles where, breaking through the capillary wall, they settle in the sarcoplasm. Here they reach maturity after moulting, so that acid-fast, pepsin resistant, infective larvae are present in the host from about the 17th day after infection. This is the pre-adult stage. Pre-adult larvae then begin to coil and become encapsulated. The cysts either persist for years, retaining full powers of infectivity, or deteriorate and undergo calcification.

The infection spreads between carnivorous and omnivorous animals. The rat often constitutes a link between wild and domestic species. Man becomes infected by the consumption of inadequately cooked pork, pork products or game.

In accordance with the life cycle of the parasite, the course of infection includes four overlapping stages, viz. those of intestinal invasion, migration of the larvae and the muscular and chronic periods.

The intestinal stage is characterized by mucosal inflammatory phenomena, swelling of the villi, vascular congestion and oedema as well as progressive infiltration of mononuclear cells, mast cells and eosinophils. As a result of intestinal invasion, absorption of food is interfered with [41, 42, 56].

The larvae lodging inside muscle cells cause basophilic degeneration of the muscle fibres, nuclear proliferation and myofibrillar lysis. The non-invaded muscle fibres also show signs of degeneration and atrophy. Simultaneously, interstitial myositis develops with hyperaemia, oedema and leukocytic infiltration, containing many eosinophils.

Following encystment there may be no reaction at all but infiltrating lymphocytes and plasma cells may be found around some of the cysts which penetrate the cyst wall and give rise to granuloma formation with macrophages and giant cells around the dying parasites.

Practically all organs and tissues may become involved by larval migration, including the heart muscle, brain, meninges, liver, kidney and lymph nodes. Injury is partly due to direct mechanical effect of the larvae, eliciting diffuse interstitial or focal infiltration, partly to a general toxic effect.

The main symptoms of trichinellosis are gastrointestinal troubles, followed by fever, muscular pain, facial or palpebral oedema, hypereosinophilia with leukocytosis and myocardial involvement which may be clinically apparent or may only cause ECG changes. In severe cases a general toxicosis, circulatory failure and central nervous symptoms may be present.

The immune response to trichinosis is very characteristic. In primary infections, expulsion of the parasite, accompanied by inflammatory phenomena takes place after about 9 to 14 days [145]. The immunological background of expulsion is very complex. An early increase of IgM producing cells and later of those producing IgG occurs in the intestinal mucosa [54]. In *Nippostrongylus brasiliensis* infection, which has been used as a model of immunological phenomena in helminth infections, granules of intestinal mast cells showed signs of depletion of biogenic amines (histamine, 5-hydroxytryptamine), acid mucopolysaccharides and basic proteins during the rapid phase of expulsion [190]. At the same time intestinal nematode infections induce a strong homocytotropic, reagin-like antibody response [204]. This weighs in favour of the hypothesis that amine release induced by a homocytotropic antibody mast cell reaction might increase the permeability of intestinal wall, thereby enabling the access of antibodies to the parasite [129]. Experiments on passive protection by cell transfer [146], on transplantation of normal or antibody-damaged helminths [70], on nude (genetically athymic) mice [246] and other studies have suggested that parasites humorally injured in the first phase of expulsion are expelled by cell-mediated mechanisms in the second phase. In lactating rats, in which lymphocyte function is deficient, no expulsion took place, although a marked infiltration of the mucosa by degranulating mast cells and eosinophils was present. Antibody induced injury of the parasites had, however, been present before the mast cells became detectable [159]. On the other hand, inhibition of the expulsion by application of anti-lymphocyte serum was accompanied by suppression of mast cell mobilization [155]. In the inflammatory response to *T. spiralis*–macrophage–eosinophil interactions (formation of rosettes) have been found. The reason for this phenomenon is probably the presence of immune complexes on the surface of macrophages [309a].

Apart from the above humoral and cell-mediated reactions, factors related to the bone marrow are also involved in the mechanism of expulsion. The expulsion of antibody-damaged worms transplanted into rats exposed to 750 rad total body irradiation required both the reconstitution of the immune function of the mesenteric lymph nodes and bone marrow cells from either an immune or non-immune donor [69].

Following expulsion the host is fully protected against reinfection. The protective response is presumably elicited by the adult helminth [63], although a subcellular, granular fraction isolated from stichocytes of the pre-adult larvae was also shown to have a marked protective effect [67]. These granules probably contain preformed secretions of the stichosome.

Another intriguing aspect of trichinellosis is the encapsulation of the larvae in muscle tissue. This process is accompanied by fulminant pathological and clinical phenomena, after which the larvae may retain infectivity in the immune host for several years. Several authors have interpreted cystic transformation as an immune phenomenon [217, 236]. The cyst wall is permeable only to small-molecular substances, e.g. certain metabolites, but not to antigen or antibody molecules. This could explain the relative absence of reactions around the encysted larvae as long as the capsule is intact and the larvae are alive.

Various procedures have been used for the immunological diagnosis of trichinellosis. The most specific test which is, however, not sufficiently sensitive, proved to be the larval microprecipitation [242]. This reaction becomes positive from the third week after infection. Metabolic antigen or worm extracts, among which acid-soluble protein is a reliable reactant [186], have been employed in many serological diagnostic tests, such as bentonite flocculation test [252], C fixation test, latex agglutination [46] and immunofluorescent antibody test [80b, 250].

Seroconversion can be detected with the immunofluorescent test using infected muscle as antigen as early as 12 days after infection [22].

Thiabendazol seems to be the drug of choice in the treatment of this condition. ACTH or corticosteroids are often given during the stage of tissue invasion.

VISCERAL LARVA MIGRANS (TOXOCARIASIS, EOSINOPHILIA-HEPATOMEGALY SYNDROME)

Toxocara canis and occasionally, *T. cati* are the causative agents.

These canine and feline ascarids are very widely spread, affecting above all young animals. In these the infection is either congenital, or acquired shortly after birth. Infection may result from ingestion of eggs containing second stage, i.e. infective larvae. The larvae hatch in the small intestine of the adequate host, penetrate the intestinal wall and migrate via the liver, lung and larynx into the small intestine, where they develop to adult worms and lay eggs. In inadequate hosts (mammals, birds) and occasionally even in adequate ones (dog, cat), a special somatic migration takes place [20].

The larvae gain access from the pulmonary to systemic circulation, and although many die in various organs, encysted larvae stay behind in somatic tissues and remain viable in a dormant state for several months or years. The development of these larvae is arrested in inadequate hosts which, therefore, harbour second stage infective larvae [143].

It is conceivable that both adequate and inadequate hosts can become infected by ingesting carcasses; on the other hand, in natural hosts, pregnancy brings about activation of dormant larvae and transplacental infection. The mechanism of this activation is not known.

Humans, especially children, living in close contact with cats and dogs become infected by eggs attached to the animal's coat or shed to the soil. Larval migration is somatic also in man.

Larval penetration across the intestinal wall is a very rapid process. In mice, larvae were found in villi and submucosa three hours after the infection and at six hours they already entered the liver [45]. The larvae are first surrounded by granuloma tissue, later by a hyaline coat. Encapsulation of the larvae may result in an enormous cellular reaction consisting of infiltrating lymphocytes and plasma cells.

Usually a number of larvae are trapped in the liver, but may often cause lesions also in the heart muscle, striated skeletal muscles, brain, kidney, lymph nodes and the eye. Severe infections frequently give rise to hypereosinophilia lasting for several months, hepatomegaly, pulmonary symptoms, fever, hyperglobulinaemia, occasionally to cerebral, ocular or cardiac involvement and to disorders of renal function. Studies on rats [209] and mice [90] in maze experiments showed abnormal behavioural patterns, decreased learning ability and EEG alterations.

The diagnosis is confirmed by biopsy or necropsy. Above all liver biopsy is conclusive. Differentiation from other larval stages also migrating in tissues is, however, essential [200a, b].

Although antibodies have been demonstrated by various methods, such as haemagglutination [92], gel diffusion [120, 143a], bentonite flocculation [249] and immunofluorescent test [194], the results have not been specific enough. The presence of a complex, heterophilic antigenic pattern in the parasite is indicated by the finding that the sera of patients showed high levels of precipitating antibodies to A and B blood group substances, elevated isohaemagglutinin titres, agglutinating antibodies to sheep erythrocytes or thermostable antiglobulins [118, 119].

The circulating antibodies do not seem to have any protective effect in humans [93]. The degree and duration of symptoms were unrelated to the level of hypergammaglobulinaemia [118].

Nevertheless, second stage infective larvae appear to be immunogenic. Fourth stage larvae implanted into the intestines of immunized puppies developed to adults in due course, whereas second stage larvae failed to develop under similar conditions [94], and on exposure to immune serum, precipitate appeared at the orifices of the larvae [111].

Both the clinical signs and histological features of this condition are indicative of hypersensitivity. An immediate hypersensitivity response has been clearly demonstrated in both animal experiments [123, 210] and human infections [112]. The IgE response has been utilized as passive cutaneous anaphylaxis test in guinea pigs to diagnose human infections [153c].

Granuloma formation around the larvae suggests that cell-mediated immunity may play a major role, but experimental evidence of this hypothesis is still lacking. A notable protective action could be achieved with extracts of infective eggs given together with complete Freund's adjuvant [124].

No specific treatment has yet been found. Thiabendazole and diethylcarbamazine have been applied with varying success.

ARTHROPOD-BORNE NEMATODES. FILARIASIS

LYMPHATIC FILARIASES (WUCHERERIASIS, BRUGIASIS)

Of the two parasites producing this disease, *W. bancrofti* is indigenous throughout the warm regions of the earth while *B. malayi* in some parts of Asia and in islands of the South Pacific. The infection is transmitted by mosquito vectors, above all Culex and Mansoni species.

Adult worms may become lodged in pelvic lymph vessels, giving rise to lymph stasis, varicose lymph vessels and lymphoedema either by mechanical obstruction or due to inflammation. The most severe lesions are caused either by worms, which die spontaneously, or as a result of chemotherapy, or by the stages preceding microfilaria production. In the latter case, the reaction is presumably elicited by the exsheathing fluid released during the third or fourth moult [256]. In these cases there is thrombolymphangitis, with conglomerates of lymphocytes and eosinophil perilymphatic infiltration. A granulomatous reaction develops with a central necrotic area which is surrounded by epitheloid and giant cells, fibroblasts and eosinophils. The process is followed by a fibrous encapsulation.

Production of the microfilariae begins about one year after the infection. The females produce masses of larvae, which show a diurnal-nocturnal life rhythm, being lodged in various organs during daytime and invading the peripheral circulation at night. The microfilariae may themselves cause a granulomatous inflammation and their aetiological involvement in 'tropical pulmonary eosinophilia' seems to be highly possible.

The first clinical signs are painful local oedemas of allergic type, followed by lymphangitis, lymphadenitis and fever recurring at periodic intervals. Obstruction of lymphatic circulation chiefly occurs in the extremities and genital organs. Hydrocele, lymph scrotum, and funiculitis are frequent, especially in wuchereriasis. Chyluria is another characteristic symptom. The process may progress to elephantiasis in the chronic stage.

W. bancrofti larval whole worm antigen in skin test reacted with high specificity and sensitivity in all microfilaria positive cases [44a]. No cross-reaction was observed with intestinal worms.

FILARIASIS OF SKIN AND/OR SUBCUTANEOUS TISSUES

Loiasis (Calabar-swellings, fugitive swellings)

The disease produced by the parasite *Loa loa* is transmitted by Chrysops fly species. It is confined to tropical Africa.

The characteristic symptoms are a 'fugitive' cutaneous swelling, acute focal hypersensitivity reaction corresponding to the migration of the parasite in the subcutis, fever and hypereosinophilia. The larval stages, the microfilariae appear in the blood only several years after the infection. It is still a matter of controversy whether or not microfilaria are involved in the aetiology of various syndromes occurring in the course of chronic loiasis [298, 300], such as cardiopathy, encephalomyelitis and nephropathy. The histological appearance of the lesions is suggestive of an allergic reaction.

Onchocerciasis (river blindness)

The causative agent is *Onchocerca volvulus*. The disease is transmitted by black flies belonging to the genus Simulium. The disease is endemic in the equatorial zone of Africa, as well as in certain riverside territories of Mexico, Guatemala, Venezuela and Colombia. The parasites live within fixed nodules—onchocercomas—found in the subcutis.

The early lesions are characterized by a marked inflammatory reaction with perivascular plasma cell infiltration, whereas later on a fibrous capsule develops around the parasite. Microfilariae escape from the nodules and start migrating through the skin.

The symptoms are either caused by adult parasites, or by microfilaria. The latter appear in the skin or in the eye.

The severe complications of onchocerciasis are caused by the larvae migrating in lymph spaces and vessels of the connective tissue. The ocular lesions may involve practically all layers of the eye. The most frequent complication is acute punctate keratitis, which may progress to sclerotizing keratitis and pannus formation. Chronic iridocyclitis and cataract may also develop. Atrophy of the retinal pigment layer, chorioidal sclerosis and even atrophy of the optic nerve have also been observed. Severe ocular lesions leading to blindness usually occur in populations whose diet is vitamin A deficient.

Tissue lesions due to microfilariae begin with an eosinophilic cell infiltration, followed by the appearance of increasing numbers of plasma cells, mononuclear cells and Russel bodies. The vessels show swelling and proliferation of endothelial cells, then hyperplasia of the media and adventitia and obliteration of the lumen may follow.

It is conceivable from the foregoing considerations that in the endemic areas a substantial part of the adult population is clinically or economically blind.

Microfilariae also produce severe scleroderma-like cutaneous lesions, owing to hyalinization of collagen and fragmentation of the elastic fibres.

Dipetalonemiasis streptocerca (acanthocheilonemiasis)

The infection caused by *Dipetalonema streptocerca* is transmitted by some species of the genus Culicoides. The parasite occurs in certain tropical regions of West Africa. The adult worms inhabit the connective tissue, whereas the microfilariae are found in the cutaneous tissue fluids. The pathogenic importance of the species has been disputed.

FILARIAS INHABITING BODY CAVITIES

Dipetalonemiasis perstans (acanthocheilonemiasis)

The disease produced by *Dipetalonema perstans* is transmitted by biting midges of the genus Culicoides. The parasite is very widely spread in large areas of Africa and in certain regions of South America. The adult stages live in the peritoneal, pleural and pericardial cavities or in the mesentery, whereas the microfilariae inhabit the blood. The pathogenic importance of the species is still unclear.

Mansonelliasis ozzardi

Simulium and Culicoides insect species transmit the infection produced by *Mansonella ozzardi*. The parasite occurs in South America. The adult worms establish themselves in body cavities, the microfilariae are found in the blood. The pathogenic importance of *M. ozzardi* is still unclear.

TROPICAL PULMONARY EOSINOPHILIA

This peculiar disease has an unclear aetiology. According to recent findings, it might be caused by microfilariae. It is characterized by fever, asthma-like symptoms, lymph node enlargement, infiltrative pulmonary lesions and eosinophilia.

There is an extremely high serum IgE level ranging from 7,000 to 56,000 U per ml. Such cases have been regarded as the main sources of human polyclonal IgE [76].

In India, where the disease is very widely spread, leukocyte adherence tests showed a good correlation with wuchereriasis bancrofti, whereas positive reactions were only infrequently obtained with Dirofilaria antigen [306]. This seems to disprove the zoonotic filariasis theory advanced to explain the origin of tropical pulmonary eosinophilia.

GENERAL CONSIDERATIONS ON FILARIASIS

The animal parasites *Brugia pahangi*, *Dirofilaria repens* and *Dirofilaria immitis* may also live in humans. These and *Litomosoides cariini*, which can be maintained in the cotton rat and the mongolian jird, have been used for experimental filariasis research.

The view that immunopathological phenomena play a major role in the pathogenesis of filariasis is increasingly advocated.

The infection mobilizes all immune mechanisms of the host. In animal experiments, the appearance of IgM and IgG antibodies was observed 6–7 weeks after the infection [102a]. On surgical transplantation of adult worms, however, such antibodies were already found after 10 days, parallel with the encapsulation of transplanted stages [102b]. These presumably anti-adult antibodies have no influence on the development of microfilaraemia. The disappearance of microfilariae from the circulation during the latent phase is presumably due to a local cell-mediated immune reaction [19a]. Microfilariae found during the latent stage in the thoracic cavity of the rat carried adherent macrophages, eosinophils and giant cells. The adherent cells could be set free by treatment with anti-thymocyte serum [19b].

These findings and the observation on the probable role of exsheating fluid in the reaction [256] indicate that the individual stages differ from one another in immunogenicity and, consequently also in pathogenicity.

A very low protection, if any, is acquired in the course of filariasis, because the parasites may persist in the host for several years or decades, and even their death elicits adverse reactions. The results of vaccination experiments in animals nevertheless suggest that protection could be achieved by active immunization.

Dogs immunized with irradiation-attenuated third stage *Brugia pahangi* larvae showed an 57 per cent decrease of the worm count, microfilaria production became completely suppressed and no pathological lesions developed in 67 per cent.

Immunodiagnostic methods have yielded contradictory results, presumably for lack of standardization of antigen and technique [153b]. The dissimilar findings may also have been due to the fact that the quality and quantity of the circulating antigens depends on the activity of the parasite, degree of microfilaraemia and intensity of the tissue reactions. This has first been shown by cutaneous tests performed with whole blood from infected persons [98]. The observation that the antibody titre is inversely related to the degree of parasitaemia can also be regarded as an indirect proof [13].

The immunofluorescent antibody test seems to be the most sensitive of the techniques used in the diagnosis of filariasis [75]. Frozen sections of a homologous or heterologous filaria species may both be used as antigen. Purification of the extracted antigens used for haemagglutination, C fixation or SAFA reactions, is desirable [255]. Cross-reactions have been observed with various helminths, such as *Trichinella spiralis*, *Ascaris lumbricoides* and *Strongyloides stercoralis* [153b].

Immunocyto-adherence has recently been introduced for the detection of filarial infection [272], and has proved more sensitive than the serological methods [232, 310].

The chemotherapy of filariasis chiefly rests on the application of diethylcarbamazine [80a]. Microfilaraemia usually ceases soon after its application, but it takes a longer time to act on adult stages. Owing to its dramatic microfilaricidal action, however, diethylcarbamazine may cause side-effects, especially in infections with *Brugia malayi, Onchocerca volvulus* and *Loa loa*. These may include high fever and shock, in general, inflammatory reaction and oedema around the lymphoid organs, in lymphatic filariasis nephrotic syndrome and meningoencephalitis in loiasis [318c], and exacerbation of ocular and cutaneous symptoms in onchocerciasis.

Allergic manifestations are the more pronounced, the higher the degree of microfilaraemia. Allergic reactions have been attributed to an immune complex disease [172]. The antigen released by the deteriorating microfilariae is believed to react with circulating antibodies and the deposition of the complexes thus formed on biological membranes may be responsible for the symptoms.

The reaction may be reduced by local and systemic administration of corticosteroids.

REFERENCES

1. Abou-Daoud, K. T.: *Amer. J. trop. Med. Hyg.* **14**, 760 (1965).
2. Aburel, E. G., Zarvos, V., Titea, and Pana, S.: *Rumanian Med. Rev.* **7**, 13 (1963).
3. Actor, P.: *Exp. Parasit.* **10**, 1 (1960).
4. Adler, S. and Gunders, A. E.: *Trans. Roy. Soc. trop. Med. Hyg.* **58**, 274 (1964).
5. Adler, S. and Sadowsky, A.: *Lancet (Lond.)* **252**, 867 (1947).
6. Ah, H. S., McCall, J. W. and Thompson, P. E.: *Proc. Third Int. Congr. Parasit.* München, **3**, 1236 (1974).
7. Alencar, J. E., Hardi, A. and Pampiglione, S.: *Parasitologie* **8**, 147 (1966).
8. Alford, C. A., Stagno, S. and Reynolds, W. D.: *Bull. N. Y. Acad. Med.* **50**, 160 (1974).
9. Ali-Khan, Z.: *Proc. Third Int. Congr. Parasit.* München, **3**, 1214 (1974).
10. Ali-Kahn, Z. and Seemayer, T. A.: *Proc. Third Int. Congr. Parasit.* München, **2**, 690 (1974).
11. Almeida, J. O.: *Bol. Ofic. Sanit. Panamer.* **55**, 133 (1963).
12. Alvarez, M., Cerisola, J. A., and Rohwedder, R. W.: *Primer Congr. Latino americanode Parasit.* Santiago de Chile, Resumenes, p. 32, 1967.
13. Ambroise-Thomas, P. and Prodhon, J.: *Proc. Third Int. Congr. Parasit.* München, **2**, 638 (1974).
14. Amrein, Y. U.: *Parasitology* **53**, 1160 (1967).
15. Andrade, Z. A., Andrade, S. G. and Sadigursky, M.: *Amer. J. trop. Med. Hyg.* **20**, 77 (1971).
16. Andrade, Z. A. and Brener, Z.: *Rev. Inst. Med. trop.* **11**, 222 (1969).
17. Ansari, N. and Mofidi, C.: *Bull. Soc. Path. exot.* **43**, 601 (1950).
18. Atchley, F. O., Aurenheimer, A. H. and Wasley, M. A.: *J. Parasit.* **49**, 313 (1963).
19a. Bagai, R. C. and Subrahmanyam, D.: *Amer. J. trop. Med. Hyg.* **17**, 833 (1968).
19b. id., *Nature (Lond.)* **228**, 682 (1970).

20. Beaver, P. C.: *J. Parasit.* **55**, 3 (1969).
21. Befus, A. D.: *Proc. Third Int. Congr. Parasit.* München, **2**, 1055 (1974).
22. Belozerov, S. N.: *Byulleten' Vsesoyuznogo Instituta Gel'mintologii im. K. I. Skryabina* No. 9. 11 (1972). cit. *Helm. Abstr.* **43**, abstr. No. 2058 (1974).
23. Berger, J. and Piekarski, G.: *Proc. Third Int. Congr. Parasit.* München, **1**, 280 (1974).
24. Beverley, J. K. A.: *Nature (Lond.)* **183**, 1348 (1959).
25. Biagi, F. F. and Buentello, L.: *Exp. Parasit.* **11**, 188 (1961).
26. Biagi, F. F., Gueyara, I. and Rodriguez, L.: *Rev. Facult. Med. Mexico* **5**, 487 (1963).
27. Boris, D. L. and Warren, K. S.: *Immunology* **24**, 511 (1973).
28. Boros, D. L., Tomford, R. and Warren, K. S.: *Proc. Third Int. Congr. Parasit.* München, **2**, 1173 (1974).
29. Boysia, F.: Thesis. New Brunswick, N. J. Rutgers. The State University, 1967.
30. Bray, R. S. and El-Nahal, H. M. S.: *Trans. roy. Soc. trop. Med. Hyg.* **60**, 423 (1966).
31. Brener, Z. and Da Costa, C. A. G.: *Proc. Third Int. Congr. Parasit.* München, **3**, 1292 (1974).
32. Brito, T. de, Gunji, J., Cammargo, M. E., Ceravolo, A. and Silva, L. C. da: *Bull. Wld Hlth Org.* **45**, 419 (1971).
33. Bruce-Chwatt, L. J.: In *Immunity to Protozoa.* Ed. by Garnham, P. C. C. Blackwell, Oxford 1963, p. 89.
34. Butcher, G. A., Cohen, S. and Mitchell, G. H.: *Proc. Third Int. Congr. Parasit.* München, **2**, 1062 (1974).
35. Butterworth, M. V., McClellan, B. and Allansmith, M.: *Nature (Lond.)* **214**, 1224 (1967).
36. Calamel, M. and Soule, C.: *Revue de Medicine Veterinaire* **123**, 1105 (1972).
37. Campbell, D. L. and Stirewalt, M. A.: *Proc. Third Int. Congr. Parasit.* München, **2**, 1170 (1974).
38. Cappuccinelli, P., Frentzel-Beyme, R. R., Sena, L. and Cavallo, G.: *Giorn. Batt. Virol. Immunol.* **64**, 162 (1971).
39. Capron, A.: *J. Parasit.* **56**, (Sect. 2) 515 (1970).
39a. id., *Rev. franç. Mal. respir.* **3**, 421 (1975).
40. Capron, A., Vernes, A., Dessaint, J. P. and Capron, M.: *Proc. Third Int. Congr. Parasit.* München, **1**, 558 (1974).
41. Castro, G. A. and Olson, L. J.: *J. Parasit.* **51**, 57 (1965).
42. Castro, G. A., Olson, L. J. and Baker, R. D.: *J. Parasit.* **53**, 595 (1967).
43. Chaffee, E. F., Bauman, P. M. and Shapilo, J. J.: *Amer. J. trop. Med. Hyg.* **3**, 905 (1954).
44. Chagas, C.: *Mem. Inst. Osw. Cruz*, **1**, 159 (1909).
44a. Chandra, R., Govila, P. and Chandra, S.: *Indian J. med. Res.* **62**, 1017 (1974).
45. Chari, S. S. and Subramanian, G.: *Indian J. Animal Sci.* **42**, 957 (1972) cit. *Helm. Abstr.* **43**, abstr. No. 521 (1974).
46. Chicoine, L., Proulx, C., Lafleur, L. and Tanner, C. E.: *Canad. J. publ. Hlth* **57**, 357 (1966).
47. Colbourne, M.: *Trans. roy. Soc. trop. Med. Hyg.* **50**, 82 (1956).
48. Colley, D. G., Magalhaes-Filho, A. and Coelho, R. de B.: *Amer. J. trop. Med. Hyg.* **21**, 558 (1972).
49. Corradetti, A.: *Med. Parasit.* **34**, 673 (1965).
50. Couvreur, J. and Desmonts, G.: *Developm. Med. Child. Neurol.* **4**, 519 (1962).
51. Crandall, C. A.: *Proc. Third Int. Congr. Parasit.* München, **2**, 1161 (1974).
52. Crandall, C. A. and Arean, V. M.: *J. Parasit.* **50**, 685 (1964).
53. Crandall, C. A., Echevarria, R. and Arean, V. M.: *Exp. Parasit.* **14**, 296 (1963).
54. Crandall, R. B., Arean, V. M., Cebra, J. J. and Crandall, C. A.: *Immunology* **12**, 147 (1967).
55. Coutts, W., Silva-Inzunza, E.: *Premier Symposium, Européen, Reims, France,* Masson and Cie, Paris 1957.
56. Cross, J. K., Partono, F., Hsu, Mei-Yuan, Ash, L. R. and Oemijati, S.: *Proc. Third Int. Congr. Parasit.* München, **2**, 613 (1974).

57. Dafalla, A. A.: *J. trop. Med. Hyg.* **75**, 109 (1972).
58. Damian, R. T.: *Amer. Naturalist* **98**, 129 (1964).
59. Dao, C., Arnaud, J. P., Petithory, J. and Brumpt, L.: *Ann. Parasit, Hum. Comp.* **48**, 23 (1973).
60. Dasgupta, A.: *Proc. Third Int. Congr. Parasit.* München, **2**, 1109 (1974).
61. Dean, D. A., Wistar, R., Murrell, K. D. and Chen, P.: *Proc. Third. Int. Congr. Parasit.* München, **2**, 1051 (1974).
62. Dekhkan-Rhodzhayeva, N. A.: In *Progress in Protozoology. 3rd Int. Congr. Protozool. Leningrad.* Publ. House "Nauka" Leningrad 1969 p. 296.
63. Denham, D. A.: *Parasitology* **56**, 754 (1966).
64. Depaux, R., Merveille, P. and Ceccaldi, J.: *Amer. Inst. Pasteur* **91**, 684 (1956).
65. Desmonts, G. and Couvreur, J.: *Bull. N. Y. Acad. Med.* **50**, 146 (1974).
66. Desowitz, R. S. and Watson, H. J. C.: *Ann. trop. Med. Parasit.* **47**, 324 (1953).
67. Despommier, D. D. and Müller, M.: *Wiad. Parazyt.* **15**, 612 (1969).
67a. Dessaint, J. P., Bout, D., Wattre, P. and Capron, A.: *Immunology* **29**, 813 (1975).
68. Dias, R. P. and Alvarenga, R. J.: *Rev. Inst. Med. trop. Sao Paulo* **15**, 60 (1973).
69. Dineen, J. K. and Kelly, J. D.: *Int. Arch. Allergy* **45**, 759 (1973).
70. Dineen, J. K., Ogilvie, B. M. and Kelly, J. D.: *Immunology* **24**, 467 (1973).
71. Echenwald, H. F.: In *Human Toxoplasmosis.* Ed. by. Siim, J. C. Munksgaard, Copenhagen, 1959. p. 41.
72a. Enders, B., Hungerer, K. D. and Zwisler, O.: *Proc. Third Int. Congr. Parasit.* München, **2**, 1141 (1974).
72b. ibid., **2**, 1142 (1974).
73. Ershow, V. S.: *Proc. Third Int. Congr. Parasit.* München, **3**, 1232 (1974).
74. Evranova, B. G.: *Uchenye Zapiski Kazanskogo, Vet. Inst.. N. E. Baumana* **107**, 193 (1970), cit. *Helm. Abstr.* **43**, abstr. No. 891 (1974).
75. Eyck, D. R.: *Amer. J. Epid.* **98**, 283 (1973).
76. Ezecke, A., Perera, A. V. B. and Hobbs, J. R.: *Clin. Allergy* **3**, 33 (1973).
77. Galliard, H.: *Helm. Abstr.* (Review article) **36**, 247 (1967).
78. Galliard, H., La Pierre, J. and Rousset, J. J.: *Clin. Parasit. Hum. Comp.* **33**, 177 (1958).
79. Galton, M.: *Transplantation* **5**, 154 (1967).
80. Garabedian, G. A., Matossian, R. M. and Suidan, F. G.: *Amer. J. trop. Med. Hyg.* **8**, 67 (1959).
80a. Gentilini, M., Pinon, J. M., Nosny, Y. and Sulahian, A.: *Rev. franç. Mal. respir.* **3**, 429 (1975).
80b. Gentilini, M., Richard-Lenoble, D., Pinon, J. M., Niel, G. and Danis, M.: *Nouv. Presse méd.* **5**, 720 (1976).
81. Gilevich, Yu. S., Astanovitskii, F. S. and Vereyutin, Yu. M.: *Klin. Khirurg.* **6**, 54 (1972), cit. *Helm. abstr.* **43**, abstr. No. 2076 (1974).
82. Gill, B. S.: *Amer. f. trop. Med. Parasit.* **58**, 473 (1964).
82a. Ginsburg, B. E., Wasserman, J., Huldt, G. and Bergstrand, A.: *Brit. med. J.* iii, 664 (1974).
83a. Glowinski, M., Steplezski, Z., Waronski, W. and Waclawezyk, H.: *Zbl. Gynäk.* **86**, 26 (1964).
83b. ibid., **88**, 24 (1966).
84. Goble, F. C., Konopka, E. A. and Boyd, J. I.: In *Protozoology, 2nd Int. Conf. Protozool. London.* Int. Congr. Ser. **91**, 54 (1965).
85a. Goldman, M.: *Amer. J. Hyg.* **58**, 319 (1953).
85b. id., *Amer. J. trop. Med. Hyg.* **15**, 694 (1966).
86. González Cappa, S. M.: *Proc. Third Int. Congr. Parasit.* München, **1**, 217 (1974).
87a. Gray, A. R.: *Seventh Int. Sci. Comm. Tryp. Res.* p. 361 (1963).
87b. id., *Amer. J. trop. Med. Parasit.* **59**, 27 (1965).
87c. id., *J. Gen. Microbiol.* **41**, 195 (1965).
88. Greenwood, B. M., Playfair, J. H. L. and Torrigiani, G.: *Clin. exp. Immunol.* **8**, 467 (1971).
88a. Grove, D. I., Burston, T. O. and Forbes, I. J.: *Clin. Allergy* **4**, 295 (1974).
89. Fabiani, M. G.: *Bull. Soc. Path. exot.* **59**, 605 (1966).
90. Favati, V., Lugetti, G. and Parenti, G.: *Ann. della Facoltà di Med. Vet. Pisa,* **24**, 308 (1971).

91. Fejér, A., Bánki, Gy., Vámos, G., Majtényi, K. and Fónyad, L.: *Orv. Hetil.* **109,** 2885 (1968).
92. Fellers, F.: *Amer. J. Dis. Child.* **86,** 767 (1953).
93. Fernando, S. T.: *Parasitology* **58,** 91 (1968).
94. Fernando, S. T., Vasudevan, B., Jegatheeswaran, T. and Sooriyamoorthi, T.: *Parasitology* **66,** 415 (1973).
95. Fife, E. H. and Kent, J. F.: *Amer. J. trop. Med. Hyg.* **9,** 512 (1960).
96. Fine, D. P., Buchanan, R. D. and Colley, D. G.: *Amer. J. Path.* **71,** 193 (1973).
97. Fletcher, S.: *J. Clin. Path.* **18,** 193 (1965).
98. Franks, M. B.: *J. Parasit.* **32,** 400 (1946).
99a. Frenkel, J. K.: *Proc. Soc. exp. Biol. Med.* **68,** 634 (1948).
99b. id., *Amer. J. trop. Med.* **2,** 390 (1953).
99c. id., *Proc. Soc. exp. Biol. Med.* **103,** 552 (1960).
99d. id., In Marcial-Rojas, R. A. (ed.): *Pathology of Protozoal and Helminthic Diseases.* The Williams et Wilkins Co., Baltimore, p. 254. 1971.
100. Frenkel, J. K., Dubey, F. P. and Miller, Nancy, L.: *Science* **167,** 893 (1970).
101. Frothingham, T. E. and Lehtimaki, E.: *Amer. J. trop. Med. Hyg.* **16,** 658 (1967).
101a. Fuhr, R.: *Dtsch. med. Wschr.* **99,** 949 (1974).
102a. Fujita, K. and Kobayashi, J.: *Jap. J. exp. Med.* **39,** 481 (1969).
102b. ibid., **39,** 585 (1969).
103. Harris, W.: *Proc. Third Int. Congr. Parasit.* München, **2,** 1165 (1974).
104. Healy, G. R.: *Health Lab. Sci.* **5,** 174 (1968).
105. Healy, G. R., Gecason, N. N. and Brandt, F.: *Proc. Third Int. Congr. Parasit.* München, **2,** 1138 (1974).
106. Heath, D. D.: *Int. J. Parasit.* **3,** 485 (1973).
107. Herman, R. and Farrel, J. P.: *Proc. Third Int. Congr. Parasit.* München, **1,** 253 (1974).
108. Herrer, A., Thatcher, V. E. and Johnson, C. M.: *J. Parasit.* **52,** 954 (1966).
109. Hoare, C. A.: *Med. Parasit.* **34,** 678 (1965).
110. Hoffmann, B.: *Wiad. Parazyt.* **12,** 349 (1966).
111. Hogarth-Scott, R. S.: *Immunology* **10,** 217 (1966).
112. Hogarth-Scott, R. S., Johansson, S. G. O. and Bennich, H.: *Clin. exp. Immunol.* **5,** 619 (1969).
113. Honigberg, B. M.: *J. Parasit.* **47,** 545 (1961).
114. Honigberg, B. M., Livingston, M. C. and Frost, J. K.: *Acta Cytol.* **10,** 353 (1966).
115. Hsu, M. F. and Hsu, S. Y. Li: *Proc. Third Int. Congr. Parasit.* München, **2,** 828 (1974).
116. Hsu, S. Y. Li, Hsu, M. F., Lust, G. L. and Davis, J. R.: *J. reticuloendothelial Soc.* **12,** 418 (1972).
117. Hume, S. O.: *Amer. J. Obstet. Gynec.* **114,** 703 (1972).
118. Huntley, C. C., Costas, M. C. and Lyerly, A.: *Pediatrics* **36,** 523 (1965).
119. Huntley, C. C., Lyerly, A. D. and Patterson, M. V.: *J. Amer. med. Ass.* **208,** 1145 (1969).
120. Huntley, C. C. and Moreland, A.: *Amer. J. trop. Med. Hyg.* **12,** 204 (1963).
121. Hussain, R., Bradbury, S. M. and Strejan, G.: *J. Immunol.* **111,** 260 (1973).
122. Hutchison, W. M., Dunachie, J. F. and Work, K.: *Acta Path. Microbiol. Scand.* **74,** 462 (1968).
123. Ivey, M. H.: *J. Parasit.* **50,** 24 (1964).
124. Izzat, N. N. and Olson, L. J.: *Canad. J. Zool.* **48,** 1063 (1970).
125. Jaaknees, H. P. and Teras, J. K.: *Wiad. Parazyt.* **12,** 385 (1966).
126. Jaaknees, H. P., Teras, J. K., Roigas, E. M. and Nigesen, U. K.: *Wiad. Parazyt.* **12,** 378 (1966).
127a. Jacobs, L.: *Amer. J. trop. Med.* **2,** 365 (1953).
127b. id., *Advanc. Parasit.* **5,** 1 (1967).
128. Jacobs, L. and Jones, F. E.: *J. infect. Dis.* **87,** 78 (1950).
129. Jarrett, W. F. H.: *J. Parasit.* **56,** (Sect. 2) 508 (1970).
130. Jarret, W. F. H., Jennings, F. W., McIntyre, W. I. M., Mulligan, W., Sharp, N. C. C. and Urquhart, G. M.: *Vet. Rec.* **70,** 451 (1958).
131. Jarret, W. F. H. and Stewart, D. C.: *Immunology* **23,** 749 (1972).
132. Joanes, A. J.: *Brit. med. J.* **2,** 1531 (1964).

133. Jenkins, J. A.: *Post-grad. med. J.* **25**, 107 (1949).
134. Jenkins, D. C. and Phillipson, R. F.: *Int. J. Parasit.* **2**, 353 (1972).
135. Jerusalem, C., Jap, P. and Eling, W.: *Advanc. exper. Med. Biol.* **15**, 391 (1971).
136. Jettmar, A. M.: *Arch. Hyg. Bakt.* **146**, 511 (1962).
137. Jira, J., Jirovec, O., Frenel, F., Blaha, R. and Bozdech, V. Z.: *Ärztl. Fortbild. Jena,* **11**, 933 (1963).
138. Johansson, S. G. O., Mellbin, T. and Vahlquist, B.: *Lancet* i, 1118 (1968).
139. Johnson, P., Neal, R. A. and Gall, D.: *Nature (Lond.)* **200**, 83 (1963).
140. Jones, M. H., Sever, J. L., Baker, T. H., Hallatt, J. G., Goldenberg, E. D., Justus, K. M., Bonnet, C., Gilkeson, M. R. and Roberts, J. M.: *Amer. J. Obstet. Gynec.* **94**, 809 (1966).
141. Laan, I. A.: *Wiad. Parazyt.* **12**, 173 (1966).
142. Lainson, R. and Bray, R. S.: *Trans. roy. Soc. trop. Med. Hyg.* **60**, 526 (1966).
143. Lamina, J.: *Dtsch. tierärztl. Wschr.* **73**, 208 (1966).
143a. id., *Dtsch. med. Wschr.* **99**, 1070 (1974).
144. Lanceley, F.: *Brit. J. vener. Dis.* **34**, 4 (1958).
145. Larsh, E. J.: *Am. J. trop. Med. Hyg.* **16**, 123 (1967).
146. Larsh, E. J. jr., Race, G. J., Goulson, H. T. and Weatherly, N. W.: *J. Parasit.* **52**, 146 (1966).
147. Leykina, E. S.: *Bull. Wld Hlth Org.* **32**, 699 (1965).
148. Leykina, E. S., Moskvin, S. N., Sokolovskaya, O. M. and Poletayeva, O. G.: *Med. Parazit.* **33**, 694 (1964).
149. Lichtenberg, F. and Mekbel, S.: *J. infect. Dis.* **110**, 246 (1962).
150. Ludwig, J. and Piekarski, G.: In *Progress in Protozoology.* Ed. by Ludvick, J., Lem, J. and Vávra, J. Czechoslovak Academy of Sciences Publ. Prague 1961, p. 369.
151. Kadubowski, R.: *Proc. Third Int. Congr. Parasit.* München, **3**, 1476 (1974).
152. Kafuko, G. W. and Burkitt, D. P.: *Int. J. Cancer* **6**, 1 (1970).
153a. Kagan, I. G.: *J. Immunol.* **80**, 396 (1958).
153b. id., *J. Parasit.* **49**, 773 (1963).
153c. id., *Clin. Pediat.* **7**, 508 (1968).
154. Kagan, I. G. and Norman, L.: *Amer. J. trop. Med. Hyg.* **12**, 346 (1963).
155. Karmanska, K., Kozar, Z., Seniuta, R. and Dugiewicz-Bulla, M.: *Acta Parasit. pol.* **21**, 173 (1973).
156. Kelly, D. R. and Schmitzer, R. J.: *J. Immunol.* **69**, 337 (1952).
157. Kelly, D. R., Schuhmacher, A. and Schmitzer, R. J.: *J. Immunol.* **71**, 40 (1954).
158. Kelly, J. D.: *Proc. Third Int. Congr. Parasit.* München, **3**, 1199 (1974).
159. Kelly, J. D. and Ogilvie, B. M.: *Int. Arch. Allergy* **43**, 497 (1972).
160. Kerr, W. R. and Robertson, M.: *Vet. J.* **97**, 351 (1941).
161. Kessel, J. V., Lewis, W. P., Ma, S. and Kim, J.: *Proc. Soc. exp. Biol. Med.* **106**, 409 (1961).
162. Khaleque, K. A.: *Pak. J. med. Res.* **4**, 234 (1965).
163. Kierszenbaum, F. and Budzko, D. B.: *Proc. Third Int. Congr. Parasit.* München, **1**, 228 (1974).
164. Kojima, S. and Ovary, Z.: *Proc. Third Int. Congr. Parasit.* München, **2**, 1066 (1974).
165. Kojima, S., Yokogawa, M. and Tada, T.: *Amer. J. trop. Med. Hyg.* **21**, 913 (1972).
166. Korte, W.: *Premier Symposium Européen, Reims,* Masson and Cie, Paris, 1597, p. 159.
167. Kott, H. and Adler, S.: *Trans. roy. Soc. trop. Med. Hyg.* **55**, 333 (1961).
168. Kozar, Z. and Soszka, S.: *Bull. Inst. mar. trop. Med.* **7**, 165 (1956).
169. Kramár, J. and Kucera, K.: *J. Hyg. Epidem.* **10**, 85 (1966).
170. Krampitz, H. E. and Disko, R.: *Nature (Lond.)* **209**, 526 (1966).
171. Kretschmar, W.: *Z. Tropenmed. Parasit.* **17**, 375 (1966).
172. Kume, S.: *Proc. Third Int. Congr. Parasit.* München, **2**, 646 (1974).
173. Maddison, S. E.: *Exp. Parasit.* **18**, 224 (1965).
174. Maddison, S. E., Kagan, I. G. and Elsdon-Dew, R.: *Amer. J. trop. Med. Hyg.* **17**, 540 (1968).
175. Maddison, S. E., Kagan, I. G. and Norman, L.: *J. Immunol.* **100**, 217 (1968).
176. Maddison, S. E., Powell, S. J. and Elsdon-Dew, R.: *Amer. J. trop. Med. Hyg.* **14**, 551 (1965).
176a. Madwar, M. A. and Voller, A.: *Brit. med. J.* i, 435 (1975).

177. Maegraith, B. G.: In *Immunity to Protozoa*. Ed. by Garnham, P. C. C., Pierce, A. E. and Roitt, I. Blackwell, Oxford 1963, p. 48.
178. Maekelt, G. A.: *Rev. venez. Sanid.* **29**, 1 (1964).
179. Mahajan, R. C., Ganguly, N. K. and Chitkara, N. L.: *Proc. Third Int. Congr. Parasit.* München, **2**, 1139 (1974).
180. Manson-Bahr, Ph. H.: *Trans. roy. Soc. trop. Med. Hyg.* **55**, 550 (1961).
181. Márquez-Monter, H.: In *Pathology of Protozoal and Helminthic Diseases*. Ed. by Marcial-Rojas, R. A. Williams et Wilkins Co., Baltimore 1971.
182. Matuszak, J. and Kuzmicki, R.: *Proc. Third Int. Congr. Parasit.* München, **2**, 777 (1974).
183. McEntegart, M. G.: *J. clin. Path.* **5**, 275 (1952).
184. McGregor, I. A. and Carrington, S. D.: *Trans. roy. Soc. trop. Med. Hyg.* **57**, 170 (1963).
185. McMillan, B.: *Proc. Third Int. Congr. Parasit.* München, **2**, 693 (1974).
186. Melcher, L. R.: *J. infect.* **73**, 31 (1943).
187. Mignoli, A.: *Reforma méd.* **40**, 577 (1924).
188. Milgram, E. A., Healy, G. R. and Kagan, I. G.: *Gastroenterology* **50**, 645 (1966).
189. Miller, H. C. and Twohy, D. W.: *Bact. Proc.* 100 (1968).
190. Miller, H. R. P. and Walshaw, R.: *Amer. J. Path.* **69**, 195 (1972).
191. Miller, Th. A.: *Proc. Third Int. Congr. Parasit.* München, **3**, 1223 (1974).
192. Mishra, N. K. and Marsh, C. L.: *Exp. Parasit.* **33**, 89 (1973).
193. Mislóczky, M., Backhausz, R. and Jurányi, R.: *Magy. Belorv. Arch.* **24**, 83 (1971).
194. Mitchell, J. R.: *Proc. Soc. exp. Biol. Med.* **117**, 267 (1964).
194a. Molinari, J. A., Cypess, R. H. and Ebersole, J. L.: *Int. Arch. Allergy* **47**, 483 (1974).
195. Montano, G. and Mcros, H.: *Bol. chil. Parasit.* **20**, 62 (1965).
196. Morseth, D. J. and Soulsby, E. J. L.: *J. Parasit.* **55**, 22 (1969).
197. Nadim, A.: *Proc. Third Int. Congr. Parasit.* München, **1**, 242 (1974).
198. Nakayama, J.: *Keio J. Med.* **13**, (1965).
199. Neal, R. A. and Miles, R. A.: *Trans. roy. Soc. trop. Med. Hyg.* **62**, 7 (1968).
200a. Nichols, R. L.: *J. Parasit.* **42**, 349 (1956).
200b. ibid., **42**, 363 (1956).
201a. Nigesen, U. K.: In *Genitourinary Trichomoniasis*. Ed. by Teras, J. K. Acad. Sci. Estonian SSR, Tallin 1963.
201b. id., Thesis, Acad. Sci. Estonian SSR, 1966.
202. Nitzulescu, V. and Sherman, I.: *Arch. Un. méd. balkan* **4**, 737 (1966).
203. O'Connor, G. R.: *Trans. Amer. opthal. Soc.* **68**, 501 (1970).
204. Ogilvie, B. M.: *Nature (Lond.)* **204**, 91 (1964).
205. Ogilvie, B. M. and Jones, V. E.: *Exp. Parasit.* **29**, 138 (1971).
206. Ogilvie, B. M., Rothwell, T. L. W., Brenner, K. C., Schmitherling, H. J., Nolan, J. and Keith, R. K.: *Int. J. Parasit.* **3**, 589 (1973).
207. Ogilvie, B. M. and Worms, M. J.: *Proc. Third Int. Congr. Parasit.* München, **2**, 776 (1974).
208a. Oliver-González, J.: *J. infect. Dis.* **95**, 86 (1954).
208b. id., *Amer. J. trop. Med. Hyg.* **6**, 384 (1957).
208c. id., *J. infect. Dis.* **107**, 94 (1960).
209. Olson, L. J. and Rose, J. E.: *J. Parasit.* **51**, 49 (1965).
210. Olson, L. J. and Schulz, C. W.: *Ann. N. Y. Acad. Sci.* **113**, 440 (1963).
211. Orr, T. S. C. and Blair, A. M.: *Life Sci.* **8**, 1073 (1969).
212. Osipova, S. O., Dekhkan-Hodjaeva, N. A. and Medvedeva, L. V.: *Proc. Third Int. Congr. Parasit.* München, **2**, 1099 (1974).
213. Ott, K. J.: Ph. D. Thesis New Brunswick, N. J. Rutgers. The State University, 1964.
214. Page, F. T. and Reeves, D. S.: *Southeast Asian J. trop. Med. Publ. Health* **4**, 256 (1973) cit. *Helm. Abstr.* **43**, abstr. No. 2095 (1974).
215. Pautrizel, R., Mattern, P. and Duret, J.: *Bull. Soc. Path. exot.* **53**, 878 (1960).
216. Pelster, B.: *Proc. Third Int. Congr. Parasit.* München, **1**, 278 (1974).
217. Perevertzeva, E. V.: *Wiad. Parazyt.* **15**, 667 (1969).
218. Petcholai, B., Benaponse, W. and Suntharsamai, P.: *Proc. Third Int. Congr. Parasit.* München, **2**, 1043 (1974).

219. Piekarski, G.: *Die Toxoplasmose*. Springer, Berlin–Heidelberg–New York 1972.
220. Piekarski, G. and Berger, J.: *Proc. Third Int. Congr. Parasit.* München, **1**, 279 (1974).
220a. Ogilvie, B. M. and Jones, V. E.: *Progr. Allergy* **17**, 129 (1973).
221. Phillips, R. S.: *Proc. Third Int. Parasit. Congr.* München, **2**, 1063 (1974).
221a. Phillips, T. M. and Draper, C. C.: *Brit. med. J.* ii, 476 (1975).
222. Pinon, N. M. and Gentilini, M.: *Nouv. Presse Méd.* **2**, 1283 (1973).
223. Pizzi, T., Niedman, G. and Jarpa, A.: *Bol. chil. Parasit.* **18**, 32 (1963).
224. Pizzi, T., Rubio, M. and Knierim, F.: *Bol. chil. Parasit.* **9**, 35 (1954).
225. Popovich, E. B.: *Vrachebnoe Delo* **8**, 145 (1972) cit. *Helm. Abstr.* **43**, No. 911 (1974).
226. Porter, J. A. and Young, M. D.: *Milit. Med.* **131**, (Suppl.) 952 (1966).
227. Powles, A. C. P.: *New Zealand Med. J.* **77**, 169 (1973). cit. *Helm. Abstr.* **43**, abstr. No. 728 (1974).
228. Rangue, J., Quilici, M., Dunan, S. and Rangue, Ph.: *Proc. Third Int. Congr. Parasit.* München, **1**, 249 (1974).
229. Realini, S. and Hofstetter, J. R.: *Schweitzer Med. Wschr.* **102**, 565 (1972).
230. Reiff, O. F. and Moraes, C. R. de: *Rev. Paulist. Med.* **80**, 151 (1972) cit. *Helm. Abstr.* **43**, abstr. No. 532 (1974).
231. Reisenhofer, U.: *Arch. Hyg. Bakt.* **146**, 628 (1963).
232. Remington, J. S., Melton, M. L. and Jacobs, L.: *J. Immunol.* **78**, 578 (1961).
233. Remington, J. S. and Miller, M. J.: *Proc. Soc. exp. Biol. Med.* **121**, 357 (1966).
234. Rezai, H. R., Behforouz, N. and Gettner, S.: *Proc. Third Int. Congr. Parasit.* München, **1**, 252 (1974).
235. Rhodes, M. B., Nayak, D. P., Kelley, G. W. jr. and Marsh, C. L.: *Exp. Parasit.* **16**, 373 (1965).
236. Ribas-Mujal, D.: In *Pathology of Protozoal and Helminthic Diseases*. Williams and Wilkins Co., Baltimore 1971.
237. Robles-Gil, J. and Perrin, M.: *Arch. Inst. Card.* Mexico, **20**, 314 (1950).
238. Rogers, W. A. and Nelson, B.: *J. Amer. med. Ass.* **195**, 685 (1966).
239. Rombert, P. C.: *Ann. Esc. Nat. Soud. Publ. Med. trop.* **5**, 291 (1971). cit. *Helm. Abstr.* **42**, abstr. No. 3102 (1973).
240. Rosenthal, F. and Nossen, H.: *Klin. Wschr.* **58**, 1093 (1921).
241. Roszkovszky, I., Prawecka, M.: *Amer. J. Obstet. Gynec.* **94**, 378 (1966).
242. Roth, H.: *Nature (Lond.)* **155**, 758 (1945).
243. Rothwell, T. L. W., Ogilvie, B. M. and Love, R. J.: *Int. J. Parasit.* **3**, 599 (1973).
244. Rowe, D. S.: *J. clin. exp. Immunol.* **3**, 63 (1968).
245. Ruitenberg, E. J. and Sleen, G. van der: *J. Parasit.* **58**, 1233 (1973).
246. Ruitenberg, E. J., Teppema, J. S. and Steerenberg, P. A.: *Proc. Third. Int. Congr. Parasit.* München, **2**, 667 (1974).
247. Rydzewski, A. K., Sulzer, A. J. and Kagan, I. G.: *Proc. Third Int. Congr. Parasit.* München, **3**, 1219 (1974).
248. Sabin, A. B.: *Advanc. Pediat.* **1**, 1 (1942).
249. Sadun, E. H. and Allain, D.: *Amer. J. trop. Med. Hyg.* **6**, 386 (1957).
250. Sadun, E. H., Anderson, R. I. and Williams, J. S.: *Exp. Parasit.* **12**, 423 (1962).
251. Sadun, E. H., Duxbury, R. E., Williams, J. S. and Anderson, R. I.: *J. Parasit.* **49**, 385 (1963).
252. Sadun, E. H. and Norman, L.: *J. Parasit.* **43**, 236 (1957).
253. Sanderson, B. E. and Ogilvie, B. M.: *Parasitology* **62**, 367 (1971).
254. Satyshev, N. I. and Kryukova, A. P.: *Probl. Reg. Gen. exp. Parasit. med. Zool.* **8**, 211 (1953).
255. Sawado, T.: *Proc. Third Int. Congr. Parasit.* München, **2**, 637 (1974).
256. Schacher, J. P. and Sahyoun, P. F.: *Trans. roy. Soc. trop. Med. Hyg.* **61**, 234 (1966).
257. Schad, G. A.: *Proc. Third Int. Congr. Parasit.* München, **2**, 772 (1974).
258. Schaffer, J. G., Shles, W. H., Radke. R. A. and Palmer, W. L.: *Amoebiasis. A Biochemical Problem*. Charles C. Thomas, Springfield Ill. 1965.
259. Seah, S. and Hucol, G.: *Proc. Third Int. Congr. Parasit.* München, **1**, 291 (1974).
260. Seed, J. R. and Weinman, D.: *Nature (Lond.)* **198**, 197 (1963).
261. Sen, H. G.: *Proc. Third Int. Congr. Parasit.* München, **2**, 775 (1974).
262. Seneca, H. and Wolf, A.: *Amer. J. trop. Med. Hyg.* **4**, 1009 (1955).
263. Senft, A. W.: *Proc. Third Int. Congr. Parasit.* München, **2**, 1157 (1974).

264. Sergent, E.: *Symp. Immunity to Protozoal Diseases.* Ed. by. Garnham P. C. C. Blackwell Sci. Publ. Oxford, 1963.
265. Shatsubayasni, H. and Akao, S.: *Amer. J. trop. Med.* **15**, 486 (1966).
266. Silverman, P. H. and Hulland, T. J.: *Res. vet. Sci.* **2**, 248 (1961).
267. Silverman, P. H. and Maneely, R. B.: *Ann. trop. Med. Parasit.* **49**, 326 (1955).
268. Singer, I., Kimble, E. T. and Ritts, R. E.: *J. infect. Dis.* **114**, 243 (1964).
269. Slais, J.: *Proc. Third Int. Congr. Parasit.* München, **2**, 582 (1974).
270. Smith, J. D.: *Parasitology* **59**, 73 (1969).
271. Smithers, S. R. and Terry, R. J.: *Trans. roy. Soc. trop. Med. Hyg.* **61**, 517 (1967).
272. Solomon, P. and Panaitescu, D.: *Proc. Third Int. Congr. Parasit.* München, **3**, 1211 (1974).
273. Soltys, M. A.: *Parasitology* **47**, 391 (1957).
274. Sommerville, R. I.: *Exp. Parasit.* **6**, 18 (1957).
275. Soulsby, E. J. L. and Stewart, D. F.: *Aust. J. agric. Res.* **11**, 595 (1960).
276. Southgate, B. A. and Manson-Bahr, P. E. C.: *J. trop. Med. Hyg.* **70**, 29 (1967).
277. Southgate, B. A. and Oriedo, B. V. E.: *J. trop. Med. Hyg.* **70**, 1 (1967).
278. Stamm, W. P.: *Proc. Third Int. Congr. Parasit.* München, **1**, 170 (1974).
279. Stein, B. and Desowitz, R. S.: *Bull. Wld Hlth Org.* **30**, 45 (1964).
280. Stepankovskaya, L. P.: *Med. Parasit.* **41**, 400 (1972).
281. Stone, W. M.: *Proc. Third Int. Congr. Parasit.* München, **2**, 771 (1974).
282. Strannegard, O. and Lycke, E.: *Acta Path. Microbiol. Scand.* **66**, 227 (1966).
283. Strickland, G. T. and Sayles, P. C.: *Proc. Third Int. Congr. Parasit.* München, **1**, 292 (1974).
284. Suslov, I. M.: *Materialy Nauchnykh Konferentsii Vsesoyuznogo Obshchestva Gel'-mintologov* 1969–1970. **23**, 273 (1971) cit. *Helm. Abstr.* **43**, abstr. No. 2604 (1974).
285. Swartzwelder, J. C. and Avant, W. H.: *Amer. J. trop. Med. Hyg.* **1**, 567 (1952).
286. Swatek, M.: *Wiad. Parazyt.* **2**, 153 (1956).
287. Taliaferro, W. H.: *Sci. Rep. 1st. sup. Sanita* **2**, 138 (1962).
288. Talis, B.: *J. Protozool.* **13**, (Suppl.) 34 (1966).
289. Tarrant, C. J., Fifer, E. H. and Anderson, R. I.: *J. Parasit.* **51**, 277 (1965).
290. Teokharov, B. A.: Progress in Protozoology. 3rd Int. Congr. Protozool. Leningrad. Publishing House "Nauka", Leningrad 1969, p. 318.
291a. Teras, J. K.: Thesis. Univ. Tartu, 1954.
291b. id., Doctoral thesis. Acad. Sci. Estonian SSR, 1964.
291c. id., *Wiad. Parazyt.* **12**, 357 (1966).
292. Teras, J. K., Nigesen, U. K., Jaakmees, H. P., Roigas, E. M. and Tompel, H. J.: *Wiad. Parazyt.* **12**, 370 (1966).
293. Teras, J. K., Roigas, E., Lenzner, H. and Nigesen, U. K.: *Proc. Third Int. Congr. Parasit.* München, **2**, 1136 (1974).
294. Terpstra, W. J., van Helden, H. P. T., Dallas, A. B. C. and Eyakuze, V. M.: *Proc. Third Int. Congr. Parasit.* München, **2**, 839 (1974).
295. Terry, R. J.: *Exp. Parasit.* **6**, 404 (1957).
296. Thalhammer, O.: *Human toxoplasmosis.* Ed. by. Siim, J. Copenhagen, 1960, p. 191.
297. Thiermann, E. and Stagno, S.: *Zbl. Bakt.* I. Abt. Orig. **219**, 249 (1972).
298. Thoulon, L.: *Bull. Soc. Path. exot.* **25**, 234 (1932).
299. Tobie, J. E. and Coatney, G. R.: *Exp. Parasit.* **11**, 128 (1961).
300. Toussaint, D. and Danis, P.: *Arch. Ophthal.* **74**, 470 (1965).
301. Trejos, A. and De Urguilla, M. A.: In *Progress in Protozoology. 2nd Int. Congr. Protozool. London, Int. Congr. Ser.* **91**, 144 (1965).
302. Turk, J. L. and Bryceson, A. D. M.: *Advanc. Immunol.* **13**, 209 (1971).
303. Varjú, L.: *Z. Parasitenk.* **28**, 175 (1966).
304. Vattuone, N. H., Gonzalez-Cappa, S. M., Menes, S. and Schmunis, G. A.: *Z. Tropenmed. Parasit.* **25**, 267 (1974).
305. Vietzke, W. M., Gelderman, A. A., Grimley, P. M. and Valsamis, M. P.: *Cancer* **21**, 816 (1968).
306. Viswanathan, R., Bagai, R. C. and Saran, R.: *Amer. Rev. Resp. Dis.* **107**, 298 (1973).
307. Vogel, H. and Minning, W.: *Zbl. Bakt. Orig. Abt. I.* **153**, 99 (1949).
308. Voller, A.: *Amer. J. trop. Med. Hyg.* **13**, 204 (1964).
309. Wadworth, C.: *Int. Arch. Allergy* **10**, 355 (1957).
309a. Walls, R. W., Hersey, P. and Quie, P. G.: *Blood* **44**, 131 (1974).

310. Waltzing, P. and Bloch-Michel, H.: *Presse Méd.* **79**, 2061 (1971).
311a. Warren, K. S.: In *Immunological Diseases.* Ed. by Samter, M. Vol. I. Little, Brown et Co., Boston 1971, p. 668.
311b. id., *Proc. Third Int. Congr. Parasit.* München, **3**, 1185 (1974).
312. Warren, K. S., Domingo, E. O. and Cowan, R. B. T.: *Amer. J. Path.* **51**, 735 (1967).
313. Weatberall, R.: *Nature (Lond.)* **5015**, 1267 (1965).
314. Weber, H. and Egger, I.: *Zbl. Bakt. Abt. I. Orig.* **212**, 155 (1969).
315. Webster, G. A. and Cameron, T. W. M.: *Canad. J. Zool.* **39**, 877 (1961).
316. Weiss, M. L.: *Proc. Third Int. Congr. Parasit.* München, **2**, 1112 (1974).
317. Williamson, J. and Brown, K. N.: *Exp. Parasit.* **15**, 44 (1964).
318a. *Wld Hlth Org. techn. Rep. Ser.*, **26**, 338 (1966).
318b. ibid., **396**, 24 (1968).
318c. ibid., **542**, 1029 (1974).
319. Yaeger, R. G. and Miller, O. N.: *Exp. Parasit.* **14**, 9 (1963).
320. Young, M. D., Eyles, D. E., Burgess, R. W. and Jeffery, G. M.: *J. Parasit.* **41**, 315 (1955).
320a. Yuan, L. and Sell, K. W.: *Immunochemistry* **11**, 235 (1974).
321. Zasukhin, D. N.: In *Progress in Protozoology.* 3rd Int. Congr. Protozool. Leningrad. Publ. House "Nauka", Leningrad 1969. p. 209.
322. Zeledon, R. W., De Monge, E. and Blanco, E.: In *Progress in Protozoology.* 2nd Int. Conf. Protozool. London Int. Congr. Ser. **91**, 133 (1965).
323. Zembrzuski, K.: *Acta Parasit. pol.* **21**, 307 (1973).

CHAPTER 80

INSECTS, MITES AND OTHER VENOMOUS ARTHROPODS CAUSING ALLERGIC OR IMMUNOLOGIC REACTIONS IN MAN

by

G. MAKARA and S. KOROSSY

GENERAL CONSIDERATIONS

CLASSIFICATION

Insects, ticks, mites, spiders and other groups of the phylum Arthropoda contain a number of species, which are of medical importance. Some of them cause allergic and toxic reactions or may give rise to immunological reactions in man. For proper orientation it is necessary to recognize or determine the groups and to identify the species of the animal involved, and to refer them into the correct place of the classification. There are around one million described species in this largest phylum of the animal kingdom, and probably three or four times that number await description and classification. The number of pests is small, only about 1,000 being of real medical importance. The identification of some arthropods may be a hard task even for experts of entomology.

Medical entomology deals with arthropods that transmit diseases or cause pathologic conditions in man. A greater part of tropical medicine deals with these and other animal parasites occurring in warmer climates.

The applied science of medical entomology began to develop at about the beginning of the 20th century, after the role of vectors had been discovered.

The knowledge of classification is indispensable, yet in addition morphology, phylogeny, biology, life histories, development, ecology, population dynamics, control measures and other fundamental aspects of arthropods of interest have to be studied. All these cannot be included in this chapter, though where it seems necessary some very brief references to the most important characteristics are given. Literature on entomology and medical entomology contain detailed information [25, 34, 64, 68, 81, 107, 136, 145a, 155, 175, 187a, 213, 219, 258, 302].

The important species and groups are listed in Table 80-I, where insects and Arachnoidea are the two large groups and there are three classes of minor interest. The more important insects belong to about 10–12 families. Only the most important genera and species could be included in the table. Obviously it would be unwise to try to include all the flies and mosquitoes which may bite man, or list all the mites which may occasionally cause allergy.

There is no final, generally accepted system of classification. In some cases different grouping and different new generic and specific names are preferred in the individual countries. In Table 80-I we adopted and retained the familiar and well established names of the taxonomic groups and specific names used in the current literature of medical entomology.

MEDICAL IMPORTANCE

Obviously the material could have been arranged in the sequence of classification, however, it seemed more appropriate to discuss it according to the ways in which arthropods cause harm to man. Thus, with regard to medical importance these are:

1. Transmitters of diseases, (a) vectors of diseases such as yellow fever, malaria, typhus, plague, filariasis, rickettsial and viral diseases, sleeping sickness;

(b) mechanical carriers of pathogenic micro-organisms transmitting enteric diseases, suppurative conditions, [107, 155, 175, 213, 219, 302] etc.;

TABLE 20-I

Arthropods of medical importance in sequence of classification

Class: CRUSTACEA

Order	Family	Genus	Species and its common name
Copepoda Cymothoidea Decapoda	Eucopepoda	Cyclops, Daphnia	*water fleas* *sea lice* *crabs, lobsters, crayfish*

Class: DIPLOPODA *millipedes*

Chilognata		Julus Polyxenus Orthoporus Rhinocrichus	R. latespargor

Class: CHILOPODA *centipedes*

		Scutigera Geophilus Lithobius Seolopendra	S. cleopatra, S. cingulata S. giganthea

Table 80-I (cont'd)

Class: A R A C H N O I D E A

Order	Family	Genus	Species *and its common name*
Scorpionidea	Buthidae	Buthus Androctonus Euscorpius Centruroides	B. afer A. australis E. europeus C. suffusus *Durango scorpion* C. vittatus, C. gertschi C. pantheriensis
scorpions	Diplocentridae	Diplocentrus	D. whitei
	Vejovidae	Vejovis Hadrurus Uroctonus	V. spinigerus *striple tailed scorpion* V. boreus H. hirsutus U. mordax *mordant scorpion*
Pedipalpida		Mastigoproctus Thelyphonus	M. gigantheus *giant whip scorpion* T. skimkewitchii
Solpugida	*sun spiders,* *wind scorpions*		

Table 80-I (cont'd)

Class: A R A C H N O I D E A *(cont'd)*

Order	Family	Genus	Species *and its common name*
Acarina:	**Argasidae** *soft ticks*	**Argas** **Ornithodorus**	A. persicus; A. reflexus *pigeon tick* O. moubata, O. turicata, O. talaje
Parasitiformes Ixodoidea *ticks*	Ixodidae *hard ticks*	Ixodes Dermacentor Haemophysalis Boophilus Rhiphicephalus Amblyomma Hyalomma	I. ricinus *castorbean tick* I. pacificus *deer tick*, I. scapularis D. andersoni *wood tick* D. occidentalis, D. variabilis H. leporis-palustris *rabbit tick* H. albipictus *winter tick* B. annulatus *Texas cattle fever tick* R. sanguineus *brown dog tick* A. americanum *lone star tick* H. aegyptieum
Acarina: *mites* Mesostigmata	Dermanyssidae *(gamasine mites)*	Dermanyssus Allodermanyssus (Lyponyssoides) Ornythonyssus (Lyponyssus)	D. avium, D. gallinae *chicken mite* A. sanguineus *house mouse mite* O. bacoti *tropical rat mite* O. bursa *tropical fowl mite*

Table 80-I (cont'd)

Class: A R A C H N O I D E A *(cont'd)*

Order	Family	Genus	Species *and its common name*
Acarina: Sarcoptiformes	Tyroglyphidae (= Acaridae)	Tyroglyphus Acarus Tyrophagus	T. longior, T. casei A. siro (= farinae) *grain mite* T. castellanii (= putrescentiae)
	Glyciphagidae	Glyciphagus Carpoglyphus	G. domesticus C. lactis
	Epidermoptidae	Dermatophagoides	D. scheremetewskyi, D. pteronyssimus
	Sarcoptidae	Sarcoptes Notoedres	S. scabiei N. cati
	Psoroptidae *mange mites*	Chorioptes Psoroptes Knemidokoptes	
Acarina: Trombidiformes	Trombiculidae *chigger mites*	Trombicula (= Trombidicula) (= Leptotrombidium)	T. autumnalis T. irritans T. alfreddugesi L. deliensis L. akamushi
	Pyemotidae	Pyemotes Cheyletidae Demodex Bryobia	P. ventricosus *grain itch mite* C. eruditus D. folliculorum *follicle mite* B. praetiosa *red spider*
	Demodicidae Tetranychidae		
Araneidea *spiders*	Theridiidae	Latrodectus	L. mactans *black widow* L. geometricus *brown widow*
	Loxoscelidae	Loxosceles	L. reclusa, L. unicolor L. arisonica, L. laeta
	Theraphosidae	Licosa Hogna Dolomedes Chiracanthium Argioge	L. tarantula H. singoriensis D. chiracantura C. inclusum A. auranta

Table 80-I (cont'd)

Class: I N S E C T A

Order	Family	Genus	Species and its common name
Blattaria	Blattidea cockroaches	Blatta Blattella Periplaneta Supella	**B.** orientalis B. germanica *German cockroach* P. americana S. supellectilium *furniture cockroach*
Manthoidea	*praying manthes*		
Othoptera	*grasshoppers*		
Psocoptera	*wood lice*		
Anoplura	*lice*	Pediculus Ptairus (= Phthyrius)	P. humanus capitis *head louse* P. humanus corporis *body louse* P. pubis *crab louse*
Mallophaga	*biting lice*		
Heteroptera	Cimicidae	Cimex	C. lectularius *bed bug* C. rotundatus *tropical bed bug* C. hemipterus *Indian bed bug* C. bonati
bugs and aphids		Oeciacus Haematosiphon	O. hirundinis *bird bug* H. inodorus *poultry bug*
	Reduviidae	Triatoma Panstrongylus Raodnius Reduvius	T. rubrofasciata, T. protracta T. sanguisuga T. megista P. megistus R. prolixus R. personatus
	Gerricidae	Benacius	B. griseus *water bug*

Table 80-I (cont'd)
Class: INSECTA (cont'd)

Order	Family	Genus	Species and its common name
Heteroptera bugs and aphids (cont'd)	Notonectidae Nepidae Tingidae lace bugs	Notonecta Nepa	N. glauca back swimmer N. cinerea water scorpion
Thysanoptera trips		Thrips Limothrips	T. tabaci L. denticornis
Coleoptera beetles	Staphylinidae rove beetles Oedemeridae Meloidae blister beetles	Paederus Atheta Sessinia Meloe Lytta Epicauta Mylabris	P. crebripunctatus A. occidentalis S. collaris, S. decolor coconut beetles M. majalis L. vesicatoria spanish fly E. flavicornis, E. solani M. variabilis
	Chrysomelidae	Diamphidia Blepharida	D. locusta B. evanida
	Disticidae Tenebrionidae mealworm beetles	Cybister Tenebrio Tribolium Blaps	C. marginatus T. molitor mealworm beetle T. confusum flour beetle B. mortisaga churchyard beetle
	Dermestidae hide beetles	Dermestes Trogoderma Anthrenus	D. lardarius bacon beetle T. granarium khapra beetle A. scrophulariae carpet beetle
Lepidoptera moths and butterflies	Lymantriidae	Lymantria Euproctis Portheria Nygmia	L. monacha nun moth-black E. chrysorrhoea brown tail moth E. flavociliata, E. flava, E. similis, E. fueralis P. similis gold tail moth N. phaeorrhoea brown tail moth
	Arctiidae	Arctia Halisitoda	H. caryae hickory tussock moth A. caja garden tiger

Table 80-1 (cont'd)
Class: I N S E C T A (cont'd)

Order	Family	Genus	Species and its common name
Lepidoptera	Thaumetopoeidae	Thaumetopoea	T. processionea *processionary caterpillar* T. pinivora, T. wilkinsoni
moths and butterflies (cont'd)	Lashiocampidae Saturniidae	Lashiocampa Automeris Hemileuca	L. quercus A. io *the io moth* H. olivae *range caterpillar*
	Megalopygidae Morphionidae	Megalopyge Lagoe Marphio	M. opercularis *puss moth*, M. lanata L. crispata *white moth* M. hercules
	Tineidae Phycitiae	Tineola Plodia Ephestia	T. bisselliella *clothes moth* P. interpunctella *Indian meal moth* E. elutella *fig moth*
	eye-frequener and blood sucking moth	Arzyophara Artitrygoides Calpe	A. interica A. cuniella C. crustigiata
Diptera: Nematocera	Psychodidae *moth flies*	Phlebotomus *sand flies, owl midges*	P. papatasii, P. perniciosus, P. major, P. vexator, P. diabolicus, P. chinensis, P. verrucarum, P. intermedius, P. lutzi
	Culicidae *mosquitoes*	Anopheles	A. maculipennis, A. superpictus, A. freeborni, A. quadrimaculatus, A. occidentalis, A. aztecus, A. claviger, A. pharaoensis, A. gambiae, A. funestus, A. culicifacies, A. minimus, A. sinensis
		Culex	C. pipiens pipiens *house mosquito* C. pipiens molestus, C. pipiens fatigans, C. pipiens quinquefasciatus, C. tarsalis

Table 80-I (cont'd)
Class: INSECTA (cont'd)

Order	Family	Genus	Species and its common name
Diptera: Nematocera (cont'd)	Culicidae *mosquitoes (cont'd)*	Aedes	A. aegypti *yellow fever mosquito,* A. vexans, A. taeniorhynchus, A. nigromaculis, A. ventrovittis, A. simpsoni, A. africanus, A. nigripes, A. impiger
		Haemagogus Mansonia Culiseta = Theobaldia Psorophora	H. spegazzini falco M. richardii, M. perturbans T. annulata C. incidens, C. inornata P. confinis, P. ciliata
	Heleidae *biting midgs, punkies*	Culicoides Leptoconops Ceratopogon Lasiohelea	C. pulicaris, C. vexans, C. canithorax, C. melleus, C. obsoletus, C. diabolicus, C. austeni, C. furans, L. torreus, L. kerteszi
	Simuliidae *black flies buffalo gnats*	Simulium Simulium-Prosimulium Simulium-Boophtora Simulium-Cnephia	S. damnosum, S. reptans, S. vittatum, S. venustum, S. arcticum, S. columbaschense P. hirtipes B. erythrocephala C. pecuarum
Diptera: Brachycera	Tabanidae *horse flies and deer flies*	Tabanus Chrysops Haematopota Pangonia Silvius	T. bovinus, T. atractus, T. stygius C. coecutiens, C. discalis C. dimidiata, C. silicea H. pluvialis P. zonata S. pollinosus, S. quadrivittatus
	Rhagionidae (= Lepidae) *snipe flies*	Symphoromyia Suragina	S. hirta, S. attripes S. longipes

Table 80-I (cont'd)

Class: I N S E C T A *(cont'd)*

Order	Family	Genus	Species *and its common name*
Diptera: Cyclorrhapha	Muscidae *muscoid flies*	Musca	M. domestica *house fly* M. autumnalis *face fly*, **M**. sorbens *lesser house fly*
		Fannia	F. canicularis *lesser house fly*
		Muscina	M. stabulans *nonbiting stable fly*
		Stomoxys	S. calcitrans *stable fly*
		Haematobia (= Siphona)	H. irritans *horn fly*
		(= Lyperosia)	H. stimulans
		Glossina *tsetse flies*	G. palpalis, G. morsitans
	Calliphoridae *blow flies*	Calliphora *bluebottles*	C. erythrocephala (= C. vicina)
		Lucilia *greenbottles* (=also Phoenicia)	L. caesar
		Cordylobia	P. sericata, P. cuprina
			C. anthropophaga *tumbu fly*,
			C. bezziana, C. megacephala
		Auchmeromyia	A. luteola *congofloor maggot*
		Callitroga (= Cochliomyia)	C. hominivorax *screw worm*
			C. macellaria
		Chrysomyia (= Cochliomyia)	C. bezziana, C. megacephala
		Protormia	P. regina, P. terra-novae
		Pollenia	P. rudis *cluster fly*
	Sarcophagidae *flesh flies*	Sarcophaga Wohlfahrtia	S. haemorrhoidalis, S. carnaria W. magnifica, W. vigil
	Chloropidae *fruit flies*	Hippelates *eye gnats*	H. flavipes, H. pallipes, H. pusio

271

Table 80-I (cont'd)

Class: INSECTA (cont'd)

Order	Family	Genus	Species and its common name
bot and warble flies	Oestridae	Oestrus Rhinoestrus	O. ovis sheep bot fly R. purpureus
	Hypodermatidae warble	Hypoderma heel flies	H. lineatum cattle grub, H. bovis Northern cattle grub
	Gasterophilidae	Gasterophilus horse bot flies	G. intestinalis (= G. equi), G. haemorrhoidalis, G. nasalis
	Cuterebridae	Cuterebra Dermatobia	D. hominis human bot fly
Pupipara	Hippoboscidae louse flies	Melophagus Hippobosca Lipoptena	M. ovinus sheep ked H. equinum L. cervi
Siphonaptera fleas	Pulicidae	Pulex Xenopsylla	P. irritans X. cheopis tropical rat flea, X. astia, X. brasiliense
		Ctenophalides Echidnophaga	C. canis dog flea, C. felis cat flea E. gallinacea
	Ceratophyllidae	Ceratophyllus Nosophyllus	N. fasciatus rat flea
	Tungidae	Tunga	T. penetrans chigoe, sand flea

Table 80-I (cont'd)

Class: I N S E C T A *(cont'd)*

Order	Family	Genus	Species and its common name
Hymenoptera	Formicidae *ants* Mirmicidae	Myrmecia Solenopsis Pogonomyrmex *harvester ants*	M. gulosa *giant bulldog ant* S. sevissima richteri *fire ant* S. geminata, S. xyloni P. barbatus, P. californicus, P. occidentalis, P. badius
	Vespidae Pompilidae	Vespa Vespula = Paravespula *wasps* Pepsis	V. crabro-crabro *yellow jacket, hornet* V. crabro germana *bald faced hornet* P. vulgaris, V. germanica, V. maculata, V. pennsylvanica P. formosa *tarantula wasp*
	Aphidae Mellitidae	Apis Halictus *sweet bees* Bombus	A. mellifera *honey bee*
	Mutilidae *velvet ants*	Dasymutilla	D. occidentalis
	Bethyloidea	Cephalonomia Sceroderma Epyris	C. gallicola S. domesticum E. californicus

2. Parasites in the tissues, in the skin, in wounds or in the intestine. There are but a few such arthropods in man. The reason for it is that they are air breathing animals.

3. Blood sucking ectoparasites, which may permanently remain on the surface of the body, like lice, or attach themselves to their human of animal host for blood meals at regular intervals, like the bed bug, mosquitoes or gnats.

4. Those causing poisoning, irritation and allergy by their bites, stings or by contact.

5. Those which are nuisances, contaminators of environment by their presence in dwellings and in food [68, 219].

Finally, there are those causing psychological effects. The effects of disgust and phobia should not be underestimated [68].

The medical importance of arthropods is far greater in the transmission of diseases than in direct effects. In this chapter, however, the indirect role has been neglected.

All of the more important insects and other arthropods causing direct harm will be dealt with according to their connections to man and his health. From this point of view allergy and immune responses cannot be separated from the venomous arthropods. The grouping corresponds to the ways in which these arthropods cause pathologic conditions. In this respect closely related species may frequently be separated from each other; e.g. some muscoid flies are only contaminators, others are eye frequenters or blood suckers, still others have parasitic larval stages causing myasis, while distant species in the orders with similar importance come into the same group of human reaction (e.g. blood sucking lice, gnats and ticks).

Animals which are adapted to parasitic life are more or less confined to special hosts. There are some species which live only in or on one host—these are called monoxenic. The human lice and itch-mite are specific parasites of man. Some others are polyxenic parasites of mammals or birds, but may accept man as a more or less adequate alternate host. Some of the blood feeders gorge almost indiscriminately on any available animal or man. Some will attack man only in the absence of their normal hosts. There are certain insects which are not parasites, but have offensive and defensive weapons and man may become accidentally the victim of their bites, stings or irritative excreta. Still others have no direct relationship with man, but man may suffer from exposure to their irritative or allergenic hairs, excreta, exuviae and secretions.

The contact between arthropods and man may be a permanent one, as in the case of true parasites: scabies mite or lice, also called stationary ectoparasites or epizoons. Sandflea or myasis-producing fly larvae have a periodic parasitic habit. Mosquitoes, bed bugs, ticks mites, and some flies attack only for a short period and are thus classified as temporary ectoparasites. Stinging scorpions, wasps, bees, etc. cause injuries only accidentally.

The practical importance of an insect is greatly influenced by its geographic distribution, population density, and the close or loose contact between man and the natural environment of the animal. Environmental, ecologic and socio-economic factors determine the range of species to which an individual is exposed. Susceptibility to infestation or attack may be also subject to changes during life.

274

It would make a huge volume to enumerate all the arthropods which have caused some harm connected with possible allergic effects in man complete with relevant details of the published material. Arthropods having a large population and a world-wide distribution are of great importance especially when they are permanently attached to man. Lice, bed bug, itch-mite are examples of this group. On the other hand, there are many other species inhabiting some limited parts of the world, or having only a low density, occurring rarely and in small numbers, or else having only little and occasional contact with man, e.g. the ectoparasites of animals, horse flies, gnats, ticks, which attack man only accidentally.

MECHANISM OF INJURIES

The mechanism and site of penetration of the irritating, allergic or toxic substances of arthropods may show great variations, of which more than one may be implicated simultaneously [134a, 150, 229a, 242d, 262c, 278b].

The closest contact is established in the course of parasitic life when the host tissues are invaded. Still, true parasites are of lesser importance and symptoms, if present, depend largely on mechanical and allergic mechanisms.

Mechanical trauma connected with the injection of harmful substances could be divided into four essential types:

1. Trauma caused by piercing, blood sucking insects
2. Biting of arthropods with two main types of offensive weapons to injure the skin: piercing tube-like mouth parts, or biting forceps-like mandibles or chelicerae
3. Injury caused by stinging arthropods
4. Penetration of hairs into the skin.

Finally, simple contact with arthropods or with their hairs, secretions, living or dead tissue may also provoke reactions either by direct toxic or irritative effect, or due to allergic sensitization.

The offensive mouth parts, as well as the defensive weapons (stings, hairs, glands) of arthropods are extremely variable. The mouth parts may have the character of primitive jaws, may be of the forceps-like mandibulate type, like those of beetles and cockroaches, or biting poison-injecting chelicerae, like those of spiders; others have sucking-licking proboscis like the house fly, or piercing-sucking mouth parts like various flies, fleas, bugs, mosquitoes, etc. The two main types of stings are the modified ovipositors of bees and other Hymenoptera, or a spine connected with a poison-gland which is the weapon of the scorpion. The bite is an offensive weapon; the salivary glands of biting insects contain enzymes and different proteins. Stings are designed primarily for defense, the structure of the venom containing organs and the venoms themselves are different from these of biting insects. Hymenoptera have injectant antigens. The two groups of 'toxins' are chemically and pharmacologically distinct, and call for different methods of therapy [282].

The site of injury is in most cases the skin, either simply the surface is contaminated through contact with the insect or its excreta or hairs, or the skin may be penetrated injecting the harmful substance into the epidermis, or transcutaneously into the subcutaneous layer. The site of penetration may be a cavity with mucous membrane, such as the intestinal or respiratory tract, or occasionally the eye or urinary tract.

The transmission of various infectious diseases introduced at the time of the bite or other injury, and secondary bacterial infections which commonly gain entry through scratching, are the most important side-effects.

VENOMS AND ALLERGENS

It is true that a spider bite is poisonous in its character and that the mite hairs have an allergic effect, nevertheless, in most cases it is difficult to sharply separate the two types of reaction. The chemical composition and pathological effect of different substances are known only in a few instances.

Irritating gland secretions, toxic glands and body fluids have mostly envenomization, irritating, vesicant, haemorrhagic, haemolytic, or neurotoxic effects. The manifestations appear almost instantly without an incubation period, and the harm is proportional to the amount of venom. Sensitization is a fairly common phenomenon caused by different enzymes and proteins of arthropods, insect secretions, insect parts, bristles, hairs, scales or cast skin. Some of them may produce anaphylactic reaction.

In a greater number of cases, however, when bites or contacts are followed by various types of local immediate- and delayed-type reactions, or systemic effects, these are due to a combined action of venomous and sensitizing substances.

The factors responsible for arthropod allergy are still rather obscure. Present knowledge regarding antigens is deficient, and the presence of specific antibodies can be proved only in the case of certain grave systemic reactions. The clinical and histological manifestations supposedly caused by antigen–antibody reaction (urticarial, Arthus-type reactions, erythema) permit no inferences as regards the mechanism itself. One has to rely on indirect proofs, such as the demonstration of the insect, or the cessation of symptoms and complaints after an application of insecticides, or in a changed milieu. It is important to know whether the time elapsing between the primary bite or sting and the appearance of clinical symptoms suffices for the development of hypersensitivity. Signs and symptoms of the anaphylactic type have been found to respond to antihistaminic and sympathomimetic drugs as well as to corticosteroids. Also clinical observations and experiments on volunteers may provide some clues.

ALLERGY AND SENSITIZATION

The first recorded case of allergic reaction to insect bite was probably the death of king Menes of Egypt in 2461 B.C. caused by allergy following a hornet sting [95]. There are few reports in the literature on deaths caused directly by arthropod bites or stings, nevertheless, in tropical and subtropical countries such fatalities occur more frequently than deaths caused by snakes, beast and other dangerous animals. The number of deaths caused by insect bite is about double of those due to snake bite in the U.S.A. [224] and ten times as many in Mexico [184]. In approximately one-third of the fatal cases an allergic mechanism is supposed to be involved, the rest is of venomous character.

Arthropods may give rise to local or systemic reactions [155]. All ages, all races and both sexes are vulnerable, but children are in general more frequently affected [95], and in ⸢diseased people the reaction may be worse than in healthy adults.

In spite of this limited knowledge, there is strong evidence that the exaggerated local reaction and the systemic effects come about on an immunological basis. This evidence is based not only on the characteristic clinical and histopathologic pictures but also indirectly on the large number of favourable therapeutic responses to injections of material of arthropod origin resulting in considerable reduction and even abolition of hypersensitivity reactions [262c]. A person having once reacted to insect contact or bite will develop a stronger reaction to the next one in about 65 per cent of the cases. Recognition of the change in the reaction intensity, or demonstration of the specific antibodies may, therefore, help in instituting measures making the next antigen–antibody reaction tolerable or to prevent a severe course. The allergic pathogenesis may play a more significant role in fatal cases than the toxic substance introduced with the arthropods' venom [207]. The most severe anaphylactic reactions are known to occur after Hymenoptera stings. Anaphylactic reactions, though mostly less severe, are also caused by black flies, bugs or by some piercing-blood sucking insects. True allergic hypersensitivity to insect proteins develops in people parasitized by mites, or in those working habitually with dead, hairy or scaled insects, or with pulverized insect parts by contact or by inhalation.

The course of naturally acquired immunity to bites and stings of arthropods is unpredictable [262c]. With some insects, such as fleas and mosquitoes, the exaggerated response subsides and soon may become minimal [135]. Certain individuals are immune and do not become hypersensitive at all [262c, 272]. Apiarists, further, people inhabiting mosquito-infested areas, as also people living in bed-bug-infested flats often become immune to these insects. On the other hand, some patients show increasingly large reactions to stings of Hymenoptera and increasingly distressing reactions to the bites of mosquitoes, flies, and fleas so that they are obliged to change their residence [262c].

Antigenic substances may be associated with saliva, venom, cuticular substance, or with the whole arthropod body itself. Each order has its special antigenic properties [298], while—within the order—antigenic identity may exist between closely related species [262a].

It is in the oral salivary secretion that the major antigen fractions of the piercing-biting insects' allergens are contained [298]. Concentrated emulsion administered i.c. may produce the clinical manifestations of hypersensitivity caused by mosquitoes [7, 276] and fleas [36a, 37]. These secretions are thought to act as haptens which, when conjugated with proteins of the skin collagen, behave as complete antigens and produce an immediate-type (weal), or delayed-type erythema response [37]. Two antigenic fractions (mol. wt. 4,000 and 1,000, respectively) have been distinguished in the oral secretion of the flea [354].

Five stages of skin reactivity could be differentiated in general as a histological response to repeated exposures to insect bites [35, 152a]. (i) Neither immediate- nor delayed-type reaction occurs when there is no poison in the injected saliva. (ii) Absence of an immune reaction, but local infiltration by lymphocytes indicating sensitization. (iii) Simultaneous infiltration by eosinophils and lymphocytes. (iv) This stage is the beginning of desensitization when infiltration by eosinophils still exists, without delayed-type reactions. (*v*) In the last stage both immediate-and delayed-type reactions subside.

As regards stinging insects, it is their venom and poison-sac which, in experiments conducted on Hymenoptera, proved to be especially significant antigens. Rabbits inoculated with the contents of the poison-sac of wasps together with Freund's adjuvant produced antibodies against 7 poison-sac, and 12 or 13 sacless body extract components [199*d*]. Antibodies produced to two of the latter group were identical with the anti-poison-sac antibodies. Inoculation with bee and yellow jacket antigen induced an antibody response only to two poison-sac components, one of which was identical with that of the body extract. It emerged from absorption tests that the specific antigen pertained to the poison-sac, a finding confirmed by experiments with pure bee venom. Members of the order Hymenoptera carry more than three body antigens. One of these is common to bees and wasps but is not present in the body of yellow jackets; an antigen common to the bee and the yellow jacket is absent from the wasp extract, whereas a third antigen contained in the extracts of the wasp and the yellow jacket does not exist in the bee. Whole-body extracts of honey bee whose stings have been removed and the non-stinging drone are likewise antigens.

There is still no conclusive evidence that the venom of stinging Hymenoptera alone is the responsible antigen [262*c*]. It is an inhomogeneous substance containing also histamine, 5-hydroxytryptamine, acetylcholine, slow reacting substance (SRS), protein-like substances with specific, non-enzymatic pharmacologic action, and enzymes [248]. The relative amounts of these substances vary from species to species, e.g. hornet venom seems to be the richest in acetylcholine [207].

It is by the presence of these potentially active substances that the non-reaginic pathway can be explained in certain cases so that such substances may be released without immunological background, especially in connection with wasp sting [274*a*]. Solenamine, a biologically active fraction, has been isolated from the venom of the fire ant [3]. Associated with the alkaline constituents of the venom, solenamine is composed of two closely related compounds (pyrrholidine and pyrrholine derivatives) and is a potent necrotoxic and haemolytic agent. Solenopsin A, an alkylated piperidine, has been isolated from the red variety of the fire ant [208].

The antigenicity of the venom has been demonstrated by gel diffusion, i.c. test, and passive transfer [263]. Specific desensitization may be successful with the use of poison-sac extract. In contrast to the protein fraction of the insects' body, the antigenicity of pure bee venom, which is characterized by tissue and/or organ specificity [298] has been doubted by some authors [59]. Chromatographic fractionation and the analysis of the major fractions have shown that the poison-sac contains a species-specific antigen suitable for the provocation of skin reaction [298].

The major protein and polysaccharide components of the integument or cuticle of insects have been examined for antigenicity [298]. Chitin, a complex insoluble polysaccharide, seems to be inactive. 'Arthropodins', i.e. water-soluble complex substances, obtainable from the endo- or procuticle [118], elicit immediate-type weal reaction in individuals possessing reaginic antibodies to them. The retention of visible quantities of cuticular material in the bite produced by ticks or other arthropods violently brushed off while their mouth parts or stinging apparatus remains, will result usually in delayed papular or nodular lesions [262*c*]. Some authors [262c] question the pathogenic significance of immediate hypersensitivity in cases of natural bite or sting. Arthropodin derived from moth larvae *(Diphania dorsalis)* has three electrophoretic fractions when examined with an antiserum produced in rabbits by immunization with the extract of flies, cockroaches and mosquito larvae. With the method of gel diffusion, the fly antigen produced four, sometimes six precipitation bands with the serum [102]. The antigenicity of sclerotin (a complex of water-insoluble pigment and amino acids, a tanned protein) is doubtful. Certain glycoproteins (e.g. resilin) have also been studied in this respect.

The whole body of the insect is often suitable as an antigen for i.c. test, and may be successfully employed for specific desensitization. Rabbits immunized with the whole-body extract of insects (bee, wasp, yellow jacket, hornet) in Freund's adjuvant produced haemagglutinating antibodies against all extracts [32]. In gel diffusion, the antisera showed four bands if wasps, three bands if bees or hornets and two bands if yellow jackets were used. Cross-reactions were not noticed except with some hornets and yellow jackets.

CLINICAL SYMPTOMS

After contact with some arthropods various forms of dermatoses are observed. In cases of arthropod parasites well characterized diseases such as scabies, myasis linearis, etc. will be observed. Biting and stinging arthropods provoke reaction by injecting the venom or the salivary secretion into the skin.

The symptoms produced primarily by poisonous venoms or simple irritating substances having no sensitizing properties, are very different and are confined to the group or species possessing that venom. The symptomatology of these reactions will be mentioned only in connection with the arthropod concerned. The allergic effects, on the other hand, follow general trends in spite of the extremely large number of species of biting and stinging arthropods, their different feeding habits, and the wide variation in the patient's reactivity to the introduced salivary secretions, irritants and allergens. These factors determine the diversity of the resulting clinical features [8, 134a, 262c, 278b].

When an insect of the sensitizing type pierces the skin, there may be no visible reaction at the site of the bite, or an urticarial weal may appear within a few minutes and persist for 3 or 4 hours. After some 24 hours this may be succeeded by an erythematous firm papule which may persist for several days, and is often replaced by a pigmented macule. Either the weal or the erythematous papule may show a central haemorrhagic punctum, which becomes more evident as the acute reaction subsides [262c]. The number and distribution of lesions depend on the type of exposure and the feeding habits of the species. New bites by the same species will often cause a recrudescence of activity in lesions already present. Bullous reactions are fairly common on the lower legs but may occur in other sites, especially in children. Rarely, haemorrhagic or ulcerated lesions, cellulitis with lymphangitis may develop. Irritation is an almost constant symptom and may be severe. Rubbing and scratching may increase the inflammatory changes, induce eczematization or vesiculation [278b], and promote secondary infection [262c]. This is often true for bites of mites, bed bugs, fleas, and lice. Some local reactions that increase in severity over a 24 to 48-hour period with erythema, swelling, tenderness, and regional adenitis are the result of infection. Patients with many simultaneous stings may show systemic symptoms of a toxic reaction.

The most common reaction to an insect sting, however, is the acute swelling which usually subsides after a day or so. The immediate reaction consists of oedema of the dermis, closely followed by perivascular infiltration of polymorphonuclears and lymphocytes [132]. After several hours eosinophils, plasma cells, and histiocytes appear. The sting canal, after a bee or wasp sting, is a minute defect in the epidermis; beneath this point a delicate necrosis is found in the dermis [180]. The surrounding loose connective tissue is oedematous, without cellular infiltration.

The type of reaction provoked by an insect bite or sting in the individual patient will depend to a large extent on previous exposures to the same or related species, but it will also be influenced by many other factors [278b]. In general, the immediate-type reaction predominates in bites by mosquitoes and in stings by bees, wasps and related insects, whereas reactions to flea bites are more commonly of the delayed type. The reactivity of the patient to the antigenic stimulus is also an important factor. Atopic subjects are particularly liable to develop immediate-type reactions, with severe, sometimes fatal, systemic manifestations. Circulatory stasis or ischaemia can increase the intensity of the local reaction.

Intensive local reaction (urtica if it is immediate, erythema if it is delayed) may indicate a state of sensitization. Nummular eczema has in some cases suggested chronic reaction to arthropods. If it is excluded that such positive skin reaction may be coincidental, an encouraging result of specific desensitizing treatment may support the causal relationship.

Lesions of hypersensitivity may vary depending on the manner of skin penetration, the quantity or quality of venom or salivary secretions introduced, and the manner of obtaining the blood meal. The lesions may be influenced by, e.g. accidental introduction of bacteria or the retention of cuticular material identified to be mouth parts or stinging apparatus [262c].

When bites are very numerous, and/or the local reaction is severe, they may be associated with generalized objective symptoms (e.g. erythema multiforme, fever) and subjective complaints (e.g. malaise). Moreover, generalized manifestations may appear without any visible local reaction.

Persistent insect bites show the following characteristics [72]: (i) lesions remain active for weeks or months after the supposed termination of the initial exposure; (ii) lesions appear also in originally intact areas; (iii) unusually large amounts of serous exudate may present a picture of pseudoeczema; (iv) if the lesions persist, they tend to disseminate around the primary trauma. The antigen may remain in situ for a long time, it may cross-react with other antigens, and also continuous occult exposure is possible.

The most characteristic form of insect bites is the manifestation known as papular urticaria [58] (syn. strophulus infantum, lichen urticatus, prurigo simplex acuta, Brocq).

According to the definition proposed by Rook [278b], papular urticaria is a chronic or recurrent eruption of weals or of firm papules or of weals surrounded by papules. There may be bullae, especially on the legs. Lesions are often grouped in clusters. The disease is frequently seasonal in incidence and afflicts predominantly children between the ages of 2 to 7. Each lesion persists for 2 to 10 days and may leave pigmentation. Apparently healed lesions may be reactivated when fresh crops appear.

Formerly endogenous infections, helminthiasis, psychological stress, chemical substances, digestive disturbances and food or drug allergies were supposed to play an aetiological and/or pathogenetical role in this disease [33a, 279, 296]. Hallam [148] called attention to the patient's environment. Subsequent investigations [278a, 279, 296] have shown that (i) the pattern of the eruption corresponds to the biting habits of the offending insect and that the seasonal incidence coincides with its peak prevalence; (ii) skin tests with the appropriate insect antigen are positive (both the immediate and the delayed type) in patients significantly more often than in control subjects [287, 296]; (iii) the histological changes in papular urticaria proved insect bites and skin test reactions to insect antigen to be strikingly similar [262c, 287]; (iv) the proper use of parasiticides is an effective treatment [50].

Papular urticaria is rare in the first year of life, since few children have as yet acquired specific sensitivity to the insect antigens [278b]. Its decreasing incidence in older children is related to specific desensitization by repeated bites. The species responsible necessarily vary with the environment. In most towns throughout the world fleas and bed bugs are important causes. In rural areas the range of species is much wider. Dog, cat and bird fleas [32a] are the usual offenders but the human flea, bed bug, mosquitoes and dog louse are sometimes incriminated [54]. The distribution of the lesions depends on the insect responsible. Recurrent impetigo may be a troublesome complication. With most free-living species the attacks are seasonal, in temperate climates being worst in the summer; with others there is no winter remission or the attacks become worse in winter (e.g. body louse). Admission to hospital always ends the attacks and moving to a new house sometimes does so. If exposure to the ectoparasite is allowed to continue, the attacks persist for an average of 3 or 4 years, perennially or recurring seasonally, but they occasionally persist into adolescence or later.

If the clinical picture is suggestive of papular urticaria, the attention of the dermatologist is nowadays usually focussed on lice and fleas from dogs, cats and human beings, less commonly on bed bugs, mosquitoes and possibly other insects. The source of infection may be the furniture and floor of the living room, even a family pet, a dog or cat (e.g. *Cheyletiella yasguri* [332] or *C. parasitivorax* [49]) mite parasite. In unsensitized human skin exposed to the *C.* mite, papules developed and faded off within several hours. After iterated exposure to the mite for some months the subjects seemed to have been sensitized to the mite and the lesions prevailed for several days [49]. In other cases harvest mites, chiggers (Trombiculidae, Dermanyssidae or Sarcoptidae) may be the causative agents of prurigo parasitaria [332].

Urticariform inflammation and oedema in the upper part of the cutis around the bite trauma are the most frequent histological findings [262c]. Histologically, the reactions to bites follow a very similar pattern, dependent on the degree and type of allergic sensitivity rather than on the species of arthropods, but with minor variations related mainly to the feeding habits [26, 75, 278b]. Oedema in the dermis is followed by perivascular infiltration with neutrophil leukocytes, later by subepidermal oedema and sometimes vesiculation. The predominance of lymphocytes supervenes subsequently [262c]. As the immediate-type sensitivity develops, eosinophils appear and gradually become predominant [200]. At the stage of the delayed-type reaction there is a diffuse dermal infiltrate consisting at first predominantly of lymphocytes but later the number of plasma cells increases. Sometimes there may be a central necrosis with round cell infiltration, walled off by fibroblasts, and marked infiltration with eosinophils [32a, 262c]. Bullous reactions [75] develop beneath a more or less intact epidermis and may be multilocular. Chronic reactions [6] persisting for months or years may show changes very similar to a delayed-type reaction but with an increased proportion of histiocytes and plasma cells. Secondary lymphoid follicles with germinal centres are sometimes formed. If remaining cuticular fractions of the feeding or stinging apparatus is present, there may also be a grossly nodular, and microscopically granulomatous lesion with many giant cells of foreign-body type. Acanthosis and hyperkeratosis, sometimes pseudo-epitheliomatous hyperplasia may occur. Reactions to remaining mouth parts, e.g. in some tick bites, may give rise to persistent granulomatous papules or nodules. In other cases the persistence of the reaction is associated with binding of the hapten to dermal collagen [37].

Persistence of reactions to bites [6] for months or years is not uncommon. Tick bites, in which broken mouth-parts may have remained, are most likely to persist, but even bites of mosquitoes and other insects may do so. A firm papule, usually between 1 and 2 cm in diameter, remains intensely irritable but acquires a warty, and sometimes pigmented, surface [278b]. The persistence of multiple bites [72] may present diagnostic problems on account of the continual activity of the original lesions and the apparent reception of new lesions at originally unaffected sites.

SYSTEMIC REACTIONS AND ANAPHYLACTIC SHOCK

Systemic reactions are occasionally preceded by increasingly large local reactions to previous stings, but many people have large local reactions to successive stings for years without ever developing systemic sensitivity. Most local reactions are simple inflammatory responses to the toxic chemical substances in the venom.

Any sensitizing substance of arthropods may provoke a high degree of hypersensitivity. Most frequently it occurs to wasp and bee stings, but bugs (Cimicides and Reduvids), lice, flies and scorpions are also known to be capable of causing anaphylaxis.

The diagnosis of systemic reaction to insect stings is usually easy on the basis of the history and physical findings. It is nevertheless likely that rapidly fatal reactions, shock fragment or anaphylactic shock are often misdiagnosed, the death being attributed for instance to heart disease [242d].

Clinically the systemic reactions may be classified into four groups of increasing severity [242d]: (i) slight general reaction (31 per cent) with generalized urticaria, itching, malaise, anxiety; (ii) moderate general reaction (38 per cent) with any of the above plus two or more of generalized oedema, constriction in chest, wheezing, abdominal pain, nausea, vomiting, dizziness; (iii) severe general reaction (20 per cent) with any of the above plus two or more of dyspnoea, dysphagia, hoarseness, confusion, feeling of impending disaster; (iv) shock reaction (11 per cent) with any of the above plus two or more of cyanosis, fall in blood pressure, collapse, incontinence, unconsciousness. The most fatal cases from insect stings occur very rapidly, within 15–30 min, so the victims have no time to seek medical aid. Reactions in such cases are as a rule of four types [207]: anaphylactic reaction; involvement of the respiratory tract; that of the vascular apparatus; and predominance of central nervous symptoms. Post-mortem examination shows marked pulmonary, laryngeal and renal oedema, acute dilatation of the heart, extensive haemorrhagic zones in the organs, tissues, body cavities, further, increased vascular permeability all over the body [343a]. The post-mortem findings in fatal cases of Hymenoptera stings are non-specific, the majority of deaths are due to anaphylaxis and only few to local reactions, e. g. glottal oedema with suffocation, from stings in the throat.

Serial intracutaneous testing with dilutions of whole insect extracts seems to be the best available method of evaluating the approximate degree of sensitivity in a given patient at a given time [242b]. Testing should be started with dilutions of 10^{-8} and both immediate- and delayed-type reactions should be looked for. Testing within 2 weeks of the acute systemic reaction is not recommended because patients may be in a refractory period, and thus give false negative reactions. In general, the more severe the sting reaction, the greater is the skin sensitivity, though there are exceptions to this rule. In rare cases, no skin sensitivity can be demonstrated even with the 1 : 100 dilution, yet clinical sensitivity is present, as shown by another allergic systemic reaction to a subsequent sting [242b]. Over 75 per cent of the patients showing systemic reactions to insect stings have a family or personal history of allergy, and they have a higher incidence of severe sting reactions.

DIAGNOSIS AND DIFFERENTIAL DIAGNOSIS

In most cases there is evidence that symptoms are caused by certain easily recognizable arthropods. Still when the animals are not seen or the reactions are doubtful, considerable difficulties may arise. The following phenomena point to the possibility of ectoparasites as causative agents: characteristic localization of the lesions, symptoms which are known to follow certain bites or stings, paroxysmal outbreak, seasonal character, connection with certain localities, demonstrable contact with some mammals or birds, increased nocturnal itching [54, 100].

Often the offender organism is elusive and yet a specific diagnosis, at least at the order level may be made from the character of the lesions and their distribution. The following should be borne in mind [262c]: (i) Flying arthropods more often bite or sting on the face and exposed upper extremities. (ii) Crawling or hopping arthropods, such as the tick and flea, attack lower extremities and accessible clothed areas. (iii) Bites of nocturnal marauders, those which attack victims during recumbency, may be found on almost any part of the body. (iv) Biting flies, mosquitoes, and bees produce single lesions, whereas those arthropods which feed more deliberately, preferring undisturbed areas (ticks), produce a cluster of lesions (fleas). (v) Minute biting or burrowing arthropods, such as mites, produce scattered and widespread eruptions with excoriation and eczematization. (vi) The seasonal incidence may offer a suggestion of the probable offending arthropods seeking mammalian blood, and the ecology will suggest their presence in certain areas at specific seasons of the year. For such information, the entomologist is an invaluable assistant in making a specific aetiological diagnosis.

On a morphological basis, reactions to bites should be differentiated from enterovirus (Coxsackie or echovirus) infection [82, 203a], accompanied by skin lesions varying from isolated weals and vesicles to confluent maculopapular and urticarial eruption appearing on the extremities and trunk. The viral lesions are frequently non-pruritic, occur most frequently in infancy and early childhood, and may be epidemic in nature, lasting for only a few days. Lesions due to arthropods are usually extremely pruritic, are unaccompanied by systemic symptoms, and follow a more prolonged and recurrent course.

No invariably reliable technique for the demonstration of specific antibodies has yet been proposed. The results of the usual serological methods (C fixation, haemagglutination, precipitation, etc.) are not convincing. The immunological response of individuals developing local and systemic reaction is supposed to be humoral, but the antibodies have not been clearly identified in the serum or tissue of the patients, nor have they been satisfactorily demonstrated by passive transfer of serum or cells either [262c].

Intracutaneous tests may give reactions of both the immediate and the delayed types, but their usefulness is reduced by the fact that certain antigens turn out to be negative in 15 to 30 per cent of clinically authentic cases of allergy (patients with obvious severe hypersensitivity, both local and systemic, may give only moderate reactions to testing with a specific extract) [262c]. Furthermore, the test may be positive in non-allergic individuals. Another limitation of these tests is that the intensity of the reaction shows little correlation with the clinical picture [262b]. Despite the limited knowledge of the nature of the antigens and the antibodies and of the immunologic mechanism involved, skin testing with an extract of the whole organism seems to be of diagnostic value [262c]. Since whole-body extract antigens have occasionally elicited violent reactions, it is advisable to begin with the scratch test; if it is negative, the i.c. test should be carried out with a 1 : 100 dilution of the extract. Cross-reactions between the whole-body, sacless-body and poison-sac extracts of the bee, wasp and yellow jacket are attributed to common antigens within the same order [262a, 300], or, else, that the given individual has been stung by various insects. Antigens specific for the order may be utilized for the preparation of stock antigens which make it possible to reduce the number of mass examinations [262a, c].

The leukocyte histamine release using Hymenoptera venoms clearly differentiates hypersensitive patients from normal controls [173a].

In sera from patients who had systemic reactions following insect stings measured by the RAST procedure the majority of sera contained IgE antibodies to either bee, yellow jacket or hornet venoms [274c]. Some sera had positive RAST reactions with 2 or 3 venoms. IgE antibodies against phospholipase A—the major allergen of honeybee venom—were found in the sera of sensitive patients [304a].

For passive cutaneous anaphylaxis (PCA), guinea pigs were injected with the serum of individuals sensitized by Hymenoptera in order to identify antibodies. Since no close correlation was found to exist between the results of the skin test [298], the precipitin test [295] and the PCA, the parallel employment of these methods has been suggested.

The passive transfer test and the absorption of passively transferable antibodies are utilized for the examination of antigenic affinity [199c]. Passive transfer of immediate hypersensitivity to antigens of mosquitoes and bed bugs has been

successfully accomplished [229a]. While bee and wasp antibodies can be completely absorbed by yellow-jacket antigen, yellow-jacket antibodies are not completely absorbable by bee antigen. The extract of the whole body contains the common antigen of the bee and wasp [13] while the sac venom does not. A minor component of the common antigen is present in the whole-body extract of the yellow
jacket. Cross-reaction is most pronounced between the wasp and the yellow jacket,
one of the common antigens being in the whole body, the other in the venom of the
sac. The use of lower laboratory animals and primates provides some information
about experimentally produced antibodies, but such information only offers a
method of identifying the antigenic substance of various arthropods and does
not reveal the antibody responsible for clinical manifestations [262c]. In experiments with rabbits the honey-bee appeared to be immunologically significantly
different from the other Hymenoptera [295].

TREATMENT AND PROPHYLAXIS

The treatment, if necessary, varies according the causative agent and the patient's reaction. Reactions of allergic nature can usually be treated with fairly satisfactory results. The immediate local symptomatic therapy is aimed at reducing
the intensity and duration of the reactions. Immediate weals appear within minutes
but usually persist for less than 1–2 hours. The irritation can be reduced by cold
compresses and analgesic applications; to allay irritation, also measures of palliative
therapy are recommended. Locally applied corticosteroids are rather recommended
for treatment of delayed reactions, long lasting papules and extensive swelling.
Various antihistamines taken orally are of questionable value, still, having certain
sedative effect, they may relieve the itching.

Marked cellulitis and lymphangitis may necessitate hospitalization and sometimes intensive antibiotic therapy.

In cases of systemic anaphylactic reaction the usual drugs should be applied
[30]: ephedrine sulphate and antihistamine orally, epinephrine subcutaneously,
and Isupral with a nebulizer followed by oral administration of corticosteroid.
In cases of quickly developing toxic or anaphylactic symptoms intravenous calcium is still a very effective drug.

The prophylaxis of insect bites has many important aspects. To avoid the attack
of arthropods various mechanical and chemical measures are advocated. Wearing
of shoes, boots, appropriate clothing — even the light colours of clothes — may play
a certain role. Bed netting and artificial ventilation of homes in tropic regions are
examples of mechanical means which might be applied for prophylaxis. Cleanliness
in and around the house and the preventive application of insecticides (dichorvos
vapour strips) may effectively reduce the danger of attack. It is not a difficult
task to eradicate infestation with lice, itch mite or other parasites, nor to clear the
house of fleas or bugs with the modern insecticides available [345e].

Outdoors repulsion of attacking insects, ticks or mites can be achieved with
odourless synthetic repellents applied on the skin or smeared on the garments or
clothes. Dimethylphthalate (D.M.P.) and diethyltoluamide are the best known
examples though they have a very limited time effect and protect only the part
of the body to which they have been applied.

Repellents advocated for oral use containing thiamine hydrochloride or anti-histamines or herb extracts are of little value. Pyrethrum-coil smoke, however, is very useful in the evenings to keep off mosquitoes and similar insects.

In cases of severe hypersensitivity to bees, wasps, horse flies, gnats, mosquitoes or mites specific desensitization (see Chapter 5 in Volume 1) of persons should be considered. Specific desensitization (specific immunizing or hyposensitizing treatment) has yielded not more than just satisfactory clinical results [240, 262c, 298, 317]. In order to prevent severe complications, desensitization should nevertheless be applied only in cases of very strong or generalized reactions. Preparations which give positive skin reaction are not necessarily efficient desensitizing vaccines [292]. Whole-body extracts, poison-sac, salivary gland or its contents are used as vaccines. Theoretically, the best results would be expected either from extracts of the whole body of insects which is supposed to contain all possible antigens or from the substance injected by the insect. The employment of polyvalent vaccines (prepared from the poison-sacs of several stinging species) has been suggested. It is fairly difficult to collect or rear a sufficient quantity from minute arthropods (e.g. sand flies, mites). Cross-reactions between families within orders may be utilized in this respect. Dosage must be individualized. In order to prevent systemic reaction the initial dose should be based on preliminary skin testing. A 1 : 10 or even 1 : 100 dilution of the suspension evoking moderate skin reaction is an optimum starting dilution. It is usually administered subcutaneously, but the combined i.c. and s.c. methods may in the long run prove most effective [262c]. The 'repository' method of treatment (water in oil emulsion) is effective, especially in case of systemic symptoms. It is debatable whether to employ mixtures prepared from the extracts of several insects that provoke grave reaction, because their use may enhance therapeutic risks [298].

The length of desensitization should be adjusted to the patient's response. It is difficult to offer a prognosis based on apparent clinical improvement because of the variability in the kind of biting and stinging arthropods from season to season and of the patient's exposure to them. Conclusions drawn from a statistical clinical survey have indicated that the prognosis after specific treatment is remarkably good [120e, 243a, 262c].

Organized control of arthropods of medical importance is carried out in most countries where vectors transmit diseases or insects cause great hygienic problems. The public health authorities are responsible and direct the control programs. Free living species cannot be completely eliminated. The modern measures of pest control need specially trained personnel, planning, equipment, economic support, and surveillance. The toxic hazards of pesticides and the insecticide resistance developing against the most effective pesticides in use should also be taken into consideration. Pest control has developed into a special science with a vast amount of information on materials and methods [345e, f].

ARTHROPODS IN RELATION TO MAN

ARTHROPOD PARASITES

The sarcoptid itch mite lives in the epidermis, sebaceous mites live in hair follicles and sebaceous glands, a number of fly larvae may live in wounds or in the subcutaneous layer of the skin, or pass the intestine, and the chigger larva burrows into the skin of the feet. These are the few parasites of man, all living near the surface where they have access to the oxygen of the air. The itch mite and follicle mites are monoxenic varieties, parasitic only in man, fly larvae and chiggers have a wide range of hosts and are accidental in humans. They are of lesser importance than the ectoparasites. There are no specific arthropod parasites in man living in the deep tissues or in body cavities (tongue worms — Linguatula — which live in the tissues, formerly regarded as Arthropods are now placed into a related separate small phylum Archipodiata).

Parasites living in tissues release their secretions and excretions into the body of the host. Some of these substances act as antigens, inducing allergic reactions. Parasites, well adapted to the host produce less harm. On the other hand, parasites, which spend the whole or a considerable part of their life cycle in a single host are profoundly influenced by the immunological reactions of the host and also by its nutritional and endocrine state [278b].

Human scabies

It is caused by the itch mite *Sarcoptes scabiei* var. *hominis*. Life history: The eggs of the human mange mite develop for about 3–4 days in the burrows where the female deposits daily more than two oval whitish eggs with an average size of 0.17×0.09 mm. The emerging larvae have three pairs of legs, and tend to wander to new sites on the skin surface and descend into hair follicles or form shallow pockets in the horny layer of the skin. After 3–4 days they moult into nymph stage with 8 legs, like the adults. They live in shallow burrows like the larvae. Another 3–4 days pass and the nymphs moult to produce either adult males or a second nymph stage which undergoes a further moulting to transform into females. Females reach maturity in about 14–17 days, measuring about 0.40×0.30 mm. The size of the males is only about half of that. After fertilization the females dig long meandering, sinuous burrows into the epidermis which are so characteristic of scabies.

The preferred sites of attack are the hands and wrists, skin folds between the fingers (60–75 per cent), and elsewhere, the elbow, shoulder blades, breast, feet and ankles, the genital region, penis, buttocks. The favoured areas show some variation with age and sex [278b]. In children under 2 years of age the palms and soles are often favoured sites. The sinuous burrow may reach the length of 1–3 cm, sometimes the mite progresses 0.05, sometimes 0.5 cm in a single day.

The incidence of scabies throughout the world has shown cyclic fluctuations. There was a noted rise during World War I, followed by a decline, and a rise beginning before the second war. A peak was reached after World War II, subsequently the disease became rare in the 1950s, however, in spite of improving socio-economic conditions it has increased considerably, especially since 1964.

Newly infected persons do not experience any itching. Sensitization begins in about 2–6 weeks. In experimental infections pruritic inflammation characterized by generalized papulovesicular exanthem started as late as the 3rd to 8th weeks after infection with the mites [155, 231c]. When the well-known stage of scabies develops, rash appears around the burrows, tiny vesicles and papules are formed and itch, worst at night, becomes so intense that it will interfere with sleep. Scratching causes weeping, bleeding and secondary infections. Only the burrows, and the vesicles at their ends are associated with the presence of the mite. The other lesions, which often dominate the clinical picture, are in connection with the degree of allergic sensitivity, with scratching, the persistence of the infection, and with secondary bacterial infection [95, 231a, 278b]. Small, urticarial papules often develop in large numbers on the abdomen, thighs and buttocks. Reddish brown, intensely irritable, indurated inflammatory nodules may persist for weeks or months after the infection has been eliminated by effective treatment [278b].

The nodules, which occasionally persist after successful treatment, rarely contain mites or ova [26a]. Histologically, they show infiltration with lymphocytes, eosinophils and histiocytes around blood vessels and sweat glands [39, 252]. Persistent scabious nodules [194] are characterized by small-cell infiltrates in all layers of the dermis. They consist mostly of lymphocytes and eosinophils. The papules appear to be due to absorption of the dilapidated products of parasitic excrements which, through the widened intercellular spaces in the epidermis and the lymph vessels of the papillary body, penetrate the dermis to produce this peculiar reaction.

The characteristic constant itching symptom of scabies, i.e. pruritus, may only in lesser part be due to movement of mites in burrows or on the skin in the warm bed; it may rather represent the subjective symptom of an '-id' reaction. Also characteristic areas without mites and eruptions become itching ('pruritus acarogenes sine materia'). This kind of itching also appears after a shorter or longer latency but persists after the extirpation of the parasites ('mnemoderma'). Scratch marks may be numerous and the rash does not correspond to the sites of the mites [231a]. In chronic stages scratching may be followed by eczematous changes. Eczema usually develops when the lesions persist owing to no or inadequate treatment.

Secondary infections may be manifest as pustulation or as impetiginous crusting. Colonization of the lesions by staphylococci and streptococci occurs soon and quite frequently [22]. Suppurative burrows do not contain mites because the animals have either migrated off or have died [155]. Pyoderma is sometimes complicated by glomerulonephritis [158]. Allergic sensitivity to secondary invading pyogenic cocci may occasionally play some part in the produced clinical syndrome.

It has been assumed [278b] that allergic sensitivity to the mite and its products plays an important role in producing the pruritus and in determining the development of the host reaction. The course of infection and the clinical picture, the suppression of the mite population, the different reactivity of reinfected persons [255a], as well as a number of experimental data all give evidence that scabies is a special kind of allergic disease, resulting in a weak partial immunity [106a, 231b].

Apparently allergic sensitivity develops rather slowly in the majority of cases but its role in the natural course of the disease is still not clear. Knowledge concerning mite antigen is scanty. Besides the body substances and products of the itch mite, also its toxic substances have recently been described as allergens [215, 240]. Intracutaneous tests with mite extracts have given equivocal results [153, 155, 231a, b]. Positive reactions were in general, only obtained from individuals infested for at least three months [67, 231b] indicating delayed-type hypersensitivity (cell-mediated immunity) [153a] probably associated with some skin sensitizing antibody (IgE) [66]. Numerous observations indicate the necessity of investigating the allergic aspects of the problem [215, 240, 257]. It has been observed that in families living under strictly hygienic conditions only certain members become afflicted; it was in some cases difficult to find the pathogen, there was moreover a disproportion between the number of demonstrable mites and the extension of the cutaneous phenomena. Clinical manifestations differing from the usual picture were seen to appear 3 to 4 weeks after the infection (time of incubation?) or 24 to 48 h after reinfection. Small burrowless nodules, sometimes also erythema, urticaria, papulovesicles and dyshidrosiform lesions appeared at unusual sites (trunk and extremities). They lasted for several weeks and the itch persisted despite careful antiscabies treatment and the prevention of reinfection. Scratching often gave rise to renewed regional or generalized lesions which may be regarded as the results of lymphogenic or haematogenic dissemination, i.e. '-id' reactions ('acarid', 'scabid'). The histological picture in this period shows abundant perivascular eosinophil infiltration and sometimes also signs of vasculitis. Eosinophilia (i.e. 4 to 21 per cent eosinophils) occurred in 41 per cent of the patients examined. Scabies is prone to relapses. Non-specific factors, like mechanical excoriation, chafing of the clothes, antiscabies treatment, may contribute to dissemination.

A relatively small number of mites may produce unpleasant generalized symptoms far from the site of the invasion. The immune response to the mite, inhabiting the epidermis is weak [155], still the population's growth is influenced by it soon after infestation is established.

The number of mites reaches a peak some 10 to 14 weeks after the infection, whereafter a further spread of the parasite is inhibited [66, 68, 318b], supposedly by some immunological response. The growth and decline of the mite population has been studied by infecting volunteers [231c]. During the first 3–4 weeks no symptoms can be observed. Thereafter the itching rash, oedema, vesicles and other typical symptoms suddenly develop; the mite population first grows slowly, then at a faster rate up to few hundred females for the next 6–8 weeks. The activity and multiplication of the mite is suppressed during the period of sensitization partly by the scratching which destroys the burrows and partly by the acute local antibody reaction destroying the mites.

The course of progress of the mite community and the human reaction are very different in reinfected persons when they have had scabies for some months and have developed a high degree of hypersensitivity. The skin reacts so strongly and immediately that the mite is usually destroyed. Local oedema and erythema develop within 24 h, this together with the effect of scratching exterminate the mite. In case of reinfection the pruritic exanthem may be apparent as soon as after 24–48 h [156]. Histological examination reveals intraepithelial vesiculation and circumscribed oedema. Supposedly, the inflammatory response in the sensitized host gives rise to conditions unfavourable to the mite [231b].

Infections by the parasite become less frequent with advancing age, further the course of the disease is milder, spontaneous improvement is more frequent in endemic areas, all pointing to the development of immunity in the course of repeated infections. Periodic fluctuations in the morbidity of scabies and its epidemiological behaviour are probably influenced also by immunobiological factors [31, 156, 257, 297b]. Patients with scabies tend to have a low serum IgA concentration; correlated with low IgA level in the skin secretions, this might predispose to sarcoptes infection [149a].

The presence of the mite can be easily demonstrated under the microscope, the female or the eggs can be traced and extracted with a needle, when the burrow is gently pricked open toward its end.

The typical clinical symptoms are fairly easy to diagnose by the itching and rash in the typical sites of the body, and also the burrows can often be seen.

Therapy of lasting success includes four steps. A hot bath is necessary to remove scaling, crusting detritus and to soften the skin. One of the potent scabicides must be applied carefully over the whole surface of the skin below the head. The most frequently applied medications are: 25 per cent benzyl benzoate emulsion, dimethylene-diphenylene disulphide diluted with paraffin oil; monosulphirane, crotonotoluidine, 1 per cent γ-benzene hexachloride (lindane); one application is sufficient with each. When the treatment is repeated within a few days, it may cause dermatitis. Sulphur ointments and polysulphide mixtures and thiosulphate have rather fallen into disuse.

At the same time the patient's soiled bed linen and underwear should be changed and disinfested by boiling.

To prevent reinfection adequate treatment of all contacts living in the same room or household is necessary. Attempts have to be made to find and eliminate the sources of infection.

The skin may remain irritable for a time. In rare cases persistent irritable nodules may require excision [278b].

Norwegian scabies

Norwegian scabies, sometimes called 'crusted scabies', is the same infestation with the itch mite *(S. scabiei* var. *hominis)* when the normal responses of the host to the parasite are impaired and modified [69, 169a, 278b]. There is a great number of horizontal burrows with incredibly large quantities of mites and ova, sometimes more than two million in one site [211].

The grossly thickened horny layer is honeycombed with cavities containing large numbers of mites. Large, warty crusts form on the hands and feet; palms and soles may be irregularly thickened and fissured. The nails are thickened and discoloured. Erythema, infiltration and scaling may generalize to erythroderma. Generalized enlargement of the superficial lymph nodes is present in some cases. Eosinophilia is usual. The condition is highly infectious. Itching is often absent or slight. The absent or reduced pruritus in mental defectives favours heavy infestation. Nutritional deficiency, particularly lack of vitamin A, has seemed to be a possible factor in some cases [126] and severe systemic disease, diabetes [176], leukaemia [101] or prolonged treatment with corticosteroids [278b] have also been implicated.

Investigations into the allergic aspects of the Norwegian scabies (the earliest to be carried out) [268, 269] showed the following results: intracutaneous inoculation with the extract of the skin-fragment containing the mite and the burrow produced positive reaction in 75 per cent of the acute cases, in 56 per cent of past cases, and had no effect on the controls. Skin tests employing erythrodermal scale extract as antigen were negative. The serum showed a reduced level of albumin and a strongly raised γ-globulin [251, 338]. In view of vasodilatation in all layers of the cutis, endarteritis, mesarteritis, perivascular infiltration and peripheral blood eosinophilia (16 per cent), it has been suggested that Norwegian scabies represents an extreme form of allergic reaction. Certain authors [290] deny the allergic nature of the anomaly.

The treatment advised for ordinary scabies is usually effective. Systemic methotrexate has been successfully used in refractory cases [341].

Mange mites acquired from animals

People having intimate contact with animals which are infected with mange mites sometimes experience transitory infections. These mites are host specific, they are unable to lodge permanently on man [278b]. Such infestations are usually self-limiting [197]. Biological races, varieties of the sarcoptic itch mite live on horses, dogs, rabbits, nearly identical with the variety living on man. Mites of other genera (Psoroptes, Notoëdres, Knemidokoptes, Otodectes) have been reliably incriminated, and others are probably capable of causing transitory symptoms [278b, 324, 348a].

Recurrent exposure can produce troublesome and puzzling lesions [278b]. Scrapings from the skin of patients have in exceptional cases shown mites and eggs. All these animal mites settle usually in the sites not favoured by the human itch mite, like the arm or the trunk or some unprotected parts of the skin. They produce disseminated eruption, strong itching, small weals or papules, follicular nodules, or occasionally papulovesicles.

It can be assumed that repeated contacts sensitize man, and symptoms are of similar allergic nature as in human scabies.

The eruption heals spontaneously within two to three weeks and it is easy to cure it with any of the usual drugs. However, symptoms may persist even after the contact with animals has ceased [250].

The follicle mites

Two species of small and slender sebaceous or follicle mites, *Demodex folliculorum* and *D. brevis* inhabit the hair follicles and sebaceous glands of man. Most workers considered these very common mites quite harmless saprophytes feeding only on the sebaceous material rather than attacking living structures of the skin [262c]. When they are found in the middle of inflamed 'blackheads' or in folliculitis necrotisans, their presence may be attributed to a foreign body reaction [141]. Nevertheless, in some cases they are associated with a rash of follicular papules. Periodic occurrence of large inflammatory lesions and a positive skin reaction to mite antigen would cast suspicion on this mite in some cases [120b, 262c]. It was supposed that antigens of the mite may diffuse into the dermis through the intact epithelium of the follicles [217] and under certain conditions have a pathogenic role. It was suggested to be responsible for diffuse erythems of the face with dryness, a nutmeg-grater appearance with follicular scales and a burning and itching sensation, or with a rash of tiny red follicular papules, i.e. rosacea-like lesions. Histological sections have suggested that rosacea granulomatosa may be a delayed-type allergy to Demodex [141]. In some suspected cases the use of balsam of Peru or sulphur ointments gave relief or cure.

Myiasis

The term myiasis is applied to various infestations, lesions and reactions at various sites of the body of man or animals caused by the lodging of living maggots. Only a few, tissue invading fly larvae are true parasites. The habits of various flies concerned are diverse, and their maggots have different food preferences [201, 204, 355, 358]. At least three groups have to be separated [278b].

1. *Obligate myiasis producers.* Their maggots can only develop in living tissues. A majority of such specific myiasis producing flies called bot flies, warble flies and srew-worm flies attack only animals, constituting a veterinary problem. Man is rarely and only accidentally a victim. A few tropical species are, however, known to regularly invade a great variety of hosts including humans. *Callitroga hominivorax* is an obligate screw-worm fly parasite in animals and man in the tropical and subtropical regions of North and South America. It is attracted by any wound; living on live tissue, it causes myiasis of the nasopharyngeal type in most cases. The flies *Chrysomyia bezziana* in Africa and southern India, and *Wohlfartia magnifica* in Europa and Central Asia have similar habits. The maggots of the African tumbu fly *Cordylobia anthropophaga* cause boil-like furuncular myiasis when penetrating unbroken skin. The bot and warble flies have a different relation to man. These are normally parasites only on certain animals; the cattle warble fly *(Hypoderma bovis)*, the sheep nostril fly *(Oestrus ovis)*, the horse bot fly *(Gasterophilus intestinalis)* and other species may rarely be accidental human parasites, and persist for a short period in the unusual host at unusual sites, mostly causing creeping eruption. *Dermatobia hominis*, the 'human bot' is a feared parasite of man and animals in Central and South Africa [302]. It has a very unusual way of reaching the host. It lays the eggs on flies, ticks or mosquitoes which transmit them to any host. The larva develops in tumorous swellings.

2. *Flies producing semiobligate myiasis* feed preferentially on necrotic tissues [34], develop normally in carcasses of dead animals or else in decaying flesh or other remains, mostly of animal origin. They will invade and feed on living tissue only when necrotic material is not available. A great number of genera—Sarcophaga, Calliphora, Phormia, Chrysomya and others—and many species of flesh and blow flies have been incriminated as accidental parasites in man. They invade open wounds, sores and ulcers causing traumatic myiasis, most frequently in the tropics, in people sleeping in the open air. The clinical picture is either a furuncular type in the skin or secondary invasion of suppurating wounds.

3. *Flies causing accidental myiasis.* These are different species of flies most frequently Muscidae living in the vicinity of human habitations or sheltering in houses. They may lay eggs in food or drink, which may also be contaminted by larvae and thus cause intestinal involvement. They may be accidentally attracted by pus or necrotizing tissue and settle in wounds or various natural cavities.

Depending on the localization of the lesions the following clinical forms may be encountered:

1. *Creeping eruption* or *myiasis linearis* [87] is a peculiar, characteristic, tortuous thread-like rather long burrow under the skin, appearing as a pale red line with a terminal vesicle causing itching, light swelling; at the moving end of the burrow the larva can be detected. It is mostly a first stage larva of oestrid fly: the horse bot fly *Gasterophilus* or cattle grub *Hypoderma*. The increasing itching and swelling indicate that these larvae start to produce in man similar immunoallergic reactions as they do in the animal hosts. Various barriers in the skin, lymph nodes and immunoglobulins were considered to be responsible for developing partial immunity against these arthropod parasites. These are physiopathological means of protection of the animal hosts against further invasion by the same or closely related species. Immunoglobulins of precipitating and non-precipitating classes are found in parasitized animals [124]. In man mild systemic symptoms and eosinophilia are observed.

2. *Follicular-type cutaneous myiasis* is produced most frequently by bot and warble flies. Larvae, penetrating the skin complete their development in subcutaneous pockets, having an external opening, then the furuncular swellings become pustular and the larvae emerge to pupate on the ground [278b, 304].

3. When flies lay their eggs or larvae at the edge of any lesion or open wound, sores, ulcers, or on diseased parts of the skin or mucous membranes, different forms of *traumatic or wound myiasis* may follow. In some cases it is a severe complication; the extensive lesion is in part the reaction to the organism and necrotic tissue, but a hypersensitivity reaction may also occur [262c]. Mild systemic symptoms and eosinophilia may point in the same direction. The presence of maggots in wounds, however, is not necessarily a serious complication, on the contrary, when they are feeding on necrotic tissue and excrete urea they may, in fact, expediate healing. This observation led at one time, after World War I, to the application of sterile 'surgical maggots' for the treatment of osteomyelitis.

4. Maggots can settle in *various cavities*. Ophthalmomyiasis is rather frequently traceable to sheep or goat bot flies struck in the eye. Conjunctivitis mostly heals spontaneously. Similarly sheep bot maggots may invade the nasal cavities of man causing severe headaches. Rhinitis may attract flesh causing symptoms of wound myiasis. Auricular and urinary myiases are mostly caused by blow fly larvae.

5. *Enteric myiasis.* Gastric and intestinal myiasis cases were published rather frequently. In a considerable number, however, it may be questioned as contamination or pseudoparasitism. The possibility of maggots to live and pass through the intestine alive, was rather doubted, since in various animal experiments such fly larvae were immobilized and killed within a comparatively short period.

Nevertheless, the symptoms are recurring attacks of acute gastric disturbances, connected with the presence of maggots, vomiting, nausea and violent pain;

diarrhoea has also been observed. The possibility cannot be excluded that in addition to the possibility of food poisoning of bacterial origin, under certain conditions (e.g. swallowed air in the stomach) some kind of toxic or allergic reactions may be caused even by the immobilized maggots.

Rectal myiasis is another way of infestation when maggots attack through the anus. The infestation by oral route can definitely be excluded in some cases. The flies frequently found are muscid flies (Fannia and Muscina spp.) Calliphoridae, Sarcophagidae or cheese skippers (Piophila).

Burrowing fleas

The sand flea, also called chigoe or jigger *(Tunga penetrans)*, inhabiting the Central American tropical and subtropical regions, also became a pest in the West Indies, Africa, Madagascar and South Asia. The larvae of this small burrowing flea develop in sandy soil, in shaded places. Fleas emerging from the cocoons are about 1 mm in length. They wait for an animal to pass by, though they highly prefer a barefoot man [34]. Once on man the females usually attach themselves to the skin under the toe nails or burrow into the soles of the feet or some other sites of the skin. The flea, in addition to causing mechanical injury, produces extreme irritation and inflammation while the flea is enveloped into the skin. It is not actually burrowing, but the peculiar — probably allergic — reaction of the skin forms in fact a hiding place around it. The females retain the eggs in their body, and as a result they swell up to the tremendous size of a small pea. The wounds are nodular swellings, which become painful and ulcerate, and rather frequently secondary infection follows. Death caused by gas gangrene or tetanus is not infrequent. The burrowed fleas can easily be removed with a needle or blade. The wearing of shoes gives proper prevention.

The stick fight flea *(Echidnophaga gallinacea)* introduced from Southern Europe to subtropical America [155] became a common pest of poultry. It may also attack man in a similar way as sand flea, attaching itself firmly to the skin. Yet it is only an accidental parasite of man, and then mostly in children.

PIERCING, BLOOD-SUCKING ARTHROPODS

In a great variety of different groups of arthropods, blood-sucking feeding habits have developed. With lice, fleas and other true ectoparasites this is the exclusive way of feeding, yet only the females of mosquitoes, gnats and other Diptera seek blood meals, since the protein of the blood is needed for egg production. There are a number of insects in which blood feeding or the licking of the mucus of the eye and wound secretions is a still developing ectoparasitic habit. This stage of adaptation is reflected in the modification and transformation of the mouth parts and also of the gland secretions, capable of preventing blood clotting and dissolving tissue cells.

There are some forms that suck only plant juices, while others live on the body fluid or blood of other insects, still others may prey on the blood of higher animals, birds and mammals. Only a few have adapted themselves to ectoparasitism on a single

294

host. Monoxenic ectoparasites of man are the human lice. Most blood-sucking arthropods may have host preference, but they may also feed on a variety of other animals, as do most of the mosquitoes. Most blood-sucking insects in the same systematic group vary in the avidity with which they feed on human blood. Man is accidentally attacked by a great variety of blood-seeking arthropods, normally feeding on animals, e.g. by horse flies, ticks, mites, etc. It may be established as a rule that the more adapted parasites tend to cause less injury to the host.

The skin is easily penetrated with the tube-like, sharp sucking-piercing mouth part of insects. This tube may be a single long rasping-piercing labellum, as in the stable fly, but usually it is formed by a bundle of very fine piercing stylets supported by a flexible labium. The stylets are strongly modified sharp mandibles, maxillae and a blade-like labrum, the lower one being a thin hypopharynx carrying the salivary duct. The salivary glands secrete proteolytic, haemolytic and other substances which prevent the clotting of blood.

The reaction of the host is primarily influenced by the composition of the saliva which is injected into the bite, and by the subsequent course of sensitization. This type of injected insect saliva contains primarily allergens, whereas that of mites and ticks has also some toxic substances.

Most larger ticks attach themselves to the skin with their chelicera mouth parts, which are then pressed deeper into the wound by muscle action. The hypostom part for sucking is slipped in afterwards. Some ticks and blood-sucking mites have comparatively short mouth parts. They need a special mechanism of feeding which can hardly be regarded as simple blood sucking. The Trombidicula larvae can push their chelicera mouth parts only about to 25 μm depth to anchor themselves. After this saliva is secreted that quickly hardens. A second secretion has a histolytic action and forms a canal in the centre of the hardened hyaline mass. This canal—called histiosyphon—serves to connect the mouth of the mite with the tissue cells of the subcutaneous tissue through the intercellular ridge. The cells at the end of the canal are dissolved by the injected proteolytic enzymes and serve as food together with the intercellular fluid containing also some blood. The response is oedema, inflammation and also some tissue necrosis. Ixodid ticks have—like Trombidiidae mites—two different saliva excreta, but no central sucking canal is formed since the anchoring chelicerae are pressed down deep enough into the tissue. Argasid ticks have only one saliva secretion of histolytic type. Their saliva, in addition to producing oedema, also causes the escape of red blood corpuscules from the capillaries in the connective tissue.

There is a difference in the mechanism of skin penetration and also in the secretions of piercing insects, and of ticks and mites; consequently, the reactions to piercing will also have distinct characteristics. Insects cause sensitization, ticks and piercing mites induce venomous long-lasting inflammatory processes.

The sensitization to saliva usually follows a similar pattern. The first bites provoke no or only a slight local reaction, but after some weeks sensitization develops with different degrees of immediate- and delayed-type reaction connected with systemic disturbances. Desensitization is a slow process.

The course of this type of reaction of allergic nature caused by blood suckers has already been mentioned in general (p. 277). Perhaps three grades could be differentiated. Lice, bed bug and anopheline mosquitoes usually do not cause any noticeable effect at the first attack. On the other hand, fleas and gnats usually cause a reaction on the first occasion, which may become quite severe after sensitization. Progressive decrease of reactions marks a process of desensitization. Ticks- and mite bites are rather venomous in character, thus hypersensitivity does not develop, nor does a real desensitization occur.

The reaction of the individuals may also vary considerably. There are some who are apparently not susceptible to insect bites, and others whose reaction is extremely severe. Bed bugs and martin bugs may cause swelling and severe irritation in some people but not in others.

The clinical picture of local immediate and delayed-type reactions is of the type of papular urticaria (see p. 280). Variations are sometimes characteristic for the insect species. At a later stage, in addition to local symptoms, systemic disturbances may be observed, such as malaise, fatigue, irritable mind, and a skin rash similar to German measles. Still later the skin becomes pigmented and hardened.

Experiments in which volunteers and guinea pigs were exposed to the bite of fleas or mosquitoes at one- or two-day intervals had the purpose of studying the acquired immunological response and the course of sensitization [36b, 37]. It was found that the initial dermal reaction was of the delayed type (7 to 14 days), which was followed by the appearance of an immediate-type reaction in the form of a weal developing within 20 to 60 min and disappearing in a few hours; the immediate-type reaction became then predominant, but it also progressively diminished until the reaction was no longer inducible. This phenomenon is looked upon as an acquired immunity. The same sequence of reactions was observed in self experiments with bed bugs [120a]: first the delayed-, then the immediate-type reaction predominated; the latter persisted, and repeated bites after five months provoked generalized urticaria and severe shock. Both types of response disappeared on desensitization. Again, others [171] observed the following sequence in human experiments with serial flea bites: (i) delayed-type inflammation for 7 to 14 days; (ii) immediate-type reaction; (iii) increased urticariform inflammation. Serial mosquito bites applied to animals [170] provoked first an immediate-type reaction, which was then followed by residual lesions.

The human lice

The head louse *(Pediculus humanus capitis)* and the body louse *(P. h. corporis)* are two closely related varieties of one species, which occur in distinct populations. They show minor morphological and more distinct physiological differences, and quite different habits. Both complete their development in about 19 days, from which about half falls to the egg and half to the nymphal stages. All sucking lice (Anoplura) are wingless, blood-sucking ectoparazites of mammals that live in continual proximity to the skin throughout their life cycle. They are highly host specific, well adapted to parasitism, and their saliva causes hypersensitivity with irritation.

The head louse inhabits the scalp mainly of children and of persons with long hair. The nits are attached onto the hairs half an inch or so from the scalp, often detected on the temporal and occipital regions. The majority of infested people usually carry only a small number of lice because they try to remove or destroy them. The reactions to the salivary antigens of the louse follow the usual course

[278b]. The pruritus induced through sensitization to the saliva varies in persons and with the time of infestation from slight itching to severe urticariform papular lesions, worst at the occiput and behind the ears. Secondary bacterial infection with Staphylococci lead to impetigo, eczematization and enlargement of the regional lymph nodes. Prolonged infestation gradually leads to habituation, and the cutaneous reactions and subjective symptoms become less pronounced in the course of the years. Several potent insecticides of low toxicity can be used to eradicate lice including 1 per cent γ-lindane emulsion, NBIN emulsion (used in the U.S.A.) and Topocide. To avoid reinfestation other members of the family or of the infested group should also be deloused [345g].

The body louse resides in the underwear and on the inner surface of clothing hiding in the seams. It is a minor problem in developed countries and in peace time when clothes are changed and washed regularly. The louse visits the skin to feed when people are resting. The majority of infested persons carry only a small number of lice, but nits can be detected in the seams of garment or sometimes attached to the hairs of the body. The great danger of body louse lies in its transmitting exanthematous typhus, trench fever and relapsing fever [345g]. The body lice saliva may give rise to similar sensitization as the head louse. In the first week there is no reaction to the bites, then minute, red, non-inflammatory points appear flush with the skin. After about a week they become papular and weal-like. The pruritus, the most prominent symptom, however, is not limited to the site of the bite, but spreads to other skin areas and is worst at the back. Parallel linear scratched excoriations in the interscapular region with bloody crusts are almost pathognomic. Prolonged persistence of these symptoms may result in the so-called vagabond's disease. Thickened, dry, scaly skin develops with postinflammatory hyperpigmentation. People feeding lice in laboratories found that periodic biting at regular intervals often results in hypersensitivity. There is also presumptive evidence of naturally acquired tolerance.

Antigen prepared from the faeces and head of Pediculi elicits delayed-type reaction in sensitized individuals. Pediculi and Pthiri may give rise to local and seldom to systemic allergy [262c].

To eradicate the infestation of larger population groups repeated application of powder insecticides (10 per cent DDT, 1 per cent Lindane, 1 per cent Malathion) is still the best measure, as it was proved at the end of World War II. To achieve immediate results, however, a combined treatment is necessary including insecticide application to the body and the delousing of all clothing and bedding by boiling, steam or dry heat, or by fumigation; in the rooms insecticide spray or fumigation should be applied to destroy the scattered hidden lice which often leave the clothes taken off at night.

The crab louse *(Pthirus pubis)* is a smaller kind of lice with broad abdomen. It moves but little, settles down usually at the pubic and perianal region grasping the hairs with strong claws, inserting its mouth parts into the skin. It may also settle on the abdomen, thighs, eyebrows and eyelashes. It is not easy to detect the small greyish insects, their nits are attached to the hairs, but the skin around where they cling to the hairs is stained with reddish brown dust of the excrements. Crab louse is mostly transmitted by intimate contact, it lives a very sedentary life and it is very sensitive away from the host.

The onset of sensitization is similar to that caused by the Pediculus lice, and is indicated by changes in the symptoms [272]. Nevertheless, the salivary antigens of the crab louse are different and the reactions are more pronounced. The fresh infestation goes unnoticed for about a week, then the slight irritation quickly turns into severe urticaria. The almost continuously injected saliva elicits an immediate urticarial and a delayed papular reaction, which causes more annoyance, itching, and burning sensation, while the sites of previous bites, whence the louse moved, also show signs of exacerbation. Extreme sensitivity can result in bullous lesions [189]. Blue-gray spots with an irregular outline, known as maculae coeruleae, are also frequently observed at the site of bites and also on the abdomen at a distance from the bites. They persist for 2–3 days, and are in connection with altered blood pigments. Heavy infestation by pubic lice accompanied by maculae coeruleae may sometimes be associated with fever, malaise, headache, lymphadenopathy and leukocytosis [286].

To eradicate the infestation the most satisfactory method is the application of insecticide dust, which does not irritate the excited skin, and repeat the treatment daily for one week. Lice on eyelashes should be removed with a fine forceps.

The bed bug

The species *Cimex lectularius* is known as the bed bug in temperate, subtropical and in some tropical zones, while *C. hemipterus* and *C. rotundatus* are more common in the moist tropics [95]. Certain other similar species are parasites on swallows, martins and bats, and may occasionally attack man [81, 278b]. The bed bugs of man will readily feed on any mammal or bird, and quite often infest laboratory animals. Bed-bug infestation has substantially decreased since the universal use of DDT, yet in some regions resistance developed, and bugs still persist in poor urban districts, slums, and also in well-heated, modern buildings.

The bed bug is a flat, reddish insect of about 0.6 cm length. It undergoes partial metamorphosis, all the five nymphal stages resembling the adults. They require a rather warm air temperature to grow and survive, the optimum being around 27 °C, and need blood meals at regular intervals, ranging from 2–10 days depending on the temperature. One female will lay 300–400 eggs, and population growth depends also upon food supply and prevailing temperature. They avoid light, and during day-time hide in cracks and crevices of the walls and furniture in a state of immobility. A full meal of blood takes about 5–10 min. The bug pierces the skin with a slender needle-like stylet which includes two canals with one duct each, one conducting the saliva, the other drawing blood. The bite causes no immediate pain and usually does not disturb the sleep of the victim. The preferred parts of body are those not tightly covered by the bed clothing. Bites are often grouped in pairs or triples fairly close together, often linear in distribution [95]. The bugs continue biting until they are able to find a capillary under the skin from which blood is tapped. In the individual not sensitized by previous exposures there may be no symptoms, only a pruritic macule indicating the site of the bite. The stages of sensitization follow the usual sequence [262c, 278b]. In sensitized subjects a succulent weal appears, surrounded by a vivid flare, or papules surmounted by haemorrhagic puncta. Some people react with a weal to the bite of *C. lectularius* while the same person may develop a papulous reaction at the site of the bite of *C.*

rotundatus [272]. The firm urticaria may transform into a lesion persisting up to 14 days; with the slightest irritation it again begins to itch intensely [95]. There may be vesicles added to the lesions and 'secondary' weals may develop nearby. If there is remission, old lesions which have disappeared are reactivated when the patient is bitten again elsewhere.

The Prausnitz–Küstner reaction may be positive if passively sensitized areas are bitten. Self experiments [120b] resulted in a delayed-type reaction followed by an immediate-type one. The latter type of reactivity persisted for more than five months, and repeated bites provoked generalized urticaria and severe shock. Both types of reaction disappeared parallel with desensitization. Some individuals are immune to the bite of bed bugs, others display an average degree of sensitivity and still others are hypersensitive. The latter develop large weals at the site of the bite with a vesicle in the centre and also more distant 'secondary' weals may develop. Oedema sometimes grows into bullae. Repeated exposure revives the past reaction to previous bites, resulting in a cumulative reaction. The time needed for the development of maximum sensitivity appears to be about 6 weeks. Persistently recurring bites confer a sort of transient immunity, and accordingly the intensity of skin reactions abates.

The bites of other Cimicid bugs are essentially similar but the reaction they elicit depends on the time and type of exposure [278b].

Haematosiphoniasis [9] is caused by 'flats' or 'mahogany flats' *(Haematosiphon indorus)*, which are pests of poultry and other birds causing eruptions usually on exposed skin, but the eruption may be generalized, polymorphic with papules. Vesicles, pustules and scabs reflecting the degree of sensitivity, the age of crops of lesions, and the amount of secondary infection may be found. It is sometimes a serious pest in the South-West U.S.A. and in Mexico.

The most effective control method against all bugs is the use of residual insecticides of prolonged action (DDT, Diazinon). The deposits of spray applied to the walls and furniture kills the insects after contact. Efficient fumigants (hydrogen cyanide, dichlorvos) also yield an immediate extermination.

Triatomid bugs

Triatomid bugs feeding on the blood of vertebrates and transmitting the American trypanosomyasis *(Schizotrypanum cruzi)* to man, occur mainly in Central and South America [34, 108, 115, 120b, 262c, 278b]. They are called conenoses, assassin bugs, vinchucas, kissing bugs, barbers, etc. These bugs, quite large in size, are often brightly coloured, fast runners and swift fliers. They hide in cracks of delapidated houses and rural dwellings or in burrows of armadillos and other small mammals around the house. They are active at night. The bites of *Triatoma megista*, the large domestic bug in Brazil and other domesticated blood-sucking species (Rhodnius, Panstrongylus spp.) are painless and leave no mark. Some prefer sucking blood through the conjunctiva.

The bite of a widely distributed species, *T. rubrofasciata* is quite different. The salivary glands contain a powerful anticoagulant. The bite leaves a large irritable itching lump, which may last for about three weeks. Certain species as *T. sanguisuga* in Mexico and Asia, and *T. protracta* on the Pacific coast have strong sensitizing saliva which may lead to severe anaphylactic reactions. *T. sanguisuga*, a notorious blood-sucking species, causes four types of kissing-bug reactions [297]: (*i*) papular lesions with a central punctum; (*ii*) grouped vesicles; (*iii*) giant urticaria-like lesions with intense oedema over a large area; (*iv*) haemorrhagic nodular to bullous lesions on hands or feet. Lymphangitis and lymphadenitis may be associated with the latter two types.

Allergic reactions [249] are usually extensive, sometimes resulting in local vesiculation and necrosis and even in generalized urticaria as well as systemic symptoms. Several species are house bugs in the rural districts of the U.S.A. 'Anaesthetic saliva' is the responsible antigen. The bite is first painless but causes after a few minutes or hours the appearance of a small weal or massive oedema, which may arise even at some distance from the bite; also stridulous laryngeal oedema, asthmatic attack or anaphylactic shock may ensue [150]. In view of the gravity and dangerous nature of the bite, desensitization with whole-body extract is the method of choice [115].

Defensive bug bites

The large order of Hemiptera including the family of Reduvid bugs, also a few blood-sucking bugs, and others feeding on plants, and some which attack other insects and suck out their vital juices, all have piercing and sucking-type mouthparts with which a number of species may inflict painful defensive bites. The painful and local irritable weal may persist for several hours, and there may be generalized urticaria [262c, 278b]. Occasionally, local vesiculation and necrosis may occur. Bug thrusts produced in self defence when handled carelessly, which are not feeding bites but are accompanied by the emission of offensive musk, cause sharp pain. Treatment of the local bite reactions, if necessary, should be in accordance with the symptoms. If itching is intense, it responds to antihistamines and local corticosteroids. Control of domestic species is fairly effective with remanent insecticide spraying, however, good housekeeping and the eradication of peridomestic small animals is also necessary.

Fleas

Fleas are all blood-sucking insects, having compressed bodies and jumping hind legs. They undergo a complete metamorphosis. The legless grubs feed on organic debris on the floor. The adult stages visit their hosts at intervals. Most fleas are monoxenic parasites of bats or other animals. There are only a few associated with human dwellings and causing annoyance. According to host preferences there are three groups: (*i*) The human flea *(Pulex irritans)*, which also readily feed on swine and other domestic animals; (*ii*) The dog flea *(Ctenocephalides canis)*, which also attacks man in many regions, and the cat flea *(C. felis)*, that similarly attacks man only occasionally, (*iii*) rodent fleas, which are more restricted to their hosts, but may accidentally suck blood from humans. Most important is the tropical rat flea *(Xenopsylla cheopis)*, the principal vector of plague and the rat flea of temperate regions *(Nosopsyllus fasciatus)*, vector of endemic murine typhus [34, 155, 219].

Infestation with fleas is in connection with a low standard of hygiene where the larvae are able to develop undisturbed on the floor. Congested communities and close contact with animals harboring fleas favour their spread, but there are also regional differences in many countries.

The sensitizing compounds of the oral secretions of fleas are somewhat different from those of most blood-sucking insects. The potent part are primarily haptens which combine with the protein of collagen tissue to form antigens. These sensitizing agents are of relatively low molecular weight and dialysable. This is an explanation why cross-sensitization is observed. People who became sensitized to any flea will also react to the bites of unusual flea species to which they could have never been exposed under normal conditions [171, 278b].

People differ greatly in their allergic reactions to flea bite. The lesions are grouped in lines or irregular clusters, have a central punctum, which, being not prominent, must be looked for. There is initially a grouping of urticarial lesions, which lasts for a few hours and is then followed by a small papule, surmounted by a vesicle [206, 262c, 349]. In contrast to urticaria, the individual lesions require several days to resolve [95]. Scratching may be followed by impetigo. The stages of sensitization and subsequent decline in sensitivity after repeated bites show the usual patterns [278b]. The sufferers are usually children or those recently exposed, such as new residents in infested areas [206] until they develop tolerance. The bite in sensitized subjects is a strongly itching weal, or vesiculation, or a papule which is often, but non invariably, centred by a haemorrhagic punctum (purpura pulicosa) depending on individual disposition and the degree of sensitization [88, 283]. Severe local reactions are unusual, but bullae occasionally develop. Sleeplessness, generalized pruritus, urticaria or delayed-type reaction with erythema multiforme-like induration and, later, discoloration are occasionally observed. In children the clinical picture is often that of papular urticaria. Of children with papular urticaria, 77 per cent were found to be sensitive to flea or bed bug antigen, whereas only 1.5 per cent of the controls showed positive reactions [51]. Flea bite produces no symptoms on the skin of newborn infants. Regularly repeated exposure of adults who react to the 'first' bites may lead to immunity [348a]. A person who is immune to the saliva of a certain flea species may, in another country, react positively to the bite of the same species.

Treatment of the flea bite—if necessary—follows the usual rules of topical and systemic anti-inflammatory therapy. Fleas, however, can be eradicated and controlled with relative ease. Still, there are some serious cases of hypersensitivity, when desensitization is indicated. The filtrate of whole-body extract may be useful [151, 207]. The results are difficult to evaluate since spontaneous desensitization may ensue after repeated natural exposure [278b].

Recommended control measures [345e] include insecticide dust (synergized pyrethrum, lindane, malathion, etc.) applied on the clothes and bedding, also similar treatment to dogs and cats, removal of all rubbish and collections of sand which are the breeding sites, cleaning the floor in the whole household, and the use of an insecticide to wash the floor, which must be regularly swept and cleaned because good housekeeping is the best prevention. When visiting flea infested areas diethyltoluamide serves as a good repellent.

The appearance of these insects is familiar to most people. The rather long slender wings, long legs and the elongate thin piercing proboscis are characteristic of all Culicidae. More than 1,600 species have been described. Only females suck blood. There is an immense literature on mosquitoes because anophelines are vectors of malaria and other diseases. *Aëdes aegypti* is a feared transmitter of yellow fever. Dengue fever, several types of filariasis and viral encephalitis are also mosquito borne diseases [25, 107, 136, 155, 175, 213, 219, 258, 302].

Different species vary in the avidity with which they feed on different hosts, and have preference to human blood. Species to attack man viciously are called anthropophilic. Only a limited number are house frequenting and bite indoors, especially *A. aegypti, Culex molestus* and a few anophelines including *A. maculipennis*. Most are troublesome in the open, woodland, parks or costal districts.

Human sweat contains certain substances attracting mosquitoes, whilst the surface lipids are repellent [212]. Mosquitoes are attracted to dark clothing, humidity and heat, especially in combination [271].

The human reaction and the clinical features of the bites of different species are extremely variable, ranging from no reaction at all, or immediate superficial and extensive soft tissue swelling to delayed reactions with indurated lesions and even vesicles and bullae occasionally progressing to necrosis [262c]. The composition of the active substances in the saliva, which are of allergenic nature, are inadequately known, but these foreign proteins acting as antigenic substances and the individual reactivity combined with the degree of acquired allergic sensitivity are the main factors determining the nature of the reactions [95]. The well adapted mosquitoes as most anthropophilic anophelines do not cause much reaction nor pain and irritation without sensitization [278b], indicating that there are no real toxic substances in the saliva. The saliva of Aëdes mosquitoes has been found to contain an anticoagulant, a haemagglutinin, as well as some toxins [234]. Different chemical entities have been shown to exist in different species and in the different regions of the mosquito's salivary glands. Bites of some species are fairly painful even at the first occasion, indicating that they contain irritative substances.

It is well known that some people suffer more than others, while certain people do not even realize that they have been bitten. As a rule, after bite or regular biting, first sensitization develops in most susceptible people, and delayed reactions, about 24 h after the bite begin to occur; these are usually itching papulae surrounded by reddening and swelling. They may persist for several days. Severe local reactions are particularly common, but anaphylactic-type generalized reactions are rare [95]. In highly sensitive subjects bullae, cellulitis and eczematization are often seen, especially on the legs. Intense haemorrhagic necrotic reactions occur but in rare instances. Further experience of biting will result sooner or later in desensitization, a tolerance, or in the case of complete immunity not even immediate weal will develop. Such a tolerance, however, is mostly confined to some species or group of mosquitoes and reactivity to others (for instance to Theobaldia) may remain to some degree.

In experiments [268] laboratory animals did not at first react to repeated bites of *Anopheles atroparvus* but then became gradually sensitized and responded by immediate and delayed-type reactions, manifested by petechial and erythematous lesions of varying intensity. The degree and persistence of sensitivity showed great individual variation. The number of eosinophilic cells was directly related to the degree of sensitization. The period of desensitization, marked by progressive decrease of the cutaneous reactions was fairly uniform.

The bites of the common European species *Culex pipiens molestus*, Anopheles and Aëdes cause small red weals, which develop into nodules that may last for several days. These lesions are itching and become especially so on being rubbed or scratched. Oedema may become vesicular (nettle rash). Scratching may lead to secondary impetiginization. Cutaneous lesions may start itching again after the lapse of 24 h (delayed-type reaction). As a rule, the bite of the female *C. pipiens molestus* causes only immediate reaction as evidenced by intracutaneous test [202]. The joint occurrence of immediate- and delayed-type reaction is twice as frequent in adults as in children. Intradermal tests with mosquito antigens showed significant immediate hypersensitivity in patients with mosquito allergy. Of the antigens prepared from the female, from the male and from the larva, the first was found to be the most potent [130], and the larval antigen the weakest. The Prausnitz–Küstner reaction may be positive if passively sensitized areas are exposed to bites. Tests regarding the antigenicity of mosquito larvae and pupae [117] showed that both were active in inducing precipitin production, and that the precipitin could be absorbed from the serum using antigenic substances prepared from another mosquito genus. Larvae are more useful for the purpose of desensitization, especially if the genus is unknown. With antisera raised in rabbits and guinea pigs with whole-body extract of male and female *C. pipiens molestus* [129] at least four (possibly six) antigen fractions common to both sexes were revealed by agar gel diffusion and immunoelectrophoresis; the precipitins were found in the IgG fraction. Similar antibodies have not been demonstrated in human sera. Successful specific desensitization has been achieved by the use of *A. aegypti* mosquito extract: response to bites was weaker or absent for periods varying from a few days to four years [229b, 276]. *Aëdes aegypti* and *C. pipiens molestus* evoke cross-immunity. Following desensitization after the bite of *C. pipiens molestus*, the skin test may remain positive in children for a very long time, even after the clinical symptoms have disappeared [317].

For therapy of usual bites a cream massage and avoiding scratching are advocated. Measures of prevention include the wearing of protective clothing and the use of repellents (dimethyl-, diethyl- or dibutyl phthalate, diethyltoluamide alone or combined with phthalate, as fluid or cream). Control measures can be directed against larval or adult stages, especially spraying in dwellings is practised [345e].

Sand-flies

More than 300 Phlebotomus species are known living in moist tropical and subtropical regions; and called sand-flies, vein cutters, gnats or midges. They are small sized, fragile, about 2–4 mm in length, have long legs, body and wings, clothed with long coarse hairs, often admixed with scales, the wings are held in angle position (erect upward and outward). They undergo a complete metamorphosis. The mouthparts are adapted for piercing and sucking. Only females suck blood on a variety of animals and on man. Their great danger lies in the transmission of diseases such as cutaneous and visceral leishmaniasis (kala-azar), the three-day or pappataci fever, and Oroya fever (Carrión's disease and verruga peruana).

By daytime they shelter in caves and dark corners and fly with short hops, and attack silently at night, seeking out ankles, wrists, knees, and elbows. A painful stinging sensation is followed by persistent pruritus. Firm, whitish weals are characteristic [95]; they persist for several days even in the absence of secondary infection. When there are many bites, systemic symptoms, such as malaise, nausea, and fever may develop.

Allergic sensitivity develops rather quickly and in cases of hypersensitivity they cause the clinical syndrome known in Israel as harara or urticaria multiformis endemica [320]. They afflict new arrivals in endemic areas. An intensely irritable eruption develops on the exposed skin in the form of papules, weals and bullae within a few days. The lesions increase in size and severity for a week or two, then gradually decrease over a period of several weeks. In subsequent seasons of sand-fly prevalence the reactions are mild or do not develop at all [99, 210].

People living in areas inhabited by sand-flies become usually tolerant or immune to their bites.

Personal prophylaxis for new arrivals can be achieved with repellents and pyrethrum sprays in the houses. Control of sand-flies is rather effective by house spraying with DDT or other residual insecticides and by destroying their breeding places (crevices in rocks and stone walls, damp cellars, drains, moist earth, animal burrows).

Biting midges

Over 400 species are known, mostly from the Holarctic region. The females of the family Ceratopogonidae are very small, gnat-like insects, called also punkies. They possess sharp piercing mouthparts, though only some of them are known to attack birds, mammals and a number of species in the genus Culicoides and Leptoconops also bite man. They bite mostly in rough open country, in warm and calm weather, near their breeding sites. In large numbers they may even prevent outdoor work in restricted areas, or constitute serious problems in costal summer resorts. They can pass through mosquito-screens.

Their feeding is fairly rapid, the bites are vicious and exceedingly unpleasant [262c]. Papules and nodules are produced, and the swelling may become vesicular and exudative healing with a red scar in particularly sensitive individuals. Irritation may persist for days or even for several weeks, and itching becomes intense in sensitized persons.

The exaggerated reaction to the bite of *Culicoides furens* (called 'no-see-ums' in Central America) showed early haemorrhagic lesions [14]. Within several hours there is widespread oedema, and after 24 h vesiculation with infiltration with eosinophils and neutrophils develops. After 48 h there are, in addition, bullous changes with more marked eosinophilic infiltration and an increased number of mononuclear cells.

For short protection repellents are useful. Control will be efficient only when breeding places, mostly marshland or mud, are treated with larvicides.

Blackflies

Simuliidae, also called buffalo gnats, turkey gnats, and coffee flies, are a world-wide terrible scourge to animals and humans, around streams and lakes, especially owing to the strong allergic reaction to bites. They are small hump-backed flies with a stout body and short legs. Their larvae are breeding in rapidly flowing steams and rivers with much oxygen content. Swarms, however, may spread over many miles. In tropical America and Africa blackflies are the vectors of onchocerciasis which often leads to blindness. In a number of other northern countries they may occur in vast swarms; some species are also common around the lake regions of the northern U.S.A. and in East Canada, and make life miserable in summer time for hunter and fisherman [34, 278b, 345b].

The blackflies have rasping, blade-like, piercing mouth parts and inflict so painful bites as no other insects do. They are feeding in daytime and only outdoors. The favoured parts are the unprotected skin on the neck, forehead, legs and wrists. It was supposed that it injects some kind of an active toxin which causes the extreme pain, and that swarming gnats are killing hundreds of horses, cattle by toxaemia from their venomous bites. The course of bites, however, seems to indicate an ana-phylactic shock in fatal cases. The normal course of the first bites is a small, usually painless ecchymosis, followed by the development of a pruritic, occasionally bleed-ing papule [143]. There is a small, but distinct haemorrhagic punctum at the site of piercing, that is not found after bites of mosquitoes or midges. Soon an itching weal develops and the area becomes oedematous. The subsequent symptoms de-pend on the degree and type of allergic sensitivity [262c]. In some individuals lesions may persist for weeks. Extreme pain, intense itching, swelling and some-times severe complications occur. Lacerating bites may bleed freely and may become secondarily infected, leading to lymphadenitis and lymphangitis. Along with local reactions there may be a general reaction, called 'blackfly fever' with headache, fever and nausea, which varies in intensity with the number of bites and the sensitivity of the individual and is usually of one or two days' duration [219]. For personal protection repellent ointments are useful for hours. To control blackflies as vectors, good results have been obtained with larvicides in the streams and rivers [345b].

Blood-sucking flies

There are a great number of the robustly built true flies which feed on blood. They are classified in different families and groups. Of the suborder Brachycera the most important are the horse and deer flies (Tabanidae), and the snipe flies (Rhagioni-dae). Some species from the large Muscidae family, notably tsetse flies, stable flies, and louse flies (Hippoboscidae) may also accidentally attack man. The tsetse flies (Glossinae) are the vectors of sleeping sickness in Africa; other flies can transmit tularaemia, anthrax or loasis. The antigenicity of their salivary gland excreta is variable.

Horse flies, deer flies, mango flies, gad-flies and clegs (Tabanidae) with more than 3,000 species of large, robust, often beautifully coloured flies, occur all over the world; their females are blood suckers of animals, but a number of species also attack man [34, 155, 219].

Tabanid flies are strictly diurnal and bite outdoors. Some of the favourite sites are the wrist, the neck or the leg. With their primitive mouth parts they inflict deep, bleeding, painful lesions.

The swelling may become extensive and lasts for days, although the delayed-type reaction varies greatly in different people. Severe immediate reactions to horse fly (Tabanus) and deer fly (Chrysops) bites are occasionally seen [278b]. Systemic symptoms may occur [262c].

Two American genera of snipe flies (Rhagionidae) include blood-sucking species behaving as deer flies, which are vicious biters, seriously annoying man in some mountain regions and along the Pacific coast and Alaska [155].

Tsetse flies are confined to tropical Africa. Both males and females are voracious blood feeders, they bite in daytime and outdoors. The bite of trypanosoma-infected flies is stated to produce more local reactions that the bites of uninfected ones, although swarms along rivers are very troublesome.

The stable fly *(Stomoxys calcitrans)* and its relatives, the horn fly *(Haematobia irritans)* and the Australian buffalo fly *(Haematobia stimulans)* are associated primarily with cattle. Both sexes attack man out of doors mainly on the legs. The stable fly may enter the houses in rainy weather. It bites with its club-shaped protruding proboscis, which is a horny beak, the lesions are painful, deep and bleeding. Allergic sensitization appears to be slight.

Louse flies (Hippobosca) are rather confined to their animal hosts. Nevertheless, some species may rarely bite man, especially in woods or persons handling animals. Their bites are very painful and the swelling reactions persist for days or weeks.

Treatment of fly bites is seldom necessary except for those in highly sensitized people, chiefly children [95].

Moths

There is very little information on the reaction of man to the blood-sucking species of moths in Africa and tropical Asia [27, 71].

Ticks

Two kinds of the large blood sucking acarines are called ticks. The hard ticks (Ixodidae) have a shield on the back and armed mouth parts visible from above, and the soft ticks (Argasidae) have no shield and their mouth part is located ventrally. Larvae, nymphs and adults attach themselves intermittently to animals or man. The period of blood sucking depends on the species and stage of development; with hard ticks it may last for some days, while soft ticks feed for short periods during the night. The approximately 800 tick species known have different host preferences. Man is not a natural host for any tick, yet a number of species may parasitize mammals and man fortuitously. Ticks are important vectors of a number of diseases of animals and men, including rickettsial infections (spotted fever), virus encephalitis and Colorado tick fever, relapsing fever, tularaemia, etc. [167, 345d].

Soft ticks visit their hosts at night, like bed bugs, while hard ticks stay in woodland and grass. Man picks them up when walking and they attack some hours later in the soft parts of the skin. Children may also be bitten on the legs and scalp.

The direct effects of tick bites, apart from loss of blood, include envenomization, injection of toxic substances, and allergic sensitization. Some ticks may produce tick paralysis. Both soft and hard ticks may cause local and systemic disturbances.

After sensitization soft ticks usually only cause a mild itching dermatosis. Some species give rise to more or less serious symptoms. The sites of bites become often necrotic and painful. Ornithodoriasis [185] is manifested as multiple, firm, crateriform nodules with haemorrhage around the central puncture wound. Intense pruritus reaches a peak about the 12th day, when the lesion begins to subside. Some Ornithodorus species, notably *O. coriaceus* in Mexico and California, the African *O. moubata*, *O. talaje* and *O. turicata* cause hard weals, swelling, irritation lasting for weeks or months, and scar formation.

The bites of most hard ticks attacking man are not serious. Little injury results from the bites of the European Ixodes or the American *Dermacentor variabilis* or *D. occidentalis*. The tendency to cause allergic reactions varies in the different species, as do also the salivary gland secretions and the penetration of the mouth parts. Some ticks secrete an anticoagulant and a toxic substance of unknown nature [278b].

The bite is painless; hence the tick is usually detected only after several hours or even days of attachment, when pruritus develops. If only the bite reactions are present, the usually small number of bites, and the presence and persistence of nodules with umbilication, necrotic centres and serous discharge may help in establishing the diagnosis [352]. The infiltrated lesion has a distinct erythematous halo. Acute inflamed pruritic areas later indurate and become ulcerous and granulomatous, or may even develop into a pseudo-epitheliomatous hyperplasy if head and mouth parts remain in the lesion. Ixodidea bites may be followed by pruritus and urticarial reaction if the host has been sensitized by previous bites [323], these may persist for a few days after the tick has been removed [278b]. In a few cases only an eczematous response was observed [352]. Persistent itching leads to lichenification. Besides local allergy [120b, 155, 221], pyrexia caused by a toxin secreted by female ticks [100] may occur. Patchy scalp alopecia has also been observed [218]. Multiple bites in berry-pickers produce the picture of papular urticaria [339].

Secondary infection is common, possibly as a result of the introduction by the tick of bacteria from the skin surface, or of the victim's own scratching of the pruritic area [262c].

Histologically [347] there is intercellular oedema causing almost complete obliteration of the basal cells in the acute stage. In the subacute stage a dense cellular infiltration, densest around the blood vessels, with lymphocytes, polymorphonuclear cells, fibroblasts, eosinophils, and large mononuclear cells extends from the reticular cutis to the subcutaneous fat. In the chronic stage the dermis is replaced by dense fibrous masses containing Langerhans' giant cells, lymphocytes, eosinophils, and mast cells.

The adult stage of castor bean tick *(Ixodes ricinus)* is thought to be dangerous and responsible for the direct skin lesions (urtica) [323]; its saliva is supposed to be antigenic [193]. In August its larvae attack individuals engaged in cranberrying and provoke epidemic strophuloid eruptions [323]. It has been supposed that erythema chronicum migrans is caused by larvae remaining in the immediate vicinity of the bite. This is supported by the observation that tick-head extract and the excised material are pathogenic to animals [193]. Used in self experiment, the excised piece of skin induced typical lesions after 6, 19 and 23 days [48]. The venom may sometimes be responsible for erythema chronicum migrans and acrodermatitis chronica atrophicans, and lymphoma-like collections of cells in the dermis. Dermal granulomata [352] may lead to lymphocytoma. The bite of *I. ricinus* may induce both disorders after a long period of incubation. It has been suggested that erythema may represent an early abortive form of acrodermatitis [218]. The mouth parts of ticks anchor them so securely to the skin that the capitulum often remains in the tissues if the tick is forcibly removed.

The nature of the tick–host interaction and the attraction of neutrophils to the site of injury has been studied [36a]. Tick salivary gland extracts have no intrinsic chemotactic activity, but can induce such an activity of human or dog serum. Activity was also generated from human C5 but not from C3. The chemotactic factor appeared to be a C5 cleavage product. C depletion of C5 in rats by cobra venom treatment greatly reduced the tissue necrosis and inflammation. This model of tissue injury is analogous to the immunological models of the Arthus reaction and acute nephrotoxic nephritis. In each case, the C system provides the chemotactic factors for neutrophils, and the ensuing damage is neutrophil dependent.

Tick paralysis occurs after a 5–6 day feeding period of the females of *Dermacentor andersoni, D. variabilis* and *Amblyomma americanum*. Humans are most susceptible and may be killed by a solitary tick. Since the year of 1900 some 300 human cases including 30 fatalities have been recorded in Canada, all due to *D. andersoni* [139]. It is a flaccid ascending paralysis without fever. Respiratory paralysis may be fatal, especially in children [1a, b]. The unknown toxin affecting the neuromotor system acts in many respects similarly to some organic insecticides. It may be detoxified easily, since rapid recovery follows upon the removal of the tick.

Acquired resistance of host to tick bites occurs in animals and man. When resistance develops, ticks either fail to attach to that host or do not feed normally. Observations prove that acquired immunity to tick bites does exist, however, only some hosts develop immunity against certain species of ticks, while others do not. Trager was the first to show the development of an acquired passively transferable immunity of the guinea pig to *D. variabilis* [328].

The mouth parts of different ticks vary in length and not all ticks in fact penetrate host tissues. Variations suggest that the relative length of the mouth parts and thickness of the epidermis are important in determining the final depth of penetration and the location of the damage produced in the dermis. *Rhipicephalus sanguineus* attaches itself to the host mainly with an adhesive cement substance, and the hypostome does not penetrate the epidermis. The reaction beneath the mouth parts develops progressively over 4–5 days. Oedema of the epidermis appears, and the dermal infiltrate becomes prominent; initially it consists of polymorphonuclear leukocytes. A cavity in the dermis develops progressively [319]. Most ticks possess longer divergent chelicerae having recurved teeth which hold so fast that if the tick is torn off by force, the capitulum is retained in the skin. Should a portion of the capitulum or the whole remain in the skin, a punch biopsy will effectively remove it.

Various means are recommended to make the tick release itself. A few drops of chloroform or ether may be most effective, then the tick's capitulum should first be pressed farther into the skin in order to release the grip of the recurved teeth, subsequently the tick can be pulled away sideways. In more tender regions a cotton-wool cover soaked in soft paraffin may be more acceptable, though removal is only possible after some hours. The supposed complete removal of the tick may not prevent a development of a prolonged and progressive tick-bite granuloma [131].

Blood-sucking mites

All active stages of gamasine-Dermanyssid mites are obligatory blood feeders mainly on birds and rodents, but they will also attack man. They wander off the hosts between blood meals. *Liponyssus sanguineus*, the American mouse mite transmits the mite-borne vesicular rickettsial pox. Other mites are vectors in the U.S.S.R. and the Far East. The ubiquitous rat mite *Ornithonyssus bacoti*, the tropical fowl mite *O. bursa* and the northern fowl mite *O. sylvarum* also bite man. The chicken mite or red poultry mite *Dermanyssus gallinae* is a common ectoparasite of fowls; it may temporarily infest human beings, similarly to a bird mite, *D. avium* [25, 107, 345d].

All these medium-sized blood-sucking mites may attack man in living quarters and induce rather extensive skin reactions, local allergic manifestations, itching, rash, and other clinical symptoms, such as an eschar at the site of the bite, or lymphadenopathy [278b, 348a].

The clinical picture varies widely according to the route and severity of infestation and the degree of the host's allergic sensitivity to the mite's antigens [278b]. The most characteristic change is a profuse eruption of small, intensely irritable weals or papules, occasionally with a central punctum, sometimes grouped and often asymmetrical, usually sparing the face and hands. Scattered superficial pruritic lesions sometimes become eczematous [262c]. In children the lesions may be vesicular.

The reactions may vary with the different species. After sensitization to the tropical rat mite, usually urticarial weals, papules or even vesicles develop [95], the fowl mites generally cause itching dermatitis [34], while chicken mite provokes small erythematous or papular, violently itching rashes [95]. Among the members of a single household exposed to the same infestation with *D. avium*, some individuals have seen to show papular urticaria, others a profuse eruption suggesting scabies but without burrows; secondary infections may complicate the clinical picture [122, 278b].

When therapy is indicated, antihistamines and corticosteroids should be preferred. Control is effective when the animal host is eliminated or freed from mites.

Cell-juice sucking mites

The larval stages of trombiculid mites, of about 0.2–0.3 mm, known as chiggers attach themselves to the skin of animals and also of man walking in low scrub, in grass, or among weeds [34, 262c, 348a]. Such mites occur over extensive parts of the world. The different species of *Leptotrombidium*, namely *L. akamushi*, *L. deliense* and other species occurring in the Far East, are also vectors of the rickettsial disease called scrub typhus or tsutsugamushi fever [34, 278b, 345d]. In other continents several other harvest or velvet mites cause scrub itch. In Europe a widely distributed species, *Trombicula autumnalis*, in America *T. alfreddugesi*, the 'red bug' and *T. irritans* [34, 155] are common. The harvest or velvet mites are red or orange in colour and have a velvety appearance.

The six-legged larva of trombiculid mites after being firmly attached to the skin by its short mouth part, first injects a digestive fluid, which hardens the epidermis, then a second fluid which forms a canal by disintegrating and digesting the cells. Thereby a canal traversing the epidermis and extending to the subcutis develops. The dissolved cells are sucked off and utilized as food. The injected fluids have both direct and sensitizing effects; the itching begins after a few hours and can be severe due to the intense and prolonged irritation, and dermatitis resembling scabies or chickenpox develops. A row of weals is often found along the line of a constriction of clothing [95, 278b].

The induced skin reactions differ according to the mite species and to the sensitization of the subject. Differences in the seasonal appearance and geographical distribution have also been noted. The North European harvest mite usually becomes attached to the ankles, thighs, groins or waist where it hides for 1–4 days [162, 219]. It provokes numerous urticarial red nodules (scrub itch) in late summer and in autumn [348a]. More generally the scratching removes the larval forms [95].

The North American *Trombicula irritans* produces local allergic and, rarely, generalized reaction. The resulting clinical picture depends [95, 265, 267, 278b, 344] on the quantity and type of clothing worn, the degree of infestation and the intensity of allergic sensitivity [34]. In the non-allergic host only slightly irritable, small, red macules develop after 1–3 h, which subside after a few days. In the sensitized host the itching gets worse, even intolerable; after 24–48 h papules and nodules appear, varying in size, often with puncta in their centres, and occasionally with vesicles [95]. There may also be marked urticarial or vesicular lesions [262c], or sometimes haemorrhagic patches [348a]. The itching gradually subsides over the next 5–6 days. Regional lymphadenitis is not unusual and some patients develop a lymphocytosis in the peripheral blood [267]. In highly allergic individuals there may be malaise and mild fever, at times with erythema multiforme-like lesions.

The lesions inflicted by the trombiculid mites are not 'bites' in the common sense of the word. Histological studies [181b] have shown variations in the degree of the secondary inflammatory response. A small hyaline mass forms around the puncture wound. The host's response is very variable and depends partly on the irritating properties of the mite's saliva and partly on the degree of allergy. In an intensely acute reaction the epidermis may show vacuolization and vesiculation, and there may be oedema and a polymorphonuclear infiltration in the dermis. Later, the lymphocytes increase in number, and chronic granulomatous changes may develop.

Antihistamines and corticosteroids have been recommended for therapy [95]. The various substances used for personal protection against chiggers are rather toxicants than true repellents [138], they provide the best protection when applied to the protective clothing, but if inadequate clothing is worn, it may be necessary to treat the skin, too.

A number of mites of other families are liable to cause irritation of allergic nature. A peculiar kind of facultative parasitism occurs with the grain itch mite *Pyemotes ventricosus* (syn. *Pediculoides* = louse mite) and with the widely distributed *Dermatophagoïdes scheremetewskyi*. Both may attach themselves to the skin of humans causing dermatitis. The grain itch mite normally is an external parasite on insect larvae, the active female often attacks man in search of a host. Epidemics of dermatitis have been recorded in America and elsewhere among people handling straw or grain, or sleeping on mattresses infected with these mites, as well as among labourers handling cotton seed. These mites often attach themselves to the skin of the chest, abdomen or back under the clothes. Dermatophagoides mite is only an accidental parasite infesting the skin, primarily on the scalp. Both cell-juice sucking mites are able to cause persistent infestation. Itching soon develops, followed by an urticarial rash, the pea-sized spots are surrounded by red areas. On the nodules vesicles may soon develop; the dermatitis sometimes resembles scabies or chickenpox. Later general symptoms, headache, vomiting, diarrhoea, rise of temperature and pain in the joints may follow in highly sensitized people [57, 113, 127]. The lesions, often numerous and distributed depending on the route and duration of exposure, are urticarial papules, sometimes surmounted by vesicles; occasionally they may be bullous.

An affliction due to *P. ventricosus* or (in straw) *Acarus tritici*, producing strongly pruritic nodules or vesicles, is wide-spread in the tropics among workers having to do with stores of cereals or provender. The said phenomena are sometimes accompanied by fever, oedema and asthmatic symptoms [348a]. The skin lesions, intensely itching, may vary from urticarial or varicelliform to eczematous [262c]. Man may be attacked by hordes of some species of *Pyemotidae*, which burrow into the epidermis and produce pale pink to bright red spots on the skin, followed by petechiae, wealing, central vesiculation, and pustulation. The lesions are accompanied by burning pruritus, fever and sweating.

The same therapy is recommended as for scabies.

ACCIDENTAL IRRITATIVE BITES

A number of insects and other arthropods may pierce the skin of man in self-defence, and at the same time inject saliva or gland secretion into the wound. These substances are more or less irritative. In the absence of previous exposure man is not allergic to these substances, still some may have rather annoying effects.

It is known that some beetles with strong mandibles and biting ants having no stings are able to bite with their beak-like mandibles, and can pour the contents of their poison glands on the region the of wounds thus produced [278b].

Thrips (Thysanoptera) are minute insects, usually yellowish brown or black in colour. Their four very narrow wings have fringes of long hairs. The majority feed on plant sap and are agricultural pests. Many species, the adults and nymphs of which may well bite man, are cosmopolitans [133]. Gardeners and agricultural workers are most frequently affected. The bites on exposed skin areas cause slight pricks developing into slightly itching pink macules or papules, these may be surrounded by a pale halo with 'whitish dots', which may persist for hours, or even for several days [24, 133, 262c, 278b]. Irritation and swelling are usually slight, but the reaction may be severe in sensitized individuals who are heavily attacked.

Members of the order Hemiptera, include the lace bug and other bugs, both terrestrial and aquatic, e.g. back swimmers and water bug. The latter bites unwary swimmers and fishermen. The lesion may persist as an irritative reaction for many hours. Most of the terrestrial members including the lace bug and its relatives produce a mild erythema which is relatively painless and may rapidly subside, leaving little or no mark of skin penetration, thus, perhaps only perplexing the victim and the consulting dermatologist [262c].

The weal bug produces swelling and redness [304]. After several days, this may lead to the development of a papilloma lasting for weeks and even months [262c].

Only one group of the class Crustacea have been reported to cause dermatitis [95]. These are organisms of the superfamily Cymothoidea (sea lice), which frequent the low waters of temperate and tropical seas and are the cause of cymothoidism (louse dermatitis). These small creatures are equipped with powerful biting parts and will quickly attach themselves to fish, but also to man's feet, or searching inquisitive hands [45]. The bite is rapid and sharp, causing punctate haemorrhage. The lesions gradually clear over a period of 5–7 days.

Venomous bites and stings

Spiders possess two-segmented chelicerae connected with the poison glands. Centipedes are provided with maxillipeds, powerful claws connected to the poison glands by a hollow tube. Both structures make forceps like bites, which serve to kill the pray insect or other small animals. Most spiders and centipedes are feared without real reason, since the mouth parts are unable to penetrate the human skin, and also the amount of their venom is small compared with the body weight of man. Only a few dozen species of the many thousand are known, which may be dangerous to humans. The principal effect is that of the venom, and the reaction depends on its nature and on the amount injected. Allergic reactions, if present, are masked by the characteristic local and general toxic symptoms.

Nevertheless, spiders and related members of this order are not only dangerous from a toxicological point of view, but are also potential sensitizers causing cutaneous lesions and sometimes also generalized reactions [120b]. In the tropics and subtropics, a few Scolopendra species may inflict a painful bite [258], which may be followed by oedema, lymphangitis and necrosis [34, 187a], a tropical species may produce, in addition to a necrotic lesion, systemic reactions such as fever, nausea, vomiting, and headache [34]. The common centipede of Europe, S. cingulata, may cause pain, swelling, and purpura over much of the bitten limb [95]. The poison is not so strong as to endanger life, and the pain diminishes rapidly. No specific therapy is available, pain can be relieved by injecting local anaesthetics.

Spiders. The most important spiders are of the comb-forked genus of Latrodectus: the black widow *(L. mactans)* occurs in the southern parts of the U.S.A.

and tropical America, the brown widow *(L. geometricus)* lives in the tropics especially in Africa. There are other species of this group in other parts of the world, which are less dangerous. The tarantulas, *Lycosa tarantula* in southern Europe, and the American tarantulas: Aphonopelme in Mexico, Sceriopelma in Panama, two Loxosceles species in the U.S.A. and Central America, *Phoneutria fera* in Brasil, two Atrax species in Australia, three species of Chiracanthium in the U.S.A. and Hawai may be dangerous or may inflict a temporarily painful but harmless bite [23].

Bites of a spider from the genus Miturga have been described in New Zealand; the symptoms are stiffness of joints, difficulty in walking and muscle cramps that persist for 45 days [342]. The most widespread species of spiders which provoke transitory local toxic phenomena, are *Hogua singoriensis*, *Dolomedes chiracantura* in Central Europe [85] and *Chiracanthium indusum* and *Argioge aurantia* in the U.S.A.

The female of *Latrodectes mactans* is glossy black, may be found in empty burrows or under stones, further in dark corners of barns, garages, store-rooms or privies. She bites man only in self-defence and is ordinarily shy and retiring [155]. The venom injected through horny fangs contains a neurotoxin 15 times as potent as that of the rattlesnake, but the dose is small in relation to the human victim's body weight.

The actual bite may not be noticed, but very soon afterwards local burning or stinging develops, to be replaced by cramp-like pain which increases to a maximum in about three hours and persists for 12–14 hours. Local swelling and two red punctae may be seen at the point of attack. Painful cramp and rigidity involve most of the muscles of the body, and the rigidity of the abdominal muscles may simulate a ruptured duodenal ulcer. The patient is restless and nauseated, and sweats profusely. The blood pressure is often slightly raised. Most cases recover spontaneously in two or three days, but the bite may be fatal in children and in the old and frail. The fatality rate in the U.S.A. exceeds 5 per cent [155].

Sedation and hot baths may be helpful [278b]. The intravenous injection of calcium gluconate relieves the muscle cramp and can be repeated. If it is obtainable, specific hyperimmune horse-serum antivenom should be given in all except in the mildest cases [95, 278b].

Human loxoscelism or necrotic arachnidism. Loxosceles reclusa and other poisonous Loxosceles, including *L. arizonica, L. unicolor,* and *L. laeta,* have been identified as the causes of necrotic arachnidism in the American continent and the West Indies [18, 235b, 284]. These yellow-brown spiders, 10–15 mm in length, occur in cupboards, bathrooms and outhouses, often biting their human victims in their home whilst they are sleeping or dressing. Their bites can be life-threatening in children, or disabling in cases of bites on the hands, face, or genitals. Clinically a sharply demarcated ulcer is produced by the venom of the spiders [40]. Microscopically, the early lesions of loxoscelism have been likened to the Arthus reaction, showing dilated capillaries filled with red blood cells, loss of vessel integrity, haemorrhage, and leukocyte infiltration [69, 303b]. The mechanism of the ulceronecrotic lesion is probably not due to the mechanism involved in the Arthus phenomenon [40], for the venom from the brown recluse spider *(L. reclusa)* when injected into the skin of rabbits causes a characteristic inflammatory necrotic ulcer; furthermore, in the rabbit the progressive haemorrhage and painful necrosis of the skin are associated with thrombocytopenia, fibrinogenaemia, and prolongation of the clotting time. Ultrastructural studies of rabbit lesions have shown early endothelial damage and thrombosis of blood vessels. Disintegration of the endothelial cells, haemorrhage, and thrombosis precede the inflammatory infiltrate and necrosis. Berger et al. [40] suggest that damage to blood vessels, activation of the clotting system, and release of local mediators of inflammation account for the characteristic clinical progression of necrotic arachnidism. The cutaneo-visceral form is produced mainly by *L. laeta* [19, 289]. Haematuria and fever are often followed by death.

Thrombocytopenia has been reported following the intravenous injection into dogs of crude extract of cephalothoraces and pure venom [94]. Some of the injected dogs developed haemolysis. Post-mortem examination of rabbits with fatal bites of Loxosceles revealed haemorrhagic involvement of the liver, small intestine and other organs [19, 303a]. Disseminated intravascular coagulation following fatal brown spider bite has been reported [337]. Fibrin degradation products found in disseminated intravascular coagulation syndromes in man were not present in rabbits with small necrotic lesions. Berger et al. [40] assume that the thrombocytopenia and lowering of fibrinogen was mainly due to a local tissue consumption coagulopathy and not to a direct intravascular thrombin-like effect of the venom. The venom of the brown recluse spider may activate C [192]. In C6-deficient rabbits the clotting time was dramatically prolonged with normal partial thromboplastin times and prothrombin times [356]. In experiments of Berger et al. [40] in rabbits there was a concomitant lowering of platelets and fibrinogen, indicating that clotting had taken place. The direct addition of venom from brown recluse spider to animal and human blood neither enhanced nor prevented clotting [179]. In skin, activators of fibrinolysis are found mainly around blood vessels in the mid and lower dermis [196].

The course of the gangrenous form of loxoscelism is apparently less severe if the antihistamine chlorpheniramine is administered intramuscularly as soon as possible after the bite [289]. Intravenously administered methylprednisolone prevented the death of rabbits from recluse spider venom [98].

Scorpions. Many scorpion species are found in subtropical and tropical regions. At the apex of the narrowed tail, where a bulbous sac is situated, we find the poison spine. The glands produce a liquid, acid in reaction, and toxins, similar in action to that of the cobra venom, but owing to its small quantity it is much less dangerous. The venom of a number of species evokes predominantly only a local reaction and does not contain neurotoxins. Six- to seven-hundred species are known, but only a limited number of the larger ones inject a sufficient quantity of poison to cause real danger [310]. However, Buthus and Centrurioides scorpions in the south-western U.S.A. and Mexico and in South America and the Buthus and Androctonus species in North Africa and the Middle East are dangerous. In Mexico in a 10-year period more than 20,000 people were recorded to have been killed by scorpions compared with about 2,000 by snakes and 274 by spiders [184, 225]. In Trinidad scorpion sting was claimed to be fatal in 4.7 per cent of the cases [136]. A higher death rate caused by scorpion stings occurs in small children [225].

Scorpion venom is primarily haemolytic, producing a local reaction consisting of a sharp burning sensation and a pronounced swelling, which may be associated with discoloration or necrosis of the skin [10, 95, 155, 278b]. The venom may contain a neurotoxin causing symptoms like nausea, tightness of thoracic muscles, salivation, sweating, abdominal cramps, restlessness, cyanosis and convulsions.

Death may occur from the direct action of the toxin on the respiratory centres [310]. The most poisonous scorpions usually produce little or no local reaction, but serious systemic symptoms [155]. The chemical composition of the North American scorpion venoms, as well as their mode of action and the clinical manifestations caused by them differ considerably from those of the Mediterranean species [282]. The less poisonous scorpions produce marked swelling which may involve the entire extremity, and may well be a hypersensitivity reaction [262c]. In the case of dangerous scorpion bites, when available specific antivenom should be administered soon after the sting is inflicted. Storage of antisera at first-aid posts is necessary where such species occur. The site of the sting has to be cauterized. A tourniquet should be applied above the site, where this is practicable. Application of an ice pack to the region of the sting prevents dissemination, it should be renewed until necessary. Morphine potentiates the lethal effect of the toxin, and must, therefore, not be given.

Stinging Hymenoptera

The colony forming wasps, hornets, bees, bumblebees and some social ants, as well as a few solitary species may sting man, occasionally causing severe symptoms in sensitized individuals. This large order of highly evolved insects, which are readily recognized by their narrow, neck-like zone, known as the petiole between the thorax and the abdomen, contains about 100,000 species, but only a few will attack man in defence and none for feeding. The sting is a complicated apparatus, a specialized ovipositor with lancets. The sharp recurved barbs of the lancets or stylets point downward and outward. The barbs of bees become embedded in the wound after being thrust into the skin. The sting (aculeus) is connected with glands and a poison sac, and the stinging involves the injection of gland secretion. Although all Hymenoptera stings are of similar nature and mechanism, there are characteristic differences among the groups and species [155]. One group kill their insect prey by stinging it; these have two poison glands: a larger acid gland, and a smaller alkaline gland at the base of the poison sac. The active substance is the combined product of the two glands, a venom producing local as well as systemic toxic and allergic symptoms, and a most severe anaphylactic shock. Another group of Hymenoptera will only paralyse their prey by the sting since they only have one formic acid gland.

The most familiar such insects are wasps, hornets, bees and stinging ants. Wasps are able to withdraw their stings. The wall of the venom sac is thick and muscular, and the venom is ejaculated by its vigorous contraction. The entire stinging apparatus of the bee is lightly attached to the abdominal organs, frequently it becomes detached and remains in the wound. The honey bee *(Apis mellifera)*, a number of bumblebees (Bombus), hornets or yellow jackets *(Vespa crabro)*, wasps *(Vespula germanica, V. vulgaris, V. maculata*, etc.) are the commonest representatives of this group. There are a number of other Vespoidea and Mutilidae which may sting. Only a few ants are provided with stinging apparatus.

The best known are the fire ants *(Solenopsis saevissima)*, harvester ants *(Pogono-myrmex barbatus* and other species) and the Australian bulldog ant *(Myrmecia gulosa)*.

The effects and importance of Hymenoptera stings depend on the kind of insect, the nature of its venom, the number of stings in a single individual, and finally on the state of sensitization of the victim. Although some fractions of the in-jected fluid are shared by most species, the majority of species have their own specific components. The effects are, as a rule, both toxic ones, and allergic. In sensitized people anaphylactic shock may occur rather frequently. The pain caused by the stings is due to the introduced venom which may be strong enough to cause severe symptoms. About 500 bee stings or about 30 stings of the Austral-ian bull-dog ants introduce a lethal dose of venom. Severe consequences are also caused by the antigens associated with the venom. On the other hand, tolerance to stings can develop.

Man is, fortuitously, the victim of these often vicious insects, which cause twice as many deaths in the U.S.A. than poisonous snakes do [256], and are responsible for many near-fatal reactions and much discomfort [262c, 278b]. About 0.4–1.0 per cent of the general population in the U.S.A. are allergic to the sting of Hymenoptera. About 20 per cent of the Americans have a hereditary disposition, and an atopic constitution, less than allergic state, was found in 56 per cent in France [80]. The Fatal Reaction Subcommittee of the Insect Sting Committee of the American Academy of Allergy has accumulated data of 495 fatal reactions recorded as being due to one or more Hymenoptera stings [29g]. The yearly number of fatal cases in the U.S.A. is at least 40. Four main patho-logical types are differentiated, viz. respiratory, vascular, anaphylactic, and neurologic. In 1 to 2 per cent the cause of the death was bacterial septicaemia, in 69 per cent respiratory tract obstruction from massive oedema and secretion. Partial respiratory obstruction contributed to the 12 per cent of cases diagnosed as anaphylactic reactions.

A considerable amount of the basic information on the nature of venom, anti-genicity of and hypersensitivity to Hymenoptera stings has been included in the introduction of this chapter (p. 278). There is a vast body of classic and recent data which shall not be discussed here. There are still many insufficiently clarified problems.

The composition of venoms is extremely complex [278b] and there are sub-stantial differences between the different groups and species [119c]. Pharmaco-logically active toxic substances and antigenic substances are both present, and the individual's reaction to the sting is determined partly by the quantity of the former and partly by the degree of acquired sensitivity to the latter.

One of the most important fractions of the bee venom, known as mellitin is a polypeptide. This is responsible for some local inflammation and also acts as an allergen. It is regarded as the therapeutical agent in medicaments containing bee venom. The bee venom also contains histamine, but other components release more histamine from the tissues. Wasp venom contains histamine, 5-hydroxytryptamine and bradykinin [220]. Hyaluronidase and lecithinase have been demonstrated in the venom of several species. Cholinesterase is present in wasp venom [340]. The venom is cholinolytic and blocks the transmission of nervous impulses in the synapses of the neuro-muscular junctions in sympathetic ganglions and in the central nervous system. The venom of the European hornet resembles that of the wasp in that it contains 5-hydroxytryptamine and histamine, but also acetylcholine in a high concentration and a different type of kinin [46].

Fire ant venom causes necrotizing lesions; systemic reactions secondary to stings [203c] and even fatalities have been reported [256b]. The venom is similar to the toxin solenamine (of the spider *Loxosceles reclusa*) but it also contains histamine, phospholipase and hyaluronidase, the deleterious and far more important components are well-known alkaloids. The sensitizing portion of the fire ant venom is probably a small peptide [283]. Bulldog ants have a venom which is chemically and pharmacologically quite the same as that of the fire ant.

The antigenic relationship between the clinically important Hymenoptera is also complex [91, 175a, 243, 278b, 330]. As a practical generalization, the antigenic components of the relatively few species investigated by modern immunological techniques and the results of skin test suggest that the venom of each species contains antigenic substances common to many other Hymenoptera, together with genus- or species-specific antigens [278b]. Bee and wasp venoms contain specific polypeptides and specific phospholipases; the latter are believed to be responsible for allergic reactions [145a]. Some of the antigens are present throughout the insect body, but probably in lower concentration than in the venom.

The injected venom [325a] contains various vasoactive chemical mediators and antigenic substances which are present not only in the extract of the poison sac but also in the body of the animals [12, 325a], although these are often cross-reactive. At the first stings the venom contains a primary toxic substance which releases histamine, and produces sharp pain, urticaria and often even haemorrhage. Once the individual has been sensitized, i.e. after the period of latency, intracutaneously negative individuals develop itching lesions at the site of the sting after 1–2 days. Each new sting induces an increasingly violent reaction: in the presence of small amounts of antibodies there may be a delayed-type reaction while in that of large amounts immediate type skin sensitivity may occur [60b].

In honey bee venom, isolated by various methods, there are at least eight antigenic protein fractions present [246]. Of these phospholipase A, mellitin (a cationic polypeptide of mol. wt. 2,840) and apamin are the three major fractions. Hyaluronidase also appears to be a potent allergen [162a, 297a].

Patients sensitive to bee stings develop immediate weal and flare and delayed reactions when the skin is tested with purified mellitin [209]. The weal and flare reaction may be immunologically non-specific, for bee venom is an anaphylactoid agent in that mellitin is a potent degranulator of mast cells and a good histamine-releasing agent [52, 121, 160]. The delayed reactions which persist for more than 4–5 h are the result of immunological hypersensitivity to the stings, as normal patients display no such reactions [209]. The demonstration of specific antibodies in rabbit sera by gel diffusion or tanned red-cell agglutination [299] is disturbed by non-immunoglobulin lipoprotein reactions even with pure bee venom [28]. Intravenous injection of bee venom into some laboratory animals may cause a fatal shock [145a], whereas the same laboratory animals are not killed by the same venom administered subcutaneously. The amount of venom involved in a bee sting or even in multiple envenomations represents only a small fraction of the minimum lethal dose calculated for man. Thus, the pharmacological activity of the bee venom is not primarily responsible for the noted human fatalities, thus, these deaths may be the result of an allergic reaction [29a]. Bee venom has antigenic properties and may also elicit anaphylactoid reaction [285]. Immunization of mice with small amounts induced both cutaneous and fatal systemic hypersensitivity to appropriate challenge with this substance [285]. All immune and anaphylactoid responses to bee venom were reproducible with mellitin. In contrast, enhanced response to phospholipase A was demonstrated only by systemic challenge of venom-immunized mice. The results suggest that mellitin, which is a membranolytic agent, is an important allergen as well as the major toxic constituent of whole bee venom. Reaginic (Layton test) and precipitable antibodies against mellitin could not be detected in the sera from any of the bee-sting-sensitive patients tested. Although phospholipase A has been shown to be antigenic [146], only the hyaluronidase constituent of the bee venom was neutralized by sera obtained from bee-keepers [28]. Moreover, no consistent correlation could be demonstrated experimentally [145a] between the severity of the reaction and the number of stings received; even single stings occurred to be fatal. Cell-mediated immunity against mellitin was not detected by the leukocyte-migration inhibition test [209]. The haemolytic and leukocyte migration inhibition activities of mellitin were associated with the intact molecule and not the carboxy-terminal heptapeptide. It is probable (since adrenalectomy rendered non-immunized mice hypersensitive to mellitin) that adrenal function plays an important role in resistance to the acute anaphylactoid response to the mellitin fraction of venom [285].

Pure venom is superior to whole body extract (WBE) in the diagnosis and treatment of bee-sting allergy [173a, 305]. Chromatography of honey bee venom (HBV) yielded four pools that contained hyaluronidase, phospholipase A, mellitin and apamin. Double antibody studies with isotope-labelled phospholipase A, and others using a RAST with phospholipase A as antigen revealed that bee-keepers' sera that have blocking activity against HBV-induced leukocyte histamine release contain anti-phospholipase A antibodies of the IgG class and bee-allergic patients have anti-phospholipase A antibodies of the IgE class. The conclusion has been drawn that phospholipase A is the major allergen of HBV.

RAST using venom and/or phospholipase A is an excellent diagnostic tool to measure insect hypersensitivity; the reaction to each of the stinging insects may be quite specific [275].

In mice immunized with bee venom, heat-labile antibodies (measured by PCA) and haemagglutinating antibodies were produced [77]. PCA reaction and haemagglutinating activity was also directed at phospholipase A.

Treatment with whole body extract produces blocking antibody the levels of which may be insufficient to prevent anaphylaxis; immunization with honey bee venom deserves an immunologically monitored trial in appropriate patients [274c, 331].

Hundred millions of people are occasionally stung by bees, wasps or other Hymenoptera, and usually only a small painful lesion accompanied by swelling and erythema follows. Unprotected parts, the head, neck and feet—in this order—are most often stung. The worst months in the U.S.A. are July and August, and the months July to September in France [80]. Polister wasp stings may occur in winter, too.

Symptoms depend on the volume of the injected substance, the quantity of toxin therein, the site of the sting (lips are the most vulnerable) but, mainly, on whether the victim has been sensitized or not [60b, 95, 262c, 278b, 325a].

The sting in non-sensitized subjects is rather unpleasant and painful, an immediate burning pain is produced, which may be severe, and is rapidly followed by swelling, weal and flare, and redness. In the absence of specific sensitivity to the antigens in the venom the local reaction subsides within a few hours.

Symptoms of the honey bee sting consist in sharp pain and marked swelling lasting several hours. The stinging apparatus may often be retained, which continues to inject venom. Symptoms of wasp stings are similar, however, the swelling is larger, the stings are often multiple, and the stinging apparatus is left behind only exceptionally [95, 262c]. The description of the histology of experimental hive bee stings [88] refer to reactions along the tract of the sting and not just at the tip. The early reaction is characterized by oedema and cellular infiltration with some patches of cytolysis. After 24 to 48 h, necrotic areas are walled off with mononuclear cells and finally surrounded by fibroblasts. Eosinophilic infiltration frequently occurs. Occasionally, the local swelling around the stings in the pharynx may be severe enough to cause death by respiratory obstruction. The direct effects of one or several stings usually does not give rise to systemic symptoms [278b], but a large number of stings may produce haemolytic, haemorrhagic and neurotoxic effects, with the main symptoms of vomiting, diarrhoea, fainting, respiratory distress and paralysis that may be fatal particularly in children [169]. After recovery from such severe symptoms, an attack of urticaria may follow on the 7th to 9th day. In cardiac patients a few stings may sometimes prove to be fatal [278b]. After a few stings secondary infections occur but rarely, also tissue injury resulting in gross necrotic changes is infrequent [262c].

Repeated stings of Hymenoptera may gradually sensitize the victim. The allergic hypersensitivity reaction thus produced is characterized by a hyperaemic oedematous local swelling and irritation, sometimes even by systemic symptoms which may last for an abnormally long time [80, 278b, 322]. The hypersensitivity is usually of the reaginic type. Pertaining experiments gave the following results: 3,000 stings induced local reaction in 11.6 per cent of the tests, mild generalized reaction in 14.3 per cent, moderately grave generalized reaction in 37.8 per cent, severe systemic reaction in 21.0 per cent and delayed type reaction in 2.4 per cent [177]. Phenomena of the serum-sickness type may arise some 10 days after the sting. Some 24 to 48 h after a bee sting a painful papulous intumescence, a sort of Arthus reaction sets in. The more severe reactions occur most frequently in atopic subjects [29a], but at least one-third of individuals developing systemic reactions give no personal or family history of atopy [293]. The localized delayed-type allergic reaction appears about 24 h following the sting, by this time the swelling and redness, the localized toxic sting reaction, has largely subsided [105]. The swelling may become massive, itching and lymphangitis are common. Systemic treatment with corticosteroids is dramatically effective, while antihistamines and epinephrine are of no value.

There are several types of generalized systemic allergic reactions elicited by the sting of honey bees, yellow jackets, hornets, wasps, fire ants and related species [262c, 298, 322]. In about 8 per cent of the cases the first stings of fire ants (i.e. those believed to be the first) are followed by anaphylaxis [60b, 203c]. Some patients do not remember the first sting, which may have happened in childhood. Generalized reaction may develop in 10 to 30 min [120a].

In the mildest generalized reactions, pruritus, urticaria, angioedema and mucous membrane swelling are the commonest symptoms. Respiratory symptoms (rhinitis. dyspnoea, cough, and wheezing which may progress to asphyxia) [322] are the most frequent concomitants of the usual local phenomena. They must not be confused with inhalant allergy [110]. Systemic reactions appear within an hour of the sting in 97 per cent of the cases [29c, 230].

In the moderate generalized reactions with increasing severity tightness in the chest, nausea and vomiting are added, and with still greater severity pallor, sweating and collapse varying in degree even to loss of consciousness with low blood pressure and rapid pulse, followed later by mild pyrexia and exceptionally by diarrhoea and polyuria [278b, 322]. The sequelae of the sting (angioedema, occasionally haemorrhage) are of medium severity. Idiosyncrasy to hymenopteran sting, i.e. generalized reaction after the anamnestically first sting [177], has been observed in 13.2 per cent of the examined cases. On the other hand, repeated stings may confer an immunity which diminishes if exposure is suspended for several months (e.g. in winter) [318]. In addition to allergic reactions, the toxic symptoms may also be favourably influenced by this transitory immunity [30].

In cases of severe generalized reactions there often may be a history of milder reaction to previous stings, but although anaphylactic symptoms tend to become more severe after each exposure, initial reactions which are purely urticarial are seldom followed by anaphylactic reactions [173]. Urticaria, angioedema with pruritus and hot flush may develop within 2 minutes. The cutaneous lesions may spread over the whole body, accompanied by general symptoms (asthma-like dyspnoea, gastrointestinal disturbance, vertigo, sudden drop of blood pressure, cessation of pulse beat, great anxiety, and even coma) [278b, 322]. In women this may be accompanied by uterine contraction. In 2.8 per cent of the cases symptoms pointing to delayed-type reaction have been observed such as hyperglobulinaemic and thrombocytopenic purpura, sanguineous diarrhoea, hepatorenal syndrome, nephrotic syndrome, necrotizing angiitis, and severe neurological changes [29a]. Atopy (66 to 73 per cent) is not a prerequisite of the anaphylactic type of hymenopteran sensitization [177, 293]. The frequency of severe reactions increases above the age of 30, a phenomenon possibly explainable by the higher number of exposures [177]. Anaphylactic shock in man presents itself most frequently (43 per cent) as an acute, allergic cardiovascular reaction, called primary anaphylactic shock or anaphylactic shock in the strict sense [164]. Oedema in the upper respiratory tract, bronchial obstruction, and acute pulmonary oedema are also common (39 per cent). The cardiovascular collapse has been attributed, at least partly, to these respiratory manifestations (secondary partial or complete anaphylactic shock) [164].

The onset of fatal reactions may be almost instantaneous and death ensues within an hour in the majority of the fatal cases [29b, 214, 227, 256b, 288]. The majority of fatal reactions occur over 40 years of age, they are very rare in childhood. Stings on the face or mucous membranes are more dangerous than those on the trunk or limbs [163]. Over 70 per cent of the victims are males, perhaps

320

because of greater exposure. As regards frequency of lethal stings, the following sequence of Hymenoptera has been established [174]: wasp, yellow jacket, honey bee, hornet. The history contained previous systemic reactions in 44 per cent of the fatal cases. Desensitizing treatment does not invariably prevent fatal complications. Swelling of the tongue, laryngeal, tracheal and bronchial oedema (respiratory obstruction) (38 per cent) and acute vascular collapse (syncope) (65 per cent) are the most frequent fatal complications [29b]. The regulation of the permeability of vessels being out of gear, the toxin gains ready access to the vital organs especially in the central nervous system [348a] and may give rise to cerebral oedema and multiple bleedings. Fatal necrotizing angiitis has apparently been induced by a wasp sting [114]. Individuals with cardiovascular and allergic diseases are particularly susceptible to fatal complications [29c,174, 214, 253]. Based on autopsy findings [29f, 164] the respiratory form (laryngeal oedema, acute pulmonary oedema, acute pulmonary distension) seems to have an especially poor prognosis. Further causes of death may include anaphylaxis, vascular collapse and infection.

When trying to assess the prognosis, the age and individual sensitivity of the patient should be considered as well as the age of the stinging insect and the season in which it had hatched [89]. However, according to experiences in the U.S.A. [29g] the number of stings, the negative or allergic histories, the type of insect and the age of patient provide but poor basis for prognosis.

In view of the possibility of fatal reactions it is extremely important to determine the immunological status. However, none of the current laboratory procedures is invariably reliable. Carefully recorded history is of great importance [353].

It is true that, in general, the results of skin tests reflect the degree of clinical sensitivity [29d, 242a, 353], although exceptions in this respect do occur. A significant number of biological false positive skin tests have been reported in non-allergic subjects, as well as occasional false negative skin tests in Hymenoptera-allergic patients who have experienced severe sting reactions [42a, 60a, 80, 242c, 292, 306]. The development of skin-sensitizing antibodies is sometimes slow (a certain length of time may be necessary for them to adhere) [60b]; a reaginic antibody is supposed to be involved in the reaction in about 50 per cent of the cases [274a]. Skin test is sometimes negative two months after the subsidence of the anaphylactic shock if commercial insect antigen extracts are used due possibly to the in appropriate testing of antigens. Pure bee venom contains a tissue-specific antigen not present in sacless body extracts. It is likewise possible that whole-body extracts do not contain a sufficient amount of the antigen [60a, 274a]. It is a limitation of the method that, though the allergy may sometimes be restricted to a single stinging insect type [60b], cross-reactions between different insects often mask the responsible antigen [116]. Comparison of results is difficult because different authors use different antigen concentrations. Skin tests performed on 380 normal persons with honey-bee extract containing 220 μg protein N per ml gave positive reactions in 38 per cent [42a]. Nevertheless, the intracutaneous test—if carried out under standard quantitative conditions—is now accepted as a satisfactory diagnostic procedure. Of course, great circumspection is needed, for the test may elicit a grave anaphylactic shock [29d].

Passive transfer is usually negative in cases in which there is only a local reaction, whereas in cases of systemic reactions, it is generally positive [60a, b]. Certain authors found the species specificity of passive transfer more pronounced than that of the skin test.

The leukocyte histamine release method [306, 353] has shown that skin sensitivity significantly correlates with leukocyte histamine release and with the severity of the reaction to Hymenoptera stings; furthermore, skin testing and leukocyte histamine release can distinguish normal subjects from Hymenoptera-allergic patients. The test is recommended for use [306] if the cutaneous test fails.

By means of the immunofluorescence test antibodies to honey bee antigens have been demonstrated in the heart and adrenal glands of three patients who died of honey bee sting while their sera contained haemagglutinating antibodies [169]. Such techniques may be of considerable medicolegal significance. Earlier attempts were made [227] to demonstrate post-mortem hymenopteran antibodies by means of the semimicro precipitin tube test and Ouchterlony's agar diffusion method.

For the most part, stings from Hymenoptera do not demand much therapeutic attention. The usual palliative drugs (local application of antiphlogistic and anti-pruritic agents) and the removal of the retained mouth parts suffice for local reactions. Antihistamine therapy is rarely necessary. Should there be conspicuous oedema, epinephrine may be employed in itself or supplemented with corticosteroids [95]. For very painful lesions application of lidocaine with epinephrine at each sting site may be considered.

To fight systemic sting reactions, the earliest possible emergency treatment is imperative. The drug of choice for therapy of acute anaphylactic reactions of any cause is epinephrine HCl (adrenaline), antihistamine and corticosteroid (the latter has no immediate effect, being effective only against late symptoms), if necessary, also oxygen mask, intravenous infusion, isopropylarterenol, aminophylline or ephedrine are useful [29b, g, 80, 89, 177, 274b, 318]. An immediate medical intervention may be of vital importance. It has been suggested that patients at risk be taught how to inject themselves with epinephrine and to keep an emergency treatment kit (antihistamine + prednisone + adrenaline) at hand [30b, 164].

Specific desensitization has proved useful and effective, it affords good protection against further stings with commercially available whole polyvalent insect body extracts in cases of both local and systemic reaction [30b, 60b, 80, 95, 104, 177, 330, 353]. It is supposed that protective antibodies of the IgG and IgM types are formed [274a]. Whole-body extract is mainly used for vaccination. It is advisable to start the treatment intracutaneously with extreme dilutions (1 : 10,000,000) and proceed with gradually increasing well-tolerated concentrations every week (i.e. in two-injection steps). The advantages of the intracutaneous injection [164] are the minimizing of the danger of initiating a generalized reaction; the avoidance of accidental intravascular application of an allergen extract, and the easy observation of local reactions. Subcutaneous 0.1 to 0.3 ml doses of 1 : 10 test concentrations may be reached in individual treatments. Booster doses should be given at intervals of 3 to 4 months.

Complete (in about 2/3 of the cases) or partial immunity (in about 1/5) to repeated stings [164, 255] may thus be achieved but for a lasting effect it must be continued indefinitely. If the patient has a rest after the injection, the effect is more favourable [274b]. In desensitized patients, cell sensitivity generally showed no change, but the antigen-neutralizing capacity of their serum was increased in about 2/3 of the cases [353]. In spite of contrary opinions [278b, 325b], the desensitizing therapy is currently accepted as the method of treatment of individuals who have had systemic allergic reactions following insect stings [274b]. It has been recommended to discontinue maintenance desensitization (usually one injection every 4 weeks) after 3 years, but this seems to be wrong [164], because after 15–27 months severe generalized reactions of the respiratory type accompanied by skin manifestations may occur. If desensitization cannot be achieved, this may be attributed to the use of an inappropriate type of Hymenoptera. Poor IgG-type blocking antibody production and/or lowering of the titre of IgE antibodies or insufficient antigen stimulation may be taken into consideration [274b]. Since the antigens are cross-reactive, also mixtures (mainly wholebody bee, hornet, wasp or yellow jacket, recently mixed stinging insect venom containing mellitin, phospholipase A and B, histamine, lecithine and mast-cell degranulating peptide) are used for desensitization [318, 353]. Also whole-body emulsified allergens have been tried [269]: two injections are administered per year, the first about the middle of April, the second three months later. Only swelling and local soreness were registered as side-effects. Of the 37 individuals thus treated, 16 sustained subsequent stings without symptoms. After desensitization therapy patients previously allergic to stings of bees, wasps or other Hymenoptera showed a repellent effect even on biting insects. Spontaneous desensitization may occur: the reaction was less strong or even absent after a repeated sting in as many as 65 per cent of the cases [274a]. Antiserum could be produced in rabbits against the venom of *Vespa orientalis*. With the serum mice could be protected against its lethal effect. The venom antigen presumably consists of nonspecific proteins of the poison sac wall or other body tissues [178].

CATERPILLARS WITH NETTLING OR STINGING BRISTLES

Different kinds of moth and butterfly (Lepidoptera) larvae and sometimes adult female moths have hairs, bristles or spines which penetrate the human skin and produce irritation, a painful dermatitis, urticaria, or even more severe symptoms. The types of reactions are different. Dermatitis caused by stinging bristles have a poisonous character, nettling hairs cause primarily allergic reactions. The symptoms are rather different when airborne hairs or scales are inhaled, penetrate into the eyes, or are swallowed and reach the intestines.

There are two main types of bristles. The one is hollow and is connected with the poison gland. The sharp, pointed, hollow bristles or spines may be scattered about the body or grouped together on processes on the dorsal or anal surface of the caterpillar. The stiff bristles are connected with a special hypodermal cell. Two distinct kinds are known [188], namely the primitive type and the augmented type; the latter occurs if the original bristle is augmented by a spine which has become evaginated. The toxic, allergic substances are the secretion of a single cell. The barbed setae release the irritant substances when the fine or coarse bristles penetrate the skin or mucous membranes [291, 326, 357a]. Only some of these substances have been studied. The toxin from the hairs of a processionary caterpillar *(Thaumetopoea wilkinsoni)* consists of some toxic proteins, carbohydrates, phospholipids, enzymes, a toxic volatile component and inorganic compounds [357b]. The most offensive substances are secreted by caterpillars in the family Saturniidae, by the range caterpillar *(Hemileuca olivae)* from New Mexico, and by the caterpillars of the io moth *(Auchmeris io)* and of the flannel moth *(Megalopyge lunata)* living in Panama. These feared caterpillars are mostly well known to the local population who avoid touching them. The hairs of many species are present not only on the caterpillars but may be transferred to the cocon, or may be present in or around the nest [278b]. The setae are re eased over the eggs by the moth, but are easily carried away by air currents, and even at considerable distances may cause outbreaks of dermatitis or urticaria.

Outbreaks of caterpillar epidemic dermatitis occur mainly in country-dwellers, and in seasons in which the offending moth is abundant [182]. Occupational exposure occurs in foresters and farmers and in those handling infested foods [140]. Christmas-trees are an occasional domestic source. Outbreaks have afflicted the crews of ships offshore because the hairs have been disseminated by the ship's ventilation system. Severe generalized dermatitis may result from the wind-blown hairs of adult moth [156, 262c].

After contact with toxic bristles of caterpillar the severity and distribution of the eruption depend mainly on the route and intensity of exposure, but there are also marked differences according to the species. In mild attacks irritation is experienced almost immediately after contact, macules, small urticarial papules and occasional vesicles develop in 30– 60 min [262c] and symptoms subside after 6–12 h. In average cases the skin reaction is characterized by a sudden burning sensation, pain, swelling, erythema and oedema, blisters, vesication, minute raised spots, red papules and itching; exceptionally, the lesions may be bullous and show deep red discolouration.

Histological examinations may show eosinophilia, leukocyte infiltration, even lymphangitis [95]. At the beginning there is infiltration with lymphocytes, histiocytes, and plasma cells. At 24 h a superficial pustule may appear, the floor of which consists of densely packed necrotic connective tissue, beneath there is a diffuse infiltrate of polymorphonuclear leukocytes, lymphocytes, and cells with small pyknotic nuclei, permeating the poorly staining connective tissue and surrounding the blood vessels. At 72 h the pustule may be found to contain many eosinophils and plasma cells in addition to the cells already noted. In the central area the epidermal floor is completely absent, and the cellular infiltrate has broken through to extend profusely into the underlying necrotic tissue.

In severe cases numbness, nausea, incapacitation, and nervous symptoms occur. The paralytic symptoms usually subside with the pain within some hours, other symptoms persist for about a day, though they may last for a week. The symptoms may vary according to the different species. For instance, in severe attacks caused by *Megalopyge opercularis*, the eruption may be extensive with diffuse oedema and severe local pain, and there may be systemic symptoms, restlessness, headache, tachycardia, and lymphadenopathy [205, 228, 235a]. The lesions slowly resolve after several days. The puss caterpillar in the southern U.S.A. causes painful papules progressing to pustules and finally to an indurated discoloured area [235a]. The pathology of the dermatitis produced experimentally with the caterpillar of *Automeris io* [262a] is characterized by a rapidly developing oedema of the dermis and subcutaneous tissues of approximately 6 h duration without necrosis. The microscopic reaction resembles that occurring to histamine [262c].

A curious occupational disease of rubber workers, called panarama, is known in Brasil. It is apparently caused by contact with caterpillars of the moth *Prelomis semirufa*. It has a chronic form causing long-term disability of the fingers. When the small dorsal hairs of the caterpillar penetrate the skin, acute oedematous inflammation and infiltration by neutrophilic leukocytes follows succeeded by fibrosis and the formation of foreign-body granulomas [97].

In the eye the hairs may cause a variety of changes, ranging from catarrhal conjunctivitis to nodular ophthalmia and even panophthalmitis. The nasal mucous membrane may also be irritated [262c].

A different type of dermatitis is observed when the moth larvae bear unhollowed hairs containing no actual poison, but causing allergic sensitivity after repeated contacts. These moth caterpillars belong to different genera, the most common ones in Europe are relatives of the gipsy moth *(Lymantria dispar)*, e.g. the brown tail moth *(Euproctis chysorrhoea)* and the garden tiger *(Arctia caja)*. The hairs and bristles are of several kinds. Some bristles are barbed and can stick in the skin. After penetration first they cause some purely mechanical irritation. In people, however, who repeatedly come into contact with these hairs, allergic sensitization occurs. Most frequently agricultural and forest workers are exposed in years of caterpillar abundance. The allergic feature of caterpillar hairs can be demonstrated by i.c. skin test [272].

Severe immediate-type allergic reactions (asthma, cyanosis, shock) occurred in silk-sensitive persons who were injected with biological agents (toxoids, vaccines, human globulin, vitamin B_{12}) probably as a result of the use of silk filters in their preparation [62, 84, 123].

Therapy is non-specific and supportive. In severe generalized reactions intravenous calcium gluconate comes into consideration [228, 235a].

SURFACE-ACTIVE ARTHROPOD SUBSTANCES

The toxic or allergenic substances of parasites, biting or stinging arthropods penetrate parenterally into the tissues, and the stinging hairs of caterpillars act by the intracutaneous route. There are, however, some arthropods which have no means of penetration, still, some possess toxic or allergenic substances, which may cause reaction through contact with the surface of the skin or more often with the mucous membranes.

Blister beetles

These insects also known as oil beetles have been known since ancient times, and were earlier used in medicine mainly for the preparation of aphrodisiac drugs. More than 100 species of the blister beetle family Meloidae are known to contain or release vesicating substances annoying man, cantharidin being the most well-known one. It is an anhydride of cantharic acid; it can be easily extracted and crystallized. It readily penetrates the epidermis. The amount of 0.1 mg is enough to produce blistering. A few hours after penetration violent irritation is felt and vesication follows. Cantharidin is excreted through the kidneys, and may produce irritation or dangerous nephritis. The Spanish fly *(Lytta vesicatoria)* is the most important species in Europe, but other Lytta species occur all over the world, e.g. *Zonabris nubica* and *Epicauta* sp. in Africa. Lesions are mostly caused only when a beetle is crushed on the skin [278b]. Momentary pain and a rapid weal formation is followed by the appearance of vesicles after 12–24 h [262c].

The cosmopolitan rove beetles (Staphylinidae), have several hundred accidentally harming species, some of them very small. The vesicant they contain is not identical with cantharidin. Blisters appear after a lapse of hours or days, then they undergo necrosis, leaving a cicatrix after healing. Phaedrus species are severe vesicating beetles in Africa [95].

There are other blister beetles: tropical species of the family Paussidae contain a powerful vesicant. The coco-nut beetles Sessinia (family Oedemeridae) in the mid-Pacific islands cause severe blistering by contact.

There are some beetles which contain powerful poison. The toxic principle of the chrysomelid beetle *Diamphidia simplex* consists of haemolytic toxalbumin. South African Bushmen use it to poison the tip of their arrowheads [95].

Contact inflammatory substances

There are a great number of arthropods which possess inflammatory properties. Contacting the skin or mucous membranes they produce slight or more or less severe symptoms. The insects and mites which live in the neighbourhood of man, the synanthropic species, frequently cause such injuries, while with free living animals the contact is only occasional and accidental. The skin is seldom penetrated by their substances which rather enter the organism through the intestines and respiratory tract. Accidentally they may get into the eye or other sense organs, or the urinary tract. Alimentary, inhalant and contact allergies caused by a number of arthropods can hardly be separated because the same mites or insects may be responsible for the reactions.

Accidental injuries of the eye and other sense organs caused by various arthropods are sometimes more severe than the skin reactions. Small flying insects or insect parts or secretions may hit the eye surface or enter the conjunctival sac. Beetles with irritative body fluids or secretions, especially minute flying Staphylinidae cause pain, severe burning and inflammation and corneal congestion. The eye becomes light sensitive or temporarily blinded. Sheep bot fly (Oestrus) may instantaneously deposit its parasitic larvae when striking the human eye, causing severe injury. There are a number of flies and a few tropical moths with specific eye frequenting habits. Eye gnats (Hippelates) are tiny flies attracted to mucous secretions. They are carriers of the contagious pink-eye conjunctivitis and also of the tropical ulcer of yaws. The pink eye caused by *Musca autumnalis*, by Hippelates and other 'face flies' is partly a simple irritative reaction, and partly the result of an allergic response to their saliva [262c].

Ingestant allergens and other ingested arthropod substances may produce various gastrointestinal symptoms. Ingested beetles with vesicating body fluid cause enteritis. The larva of the churchyard beetle (Blaps) provokes enteric symptoms when drinking contaminated water. The ingestion of meal prepared with flour infested with insects, among others with the meal worm *Tenebrio molitor* is fairly common. The insect, or its products may act as intestinal allergens. Cockroaches are regarded to be ingestants [5]. The most incriminated arthropods are the common mites in stored food, causing both contact allergies on the skin and enteric reactions.

Skin irritative arthropods

Millipeds feed on decaying vegetable matter. Some tropical species have 'repugnatorial glands' [262c] and exude an irritant substance [149]. In the species occurring in temperate regions [155], the poison produces vesicular dermatitis, mostly not severe.

The minute plankton of the ocean and inland bodies of waters as well as of ponds and pools include Copepoda (brine shrimp) and Daphnia (fairy shrimp). These often abound in great numbers and may certainly act as contactants. Although no dermatologic lesions have been clearly identified with such contactants, in routine tests with arthropod extracts often large skin reactions are elicited, suggesting that a causal relationship to urticarial and eczematous lesions among some bathers may exist [262c].

Mallophaga or biting lice infest chiefly fowl and domesticated mammals, and only exceptionally man. Their mouth parts are too feeble to penetrate deeply into the human skin, however, their oral secretion may account for the minor irritative effect and infrequent urticarial reactions [262c].

Many species of the large and colourful Mygalomorph spiders (family Theraphosidae) known as tarantules in the U.S.A. and other parts of the western hemisphere, and smaller hairy spiders elsewhere, possess urticating hairs and produce pruritic papular lesions, which may persist for several weeks [23].

In Japan, the house entering stink bugs (Pentatomids) constitute in winter a serious nuisance by their offensive smell causing vomiting, conjunctivitis and dermatitis. Contact dermatitis of bee-keepers may occur due to substances in the beeswax.

Several species of beetles contain in their bodies powerful irritants, others have irritative gland secretions, or hairs which may cause an apparently allergic dermatitis [278b, 321]. The common carpet beetle *(Anthrenus scrophulariae)* and the rust-red flour beetle *(Tribolium castaneum)* have been reported to cause dermatitis [86, 346].

Various mites living in foodstuffs have caused dermatitis in sensitized people. Some of these mites attach themselves to the skin (see p. 311) as the grain itch mite *(Pyemotes ventricosus)*, others are associated with a wide variety of food and stored products.

Cockroaches

Blattidea contain about 4,000 species, of which a few hundred are domiciliary pests. They have primitive chewing mouth parts, feed on almost anything edible, from debris to man's food. Due to their filthy habits they may act as mechanical transmitters of various germs. They are not only domestic food visiting pests, spoiling food by dropping excrement on it, and disgusting with their smell, but certain species also produce allergenic and irritating secretions. *Eurycotis floridiana* emits irritative odourous secretions, which have a persistent and characteristic smell, irritating to some individuals. The blister-raising properties have been attributed to their cuticular grease and to a discharge from their mouth [345c]. Their contact with human skin will cause pruritus and even urticarial reactions linear in character, following their paths [262c]. Oedema of eyelids have been attributed to cockroaches.

Cockroaches seem to have surface-active substances of very strong allergenic power. Their principal victims are children living under poor hygienic conditions who have become sensitized by the antigens contained in the gland secretions, in the saliva, faeces and body tissues of the insect (through contact, inhalation, ingestion or injection) [42b].

The body extract of the cosmopolitan German cockroach *(Blattella germanica)* and its faeces have been applied as antigens to allergic individuals in scratch and intracutaneous tests [119b]. They elicited immediate-type action, the frequency of which has been found to vary from country to country ranging from 28 to 75 per cent [42c, d, 79, 83]. Approximately half of the children allergic to house dust were found to react to cockroach extract [79], as compared with the 4–11 per cent among non-allergic controls. The faecal allergen acts in a dual capacity as an ingesta (contamination of human food) and as an inhalant (when its dried granules are incorporated in house dust) [42d, 79].

Some cases of respiratory allergy to the American cockroach *(Periplaneta americana)* have been described [42e, 232]. The haemolymph protein of the American cockroach contains five major plasma fractions, some being species-specific [316]. It has been found that the American cockroach and an other large species normally excrete compounds which are either mutagenic or carcinogenic [345c]. These acid compounds are tryptophan derivates, present in the excrements in consistent quantities, and the dropping of faecal material on food represents a potential hazard.

In spite of the information available about the presence of allergen and other harmful substances in cockroaches, our knowledge is far from being complete and it is very difficult to evaluate their actual significance.

Owing to their hiding habits in day time, unsuspected large numbers are prevalent all over the world and the control measures with any insecticide treatment will show gratifying number of corpses, but seldom achieve complete eradication, unless repeated systematically.

Sarcoptiform mites

Mites, belonging mainly to the family Acaridae (syn. Tyroglyphidae and Glyciphagidae), are pests of stores, warehouses, and grain mills, which may cause severe dermatitis in workers handling stored organic products [278b]. They are particularly common in hay, grains, crude sugar, dried fruits, cheese, and cereals [34].

Tyroglyphid mites are very tiny, and live in flour, grain, dried meat, cheese and dried fruits [68]. They multiply extremely rapidly. *Acarus siro*, the grain or cheese mite, also occurs in stored vanilla pods. *Tyroglyphus castellanii* causes copra itch, but is also found in cheese. *Tyroglyphus longior* is a cheese mite. Many other species of tyroglyphid mites have been associated with dermatitis from stored products [198, 254, 270]. In contact with man they cause allergic reactions commonly referred to as 'grocer's itch', 'copra itch', 'miller's itch', etc. [34]. Mites on cheese and vegetables are ingested and, when numerous, cause gastrointestinal symptoms. Eggs and mites in all stages of development are often found in the faeces. A famous German cheese is said to owe its delicious flavour to the myriads of mites deliberately seeded in it. Individuals so invaded invariably have some gastrointestinal disturbances. Mites have also been reported to occur the lungs, ears, and urinary tract.

The flour mite *(Acarus siro)*, one of the best-known species, gives rise to local allergic phenomena on the uncovered skin surface. Pruritus may appear in itself or associated with papular or papulovesicular itching eruptions. Infestation may be the result of occupational exposure in workers in supply stores or in grocers engaged in the assortment and packing of mite-infested cereals and fruits as well as those who are staying in Tyroglyphus-infested storehouses or in thatched premises. Sensitization is usually brought about by repeated infestation [95, 348a]. Repeated contact with the mite-infested material causes persistent urticarial manifestations or bronchial asthma [95]. Sensitization (especially in the form of dermatitis) may be due to the cheese mite *T. longior* [112] and *A. siro*. On subjects working in the cheese making industry the intracutaneous test with *A. siro* extract was positive in 45 per cent and anti-Acarus precipitins in sera were demonstrable in 49 per cent [239a]. Epicutaneous test with the dried dust of the mites elicits erythema, while the living animal, placed on the skin and kept there under a watch glass for 12 h, provokes strong pruritus, punctiform erythema and papules.

The house or grocery mite *(Glyciphagus domesticus)* may be present in enormous numbers on dried fruit, skins or feathers and cause dermatitis.

The pathogenesis of the dermatitis [191] is generally considered to be an allergic reaction to mites [278b], living or dead, their excreta and their moulted skins. Dockers and warehouse labourers handling stored products are most exposed, but shopkeepers and housewives, too, are occasionally affected. A heavily infested cargo may cause serious outbreaks. In industrial outbreaks the cause is readily suspected, but in sporadic cases it is easily overlooked.

The clinical picture is dominated by an acute papular or papulovesicular eczematous dermatitis involving the hands, forearms, face and neck and any exposed skin. The dermatitis is diffuse and may be severe. Irritation is usually intense.

Prophylaxis involves avoiding infested foodstuffs. No treatment is necessary, as the disease is self-limiting; if pruritus is severe, antihistamines are valuable [95].

Inhalant allergens of arthropods

A number of insect hairs, scales, dust of fragment, particles of wings or body act as inhalant allergens and may cause allergy, especially bronchial asthma and hay fever in humans. Such proven cases, however, are rarities. A world-wide rise in the incidence of respiratory allergies is noted, with particular reference to allergy caused by house dust mites, mainly Tyroglyphid mites.

Among insects, moths (Lepidoptera), caddis-flies (Trichoptera), mayflies (Ephemeroptera) aphids and rarely locusts are known as possible sensitizers. Residents on the shores of lakes where cast skins of mayflies abound may suffer from allergic asthma [155].

Caddis-fly contains an antigen of peptide nature (mol. wt. about 3,000), which induces in rabbits the production of antiserum giving 7 to 9 precipitation lines [199a]. Also the production of haemagglutinating and skin sensitizing antibodies has been demonstrated, neither of which is correlated with the degree of clinical hypersensitivity [199b].

House dust mites

These mites may be important factors in some cases of bronchial asthma, especially nocturnal asthma attacks, perennial asthma or rhinitis. House dust has been found to contain mites, which may act as allergens and produce cutaneous and respiratory allergies. There is a vast amount of information and experimental evidence that mites seem to be more important in most regions than allergens originating from other animals or fungi [308].

House dust (clothing, bedding, floor dust, upholstery, skin scrapings) [159] is a conglomerate, the composition of which is subject to seasonal periodicity and depends—rather quantitatively than qualitatively—on geographical and meteorological factors, on the dampness and temperature of houses and different habitats, etc. [236].

More than 35 species of mites have so far been isolated from house dust [239]. The majority of these Sarcoptiform mites belong to the family Psoroptidae, and Tyroglyphidae. In different regions different species seem to have significance, and different clinical pictures are attributed to them.

In England the order of their frequency has been found as follows [159]: *Dermatophagoïdes pteronyssinus*, *Glyciphagus* spp., *Cheyletiella* and *Cheyletophanes* spp., *Gohiera fusca*, *Tyrophagus* spp., *Euroglyphus maynei*, *Tarsonemoïdes* and *Pygmephorus* spp., *D. farinae*. In Finland *D. pteronyssinus*, *D. farinae* and *Euroglyphus maynei* were found [312] to form the bulk (92 per cent) of the mite population present in house dust. In the German Democratic Republic the most important mite allergen sources are as follows: *D. pteronyssinus*, *D. farinae*, *Euroglyphus maynei* and *Glycyphagus domesticus* [183]. The house dust mites live in flats with damp flooring or walls, but also old kapok mattresses, old feathers and furniture may abound in them [223]. The mite densities were greater in unheated wooden houses than in those of stone or wood with central heating [312, 332b]. The material of the mattress did not seem to have any influence on the quantity or quality of the mite findings [312]. National differences in housekeeping practice may play a role in the diversity of data. The preferred food of these mites is dander. They grow well on human dander and many types of animal dander [335]. The allergenicity of house dust is directly related to the number of mites and presumably to their faecal pellets. It is possible that the mites gain access to house dust by being carried on the hair or the scales of pets.

Inhaled with the air the dry excreta of these mites may elicit allergic phenom-

330

ena mainly in the respiratory tract [334, 336]. House dust mites causing asthma-like attacks (even in children), are sometimes responsible for atopic dermatitis, chronic urticaria and may induce even megalerythema epidemicum (erythema toxicum) [264]. Occasionally a causal relationship is supposed [245] between cot death, atopy and the presence of house dust mites in the bedding of the dead infant.

In house dust animal and plant constituents such as serum albumin and immunoglobulin, human dandruff, feathers, kapok, cotton linters, hay and wool may be present [44]. On the other hand, in the mite extracts only mite and nutrient medium constituents (powdered human dandruff and dried baker's yeast) are present. It was thus possible to prepare allergens from *D. pteronyssinus, Glyciphagus destructor* and *Tyrophagus putrescentiae* and to detect precipitins in the sera of sensitized rabbits as well as in human sera [11]. It seems that the house dust allergens are (*i*) degradation products of house dust components that arise more easily in the alimentary tract of mites from house dust [332a] or (*ii*) into which lysine-sugar structures enter as a result of degradation of the medium promoted by mites.

No distinction will be made between the various species of house dust mites (*D. pteronyssinus, D. farinae, Euroglyphus maynei*) because all are supposed to contain the same allergen [333b]. Obviously, the immunological responses induced by house dust are complex and probably variable, owing to the different physicochemical characteristics of house dust constituents.

D. pteronyssinus has been used as antigen for both i.c. and inhalant tests. Applied to persons suffering from house dust allergy it gave positive reaction in 80 per cent or more [350]. That house dust mites are antigens is moreover evident from the histamine release by peripheral leukocytes and from the lymphocyte transformation test [17a]. The antigenic properties of *D. pteronyssinus* have recently been studied in five ways. The incidence of positive reactions was as follows: skin 67 per cent, nasal mucosa 86 per cent, bronchi 86 per cent, leukocytes 90 per cent, passively sensitized normal human lung tissue 100 per cent [226]. However, the pathogenetic role of the mite has not yet been identified.

An antigenic similarity of the Dermatophagoides allergen and the acarian antigens could be demonstrated by using the agar immunodiffusion technique [11]. Coexistence of precipitins and reagins in patients presenting with characteristic features of allergy is possible. According to others [186], in the sera of rabbits immunized with mite extracts immunodiffusion analysis revealed a major line of antigenic identity between mite, dust, and human dander, but this antigen was not a major allergen common to dust and mite. On the other hand, it was found that at least one antigen was common to house dust, dust mite, and human scales, but human epithelial cells were shown to possess antigens clearly distinct from those of both *D. pteronyssinus* and *D. farinae* [92]. By the micro-Ouchterlony technique of Crowle, and counter-immunoelectrophoresis of Gocke and Howe, anti-dust antibodies were found in the serum of all the house dust sensitive and non-atopic individuals tested [277]. House dust extract induced significant thymidine incorporation into lymphocytes from house dust sensitive as well as non-allergic individuals. An *in vitro* response to mite extract, even if less marked, was also seen in most of mite sensitive persons. Type III allergic reactions have been suspected to cause the 'late' bronchial obstructive reactions due to inhalation of house dust [55]. Delayed and Arthus-type cutaneous reactions have been demonstrated [65] by skin biopsy in house dust sensitive patients. In particular, delayed-type reactions appeared to be related to fraction S III obtained by fractionating the house dust extract on DEAE-cellulose and Sephadex G-75 [144]. On the other hand, unfractionated house dust extract as well as S I fraction induced cutaneous reactions characterized by a predominantly polymorphonuclear infiltrate [65].

D. culinae is responsible for another house dust allergen demonstrable by positive nasal and bronchial challenge reactions [261]. In prick tests carried out in France positive reactions were obtained equally in 81.8 per cent with house dust and *D. culinae* [307]. Atopic patients resident in Cairo were found to be sensitive to Cairo dust, which contains a large amount of the mite *D. culinae*, whereas British atopic patients displayed higher sensitivity to British house dust [105]. Immediate-type skin reaction caused by *D. culinae* is correlated with the IgE antibody level in patients suffering from house dust allergy [313].

D. farinae contains a protein antigen similar to that present in house dust. *D. farinae* have been found to be most abundant in North America. Reactions to these mites have been shown to be very common in England, both in adults and in children [53]. In France, reactions to *D. farinae* were positive in 59 per cent of the house dust positive patients suffering from asthma bronchiale or vasomotor rhinitis, while 86 per cent of the *D. farinae* positive subjects gave a positive reaction to house dust [78]. *D. farinae* was found to play an important role in Egypt as well [260]. It grows readily in dog meal plus yeast. Reagin can be absorbed with *D. farinae* from the serum of individuals suffering from house dust allergy [237a]. *D. farinae* mite body fluids have been separated by polyacrylamide gel electrophoresis; it has been suggested that there may be as few as 2, and as many as 5 allergens in or on *D. farinae* mite, which are capable of producing immediate-type responses in human [349a]. The intensity of the precipitin line detected by radioimmunoelectrophoresis did not correlate with the relative concentration of the IgE antibodies as determined by RAST [178a]. IgG antibodies to mite were found in 3 out of 37 sera (as a sign of hyposensitization?).

Specific IgE antibodies against *Dermatophagoides* spp. were encountered in Scandinavian and British patients [165, 315]. A positive correlation has been established between the said antibodies on the one hand, and the clinical course, the result of the prick test, that of the nasal test and of the test carried out with compound 48/80, on the other. There are, however, inconsistent data, viz. no significant correlation has been found [314] between specific IgE levels to *Dermatophagoides* spp. or between total IgE levels and the age of patient, age at onset, and the duration, severity and frequency of symptoms.

Patients with bronchial asthma whose sera were shown to be positive by RAST to house dust or mite extracts reacted positively to inhalation provocation tests with these substances [238]. In general, when the RAST was negative, the inhalation provocation test was also negative. The end point of i.c. test titration with the mite extract *D. farinae* correlated well with the level of specific IgE to mite as determined by RAST, thereby indicating that the end point of i.c. testing provides a good indication of the serum level of allergen-specific IgE. The lowest concentration of anti-IgE producing a positive skin reaction did not, however, correlate well with the IgE level in the serum.

Two Glyciphagus species, *G. destructor* and *G. domesticus*, have been thoroughly studied. Glyciphagus species were found to make up only 1 per cent of all mites in Birmingham [53]. Data regarding *Euroglyphus maynei*, frequently present in house dust, are scanty [334]. Investigation of mattress dust in Birmingham revealed a high frequency of *E. maynei* [53]. This applies also to the fruit-tree red spider mite *(Panonychus ulni)*, the glass-house (or hop) red spider mite *(Tetranychus urticae)* and the chicken mite *(Dermanyssus gallinae)* [41].

Comparative skin tests made in England gave the following frequency sequence in respect of house dust allergy [61]: *D. culinae*, 96.2 per cent; *D. pteronyssinus*, 84.3 per cent; house dust, 73.5 per cent; *G. destructor*, 57.4 per cent; *G. domesticus* 35.6 per cent. In the Netherlands [333a], *D. pteronyssinus* and house dust proved equivalent in skin tests. In Denmark [5], the sequence in respect of atopic dermatitis, as determined by positive prick tests, was as follows: *D. culinae*, 46.6 per cent; *D. pteronyssinus*, 40 per cent, house dust, 30 per cent. Six species were studied in Japan, and each was found to represent a special characteristic antigen [239]. *D. farinae* was the most potent and had the widest antigenic range in common with the other species. House dust allergy in South Hungary is mostly due to mites, whereas (in the capital and in other towns with many old buildings) fungi and moulds are most frequently responsible [147].

Desensitization in house dust allergy has been achieved with different mite extracts, especially with *D. pteronyssinus* extract [333a]. The early results include alleviation of skin reactions and eosinophilia, and the appearance of blocking antibodies. Bronchial challenge showed a significant increase in bronchial tolerance to mite antigen [17b]. Both the total and the specific serum IgE to *D. pteronyssinus* was found to be increased [17b, 103]. More effective desensitization has been reported with mite extracts than with the whole house dust extract [333a]. Very good results were achieved with pyridine extracted, alum precipitated mite fortified house dust. Prolonged careful treatment (never less than six months) seems to be necessary [44a].

Some authors did [103] others did not [17b] achieve improvement in hypersensitivity as measured by the nasal test. In some cases the specific IgG antibodies increased significantly but there was no evidence of any connection with clinical improvement [103]. The lymphocyte transformation test and the liberation of leukocyte migration inhibitory factor showed no difference between the treated and the control groups.

In the mechanism of successful desensitization the following factors have been incriminated [17b]: development of blocking antibodies, change in the affinity of IgE antibodies for different tissues; a competition between non-specific IgE (produced in excess) and allergens-specific IgE. The efficacy of desensitization emphasizes the important role played by tyroglyphid mites in domestic dust [44a].

As for prevention it is essential to keep the houses clean and dry, to eliminate the mites; ultraviolet irradiation for 2h, the use of vacuum-cleaner and the spraying of mattresses and bedrooms with acaricids are effective measures.

REFERENCES

1a. Abbot, K. H.: *Proc. Staff Meet. Mayo Clin.* **18**, 39 (1942).
1b. ibid., **18**, 59 (1942).
2. Adrouny, G. A.: *Bull. Tulane Univ. Med. Fac.* **25**, 67 (1966).
3. Adrouny, G. A., Derbes, V. J. and Jung, F. C.: *Arch. Derm.* **75**, 475 (1957).
4. Alani, M. M. : *J. Natl. Med. Assoc.* **64**, 302 (1972).
5. Alani, M. and Hjorth, N.: *Acta allerg.* (*Kbh.*) **25**, 41 (1970).
6. Allen, A. C.: *Amer. J. Path.* **24**, 367 (1948).
7. Allen, J. R. and West, A. S.: *Mosquito News* **22**, 157 (1962).
8. Allington, H. V. and Allington, R. R.: *J. Amer. med. Ass.* **155**, 240 (1954).
9. Andrade, R. N.: In *Handbook of Tropical Dermatology.* Vol. II. Ed. by Simons, R. D. G. P. Elsevier, Amsterdam 1953, p. 905.
10. Anseri, M. Y.: *Brit. med. J.* ii, 338 (1948).
11. Aranjo-Fontaine, A., Wagner, M., Moreau, G. and Basset, A.: *Rev. franç. Allergol.* **12**, 231 (1972).
12. Arbesman, C. E., Langlois, C., Bronson, P. and Shulman, S.: *J. Allergy* **38**, 1 (1966).
13. Arbesman, C. E., Langlois, C. and Shulman, S.: *J. Allergy* **36**, 147 (1965).
14. Arean, V. M. and Fox, L.: *Amer. J. clin. Path.* **25**, 1359 (1955).
15. Artemov, N. M.: *Proc. XIII. Int. Congr. of Entom. Moscow.* Vol. III. Publishing House Nauka, Leningrad, 1972, p. 284.
16. Arthur, D.: *Adv. Parasit.* **3**, 249 (1965).
17a. Assem, E. S. K. and McAllen, M. K.: *Brit. med. J.* ii, 504 (1970).
17b. id., *Clin. Allergy* **3**, 161 (1973).
18. Atkins, J. A., Wingo, C. W. and Sodeman, V. A.: *Science* **126**, 73 (1957).
19. Atkins, J. A., Wingo, C. W., Sodeman, W. A. and Flynn, J. E.: *Amer. J. trop. Med. Hyg.* **7**, 165 (1968).
20. Ayala, L.: *Minerva derm.* **42**, 593 (1967).
21. Ayres, S. and Ayres, S.: *Arch. Derm.* **83**, 816 (1961).
22. Bacon, D. F. and Morples, M. J.: *Trans. Roy. soc. trop. Med. Hyg.* **49**, 76 (1955).
23. Baerg, W. J.: *The Tarantula.* University of Kansas Press, Kansas 1958.
24. Bailey, S. F.: *Canad. Ent.* **68**, 95 (1936).
25. Baker, E. W. and Wharton, G. W.: *An Introduction to Acarology.* Macmillan, New York 1952.
26. Bandman, H.-J. and Bosse, K.: *Arch. klin. exp. Derm.* **231**, 59 (1967).
26a. Barthelmes, H. and Barthelmes, R.: *Derm. Mschr.* **160**, 573 (1974).
27. Bauzinger, H.: *Fauna* **1**, 3 (1971).
28. Barker, S. A., Mitchel, A. W., Walton, K. W. and Weston, P. D.: *Clin. chim. Acta,* **13**, 582 (1966).
29a. Barnard, J. H.: *J. Allergy* **40**, 107 (1967).
29b. ibid., **43**, 159 (1969).
29c. ibid., **45**, 92 (1970).
29d. ibid., **45**, 120 (1970).
29e. id., *Ann. Allergy* **29**, 372 (1971).
29f. id., *J. Allergy clin. Immunol.* **51**, 97 (1973).
29g. ibid., **52**, 259 (1973).
30a. Barr, S. E.: *Ann. Allergy* **29**, 49 (1971).
30b. id., *J. Amer. med. Ass.* **228**, 718 (1974).
31. Barthelmes, R., Sönnichsen, N. and Barthelmes, H.: *Derm. Mschr.* **156**, 881 (1970).
32. Baugh, A. T., Favrot, L., Thomas, O. C., Dukes, C. D. and McGovern, J. P.: *Ann. Allergy* **23**, 430 (1965).
32a. Bazex, A., Bazex, J., Broussy, F. and Balas, D.: *Bull. Soc. franç. Derm. Syph.* **82**, 369 (1975).
33a. Bazex, A. and Dupré, A.: *Ann. Derm. Syph.* **92**, 371 (1965).
33b. id., *Derm. Vener.* (*Sofia*) **6**, 217 (1967).
34. Beck, J. W. and Barrett-Connor: *Medical Parasitology* Mosby, Saint Louis 1971.
35. Benjamini, E. and Feingold, B. F.: In *Immunity to Parasitic Animals.* Ed. by Jackson, G. J., Herman, R. and Singer, I. Vol. II. Appleton-Century-Crofts, New York 1970, p. 1061.
36a. Benjamini, E., Feingold, B. F. and Kartman L.: *Nature* **188**, 959 (1960).

36b. id., *Exp. Parasit.* **10**, 214 (1960).

36c. id., *Proc. Soc. exp. Biol. N. Y.* **108**, 700 (1961).

37. Benjamini, E., Feingold, B. F., Young, J. D., Kartman, L. and Shimizu, M.: *Exp. Parasit.* **13**, 143 (1963).

38. Berenberg, J. L., Ward, P. A. and Sonenshine, D. E.: *J. Immunol.* **109**, 451 (1972).

39. Berge, T. and Krook, G.: *Acta derm.-venereol.* **47**, 20 (1967).

40. Berger, R. S., Adelstein, E. H. and Anderson, Ph. C.: *J. invest. Derm.* **61**, 142 (1973).

41. Bernecker, Chr.: *Acta allerg.* **25**, 392 (1970).

42a. Bernton, H. S. and Brown, H.: *J. Allergy* **36**, 315 (1965).

42b. id., *Sth. med. J.* **62**, 1207 (1969).

42c. id., *Ann. Allergy* **28**, 175 (1970).

42d. ibid., **28**, 543 (1970).

42e. id., *Brit. J. Dis. Chest* **66**, 61 (1972).

43. Berrens, L.: *Progr. Allergy* **14**, 259 (1970).

43a. Berrens, L., van Bronswijk, J. E. M. H., Young, E. and van Dijk, A. G.: *Acta allergol.* **30**, 390 (1975).

44. Berrens, L. and Versie, R.: *Acta allerg.* **22**, 347 (1967).

44a. Bessot, J.-Cl., Moreau, G., Lenz, D., Parini, J.-P., Aranjo-Fontaine, A. and Pauli, G.: *Rev. franç. Allergol. Immunol. clin.* **15**, 73 (1975).

45. Best, W. C. and Sablan, R. G.: *Arch. Derm.* **90**, 177 (1964).

46. Bhoola, K. D., Calle, J. D. and Schachter, M.: *J. Physiol. (London)* **159**, 167 (1961).

47. Billiotti, G.: *Clin. Allergy* **2**, 109 (1972).

48. Binder, E., Doepfmer, R. and Hornstein, O.: *Klin. Wschr.* **33**, 727 (1955).

49. Bjarke, T., Hellgren, L. and Orstadius, K.: *Acta derm.-venereol.* **53**, 217 (1973).

50. Blank, H., Shaffer, B., Spencer, M. and Marsh, W. C.: *Pediatrics* **5**, 408 (1950).

51. Blank, H., Shaffer, B., Spencer, M. C. and Marsh, W. C.: *Pediatrics* **5**, 408 (1950).

52. Bloom, G. D. and Haegermark, O.: *Acta physiol. scand.* **71**, 257 (1967).

53. Blythe, M. E., Williams, J. D. and Morrison Smith, J.: *Clin. Allergy* **4**, 25 (1974).

54. Bolam, R. M.: *Brit. J. Derm.* **70**, 368 (1958).

55. Booij-Noord, H., Orie, N. G. M. and DeVries, K.: *J. Allergy clin. Immunol.* **48**, 344 (1971).

56. Booth, B. H. and Jones, R. W.: *J. Amer. med. Ass.* **150**, 1575 (1952).

57. Born, W.: *Z. Haut.-Geschl. Kr.* **20**, 33 (1956).

58. Braun-Falco, O.: *Med. Welt* **11**, 1371 (1961).

59. Brown, E. A.: *Rev. Allergy* **23**, 385 (1969).

60a. Brown, H. and Bernton, H. S.: *J. Allergy* **44**, 146 (1969).

60b. id., *Arch. intern. Med.* **125**, 665 (1970).

60c. id., *Med. Ann. D. C.* **40**, 246 (1971).

61. Brown, H. M. and Filar, J. L.: *Brit. med. J.* iii, 646 (1968).

62. Brown, S. F.: *J. Amer. med. Ass.* **165**, 2178 (1957).

63. Browne, S. G.: *Brit. med. J.* ii, 1290 (1960).

64. Brues, C. T. Melander, A. L. and Carpenter F. M.: *Classification of Insects.* Mus. Comp. Zool. Vol. 108. Cambridge, Massachusets 1954.

65. Buffe, D., Burtin, P., Verley, J.-M. and Kourilsky, R.: *Ann. Inst. Pasteur* **105**, 1037 (1963).

66. Burgess, I.: *Brit. J. Derm.* **88**, 519 (1973).

67. Burks, J. W., jr., Jung, R. C. and George, W. M.: *Arch. Derm.* **74**, 131 (1956).

68. Busvine, I. R.: *Insects and Hygiene,* Methuen and Co. Ltd. London.

69. Butz, W. C., Stacy, L. D. and Heryford, N. N.: *Arch. Pathol.* **91**, 97 (1971).

70. Burton, P. A.: *London School Hyg. Trop. Med.* Mem. 10 (1955).

71. Büttiker, W.: *Proc. XIII. Intern. Congr. Entom. Moscow.* Vol. III. Publishing House Nauka, Leningrad 1972.

72. Calnan, C. D.: *Trans. St. John's Hosp. derm. Soc. N. S.* **55**, 198 (1969).

73. Canizares, O. and Shatin, H.: *Arch. Derm.* **68**, 157 (1953).

74. Caro, M. R., Derbes, V. J. and Jung, R.: *Arch. Derm.* **75**, 475 (1957).

75. Carteaud, A., Hewitt, J. and Tabernat, J.: *Presse méd.* **63**, 186 (1955).

76. Chafee, F. H.: *Acta Allerg.* **25**, 292 (1970).

77. Charavejasarn, C. C., Wypych, J. I., Reisman, R. E. and Arbesman, C. E.: *J. Allergy clin. Immunol.* **53**, 104 (1974).

78. Charpin, J., Autran, P., Penaud, A., Nourrit, J. and Razzouk, H.: *Nouv. Presse méd.* **1**, 859 (1972).
79. Chehreh, M. N., Griffith, C. E. and Scott, R. B.: *Med. News* **225**, 355 (1973).
80. Cheminat, J., Brun, J., Grouffal, C., Petit, R. and Molina, Cl.: *Rev. franç. Allergol.* **12**, 239 (1972).
81. Cheng, T. C.: *The Biology of Animal Parasites.* Saunders, Philadelphia 1964, p. 628.
82. Cherry, J. D., Lerner, A. M., Klein, J. O. and Findland, M.: *Pediatrics* **31**, 198 (1963).
83. Choovivathanavanich, P., Suwanprateep, P. and Kanthavichitra, N.: *Lancet* **ii**, 1362 (1970).
84. Coleman, M.: *J. Allergy* **28**, 494 (1957).
85. Coltoiu, A., Mateescu, D. and Diaconu, J.: *Derm.-Vener. (Buc.)* **13**, 343 (1968).
86. Cormia, F. E. and Lewis, G. M.: *N. Y. St. J. Med.* **48**, 2037 (1948).
86a. Conwell, P. B.: *The Cockroach.* Hutchinson, London 1968, p. 391.
87. Craig, G. E.: *Canad. med. Ass. J.* **80**, 828 (1959).
88. Crewe, W. and Gordon, R. M.: *Ann. trop. Med. Parasit.* **43**, 341 (1949).
89. Cseplák, Gy., Szekér, K., Magyari, I. and Bodzás, M.: *Orv. Hetil.* **115**, 569 (1974).
90. Cunnington, A. M.: *Clin. Allergy* **1**, 447 (1971).
91. Dao, L.: *Derm. internat.* **6**, 144 (1967).
92. Dasgupta, A. and Cuncliffe, A. C.: *Clin. exp. Immunol.* **6**, 891 (1970).
93. Dekker, H.: *J. Allergy Clin. Immunol.* **48**, 251 (1971).
94. Denny, W. F., Dillaha, C. J. and Morgan, P. N.: *J. Lab. clin. Med.* **64**, 291 (1964).
95. Derbes, V. J.: In *Dermatology in General Medicine.* Ed. by Fitzpatrick, Th. B., Arndt, K. A., Clark, W. H., jr., Eisen, A. Z., Van Scott, E. J. and Vaughan, J. H. McGraw-Hill, New York 1971, p. 1940.
96. Desch, C. and Nutting, W. B.: *J. Parasit.* **58**, 169 (1972).
97. Dias, L. B. and Azevedo, M. C.: *Boll. Ofic. Sanit. Panam.* **75**, 197 (1973).
98. Dillaha, C. J., Jansen, G. T., Honeycutt, W. M. and Hayden, C. R.: *J. Amer. med. Ass.* **188**, 33 (1964).
99. Dostrovsky, A.: *Handbook of Tropical Dermatology.* Ed. by Simons, R. D. G. P. Elsevier, Amsterdam 1953, p. 889.
100. Dostrovsky, A. and Even-Paz, Z.: *Arch. Derm.* **84**, 750 (1961).
101. Dostrovsky, A., Raubitschek, F. and Sagher, F.: *Dermatologica* **113**, 26 (1956).
102. Downe, A. E. R.: *Canad. J. Zool.* **40**, 957 (1962).
103. D'Sousa, M. F., Wells, I. D., Tai, E., Palmer, F., Overell, B. G., McGrath, I. T. and Megson, M.: *Clin. Allergy* **3**, 177 (1973).
104. Eichenberger, H.: *Dermatologica* **132**, 68 (1966).
105. El Hefny, A. and Frankland, A. W.: *VIII. Europ. Congr. Allergol., Marseille 1971.* Excerpta Med. Int. Congr. Series No. 235, p. 177.
106. Epstein, E.: *J. Amer. med. Ass.* **222**, 1309 (1972).
106a. Espy, P. D. and Jolly, H. W., jr.: *Arch. Derm. (Chic.)* **112**, 193 (1976).
107. Faust, B. and Russel, P.: *Clinical Parasitology.* 7th ed. Lea and Febiger, Philadelphia 1964.
108. Favorite, E. G.: *Publ. Hlth. Rep. (Wash.)* **73**, 445 (1958).
109. Feder, I. A.: *J. Amer. med. Ass.* **126**, 293 (1944).
110. Feinberg, S. M., Feinberg, A. R. and Pruzansky, J. J.: *III. Int. Congr. Allergol.* Flammarion, Paris 1958, p. 293.
111. Feingold, B., Benjamini, E. and Michaeli, D.: *Ann. Rev. Entom.* **13**, 137 (1968).
112. Fields, J. P., Hoke, A. W. and Crone, P. C.: *Arch. Derm.* **98**, 669 (1968).
113. Fine, R. M. and Scott, H. G.: *Sth. med. J. (Nashville)* **58**, 416 (1965).
114. Fogel, B. J., Weinberg, T. and Markowitz, M.: *Amer. J. Dis. Child.* **114**, 325 (1967).
115. Ford Wolf, A.: *Ann. Allergy* **27**, 271 (1969).
116. Foubert, E. L. and Stier, R. A.: *J. Allergy* **39**, 13 (1958).
117. Fox, I. and Bayona, I. G.: *Derm. int. (Philadelphia)* **5**, 125 (1966).
118. Frankel, G. and Rudall, K. M.: *Proc. roy. Soc.* **129**, 1 (1940).
119a. Frankland, A. W.: *Int. Arch. Allergy* **6**, 180 (1955).
119b. id., *Allergie Asthma* **1**, 229 (1955).
119c. Franklin, R. and Baer, H.: *Ann. Allergy* **55**, 285 (1975).
120a. Frazier, C. A.: *Ann. Allergy* **23**, 37 (1965).
120b. id., *Arch. Derm.* **100**, 127 (1969).

120c. id., *Insect Allergy; Allergic and Toxic Reactions to Insects and Other Arthropods.* Warren H. Green Inc., St. Louis 1969, p. 493.
120d. id., *F. Asthma Res.* **10**, 3 (1972).
120e. id., **32**, 200 (1974).
121. Fredholm, B. and Haegermark, O.: *Acta physiol. scand.* **71**, 357 (1967).
122. Frenken, J. H.: *Dermatologica* **125**, 322 (1962).
123. Friedman, H. J., Bowman, K., Fried, R. and Weitz, M.: *J. Allergy* **28**, 489 (1957).
124. Gaafar, S. O.: In *Immunity to Animal Parasites.* Ed. by Soulsby E. J. L. Academic Press, New York 1972.
125. Garin, N. S. and Grabareo P. A.: *Meditsinskaya Parat. i Paras. i Bolasi* **41**, 372 (1970).
126. George, W. M.: *Arch. Derm.* **78**, 320 (1958).
127. Glass, F. A.: *Indian med. Surg.* **17**, 95 (1948).
128. Goethe, H., Brett, R. and Weidner, H.: *Z. Tropenmed. Parasitol.* **18**, 5 (1967).
129. Gold, D. and Lengy, J.: *Int. Arch. Allergy* **34**, 571 (1968).
130. Gold, D., Lengy, J., Lass, N. and Tager, A.: *Int. Arch. Allergy* **31**, 274 (1967).
131. Goldman, L.: *Amer. J. trop. Med. Hyg.* **12**, 246 (1963).
132. Goldman, L., Rockwell, E. M. and Richfield, D. F.: *Amer. J. trop. Med. Hyg.* **1**, 514 (1952).
133. Goldstein, N. and Skipworth, G. B.: *J. Amer. med. Ass.* **203**, 53 (1968).
134a. Gordon, R. M.: In *Modern Trends in Dermatology.* Ed. by MacKenna, R. M. B. Butterworths, London 1948, p. 186.
134b. id., *Brit. med. J.* **ii**, 316 (1950).
135. Gordon, R. M. and Crewe, W.: *Ann. Trop. Med. Parasit.* **42**, 334 (1948).
136. Gordon, R. M. and Lavoipierre, M. M. J.: *Entomology for Students of Medicine.* Blackwell, Oxford 1962, p. 147.
137. Gorhan, J. R. and Rheney, T. B.: *J. Amer. med. Ass.* **206**, 1958 (1968).
138. Gouck, H. K.: *Arch. Derm.* **93**, 112 (1966).
139. Gregson, J. D.: In *WHO Seminar on the Ecology, Biology and Control of Ticks and Mites*, WHO/UBC/68.57 1968, p. 37.
140. Grosdanov, A.: *Berufsderm.* **7**, 30 (1959).
141. Grosshans, E. M., Kremer, M. and Maleville, J.: *Hautarzt* **25**, 166 (1974).
142. Grütz, O.: *Dermatologia (Basel)* **97**, 279 (1948).
143. Gudgel, E. F. and Grauer, F. H.: *Arch. Derm.* **70**, 609 (1954).
144. Guibert, L. and Causse Combes, R.: *Ann. Inst. Pasteur* **103**, 579 (1962).
145. Habermann, E.: In *Venomous Animals and their Venoms.* Vol. III. Ed. by Bucherl and Buckley, E. E. Academic Press, New York 1971.
145b. Habermann, E.: *Science* **177**, 314 (1972).
146a. Habermann, E. and El Karemi, M. M. A.: *Nature* **168**, 1349 (1956).
147. Hajós, M.-K.: *Lancet* **i**, 1404 (1970).
148. Hallam, R.: *Brit. J. Derm.* **44**, 117 (1932).
149. Halstead, W. B. and Ryckman, R.: *Med. Arts Sci.* **3**, 16 (1949).
149a. Hancock, B. W. and Ward, M.: *J. invest. Derm.* **63**, 482 (1974).
150. Harman, R.: *Practitioner* **206**, 595 (1971).
151. Hatoff, A.: *J. Amer. med. Ass.* **130**, 850 (1946).
152a. Hecht, O.: *Zool. Anz.* **3-4**, 94 (1930).
152b. id., *Zbl. Haut u. Geschl.-Kr.* **44**, 241 (1933).
153. Heilesen, B.: *Acta derm.-venereol.* **26**, Suppl. 14 (1946).
153a. Hejazi, N. and Mehregan, A. H.: *Arch. Derm. (Chic.)* **111**, 37 (1975).
154. Hellmut, A.: *Ztschr. Immun.forsch.* **105**, 241 (1940).
155. Herms, W. B. and James, M. T.: *Medical Entomology.* Macmillan, New York 1961.
156. Herrmann, W. P.: *Landarzt* **48**, 1215 (1972).
157. Herrmann, W. P. and Steigleder, G. K.: *Dtsch. med. Wschr.* **92**, 1557 (1967).
158. Hersch, C.: *Sth. Afr. med. J.* **i**, 29 (1967).
159. Hewitt, M., Barrow, G. I., Miller, D. C., Turk, F. and Turk, S.: *Brit. J. Derm.* **89**, 401 (1973)
160. Higginbotham, R. D. and Karnella, S.: *J. Immunol.* **106**, 233 (1971).
161. Higuchi, K. and Urabe, H.: *Hautarzt* **10**, 79 (1959).
162. Hoeppli, R. and Schumacher, H. H.: *Z. Tropenmed. Parasit.* **13**, 419 (1962).
162a. Hoffman, D. R. and Shipman, W. H.: *J. Allergy* **55**, 73 (1975).

163. Hoigné, R.: *Schweiz. med. Wschr.* **95,** 1731 (1965).
164. Hoigné, R., Klein, U., Fahrer, H. and Müller, U.: *Schweiz. med. Wschr.* **104,** 221 (1974).
165. Holford-Strevens, V., Wilde, L., Milne, J. F. and Pepys, J.: *Clin. exp. Immunol.* **6,** 49 (1970).
166. Holtschmidt, J.: *Hautarzt* **3,** 267 (1952).
167. Hoogstraal, H.: *Ann. Rev. Entom.* **11,** 261 (1966). **12,** 377 (1967).
168. Hoseu, H. I.,: *Ann. Allergy* **28,** 596 (1970).
169. Huang, I., Bernton, H. S., Stauch, J. and Brown, H.: *J. Allergy* **47,** 198 (1971).
169a. Hubler, W. R., jr.: *Arch. Derm. (Chic.)* **112,** 179 (1976).
170. Hudson, A., McKiel, J. A., West, A. S. and Bourns, T. K. R.: *Mosquito News* **18,** 249 (1958).
171. Hudson, B. W., Feingold, B. F. and Kortman, L.: *Exp. Parasit.* **9,** 151 (1960).
172. Hughes, T. E.: *Mites.* Athlone Press, London 1959.
173. Hunt, B. R. and Edwards, P.: *Canad. med. Ass. J.* **63,** 69 (1951).
173a. Hunt, K. J., Sobotka, A., Valentine, M. D., Zeleznick, L. D. and Lichtenstein, L. M.: *J. Allergy clin. Immunol.* **55,** 74 (1975).
174. Hunt, W. B., jr. and McLean, D. C.: *Ann. Allergy* **28,** 64 (1970).
175. Hunter, G. W., Frye, W. W. and Schwarzwelder J. C.: *A Manual of Tropical Medicine,* 4th ed. Saunders, Philadelphia–London 1966, p. 931.
175a. Ilea, V., Okazaki, T., Wypych, J. I., Reisman, R. E. and Arbesman, C. E.: *J. Allergy* **55,** 74 (1975).
176. Ingram, J. T.: *Brit. J. Derm.* **63,** 311 (1951).
177. Insect Allergy Committee of the American Academy of Allergy: *J. Amer. med. Ass.* **193,** 115 (1965).
178. Ishay, J., Gitler, S. and Fischl, J.: *Acta allerg. (Kbh.)* 26, 286 (1971).
178a. Ito, K.: *Acta allergol.* **30,** 194 (1975).
179. Jansen, G. T., Morgan, P. N., McQueen, J. N. and Bennett, W. E.: *Sth. Med. J.* **64,** 1194 (1971).
180. Jensen, O. M.: *Acta path. microbiol. scand.* **54,** 9 (1962).
181a. Jones, B. M.: *New Biol.* **21,** 74 (1956).
181b. id., *Parasitology* **40,** 247 (1950).
182. Jones, D. L. and Miller, J. H.: *Arch. Derm.* **79,** 81 (1959).
183. Karg, W.: *Allergie Asthma* **19,** 81 (1973).
184. Karlsson, E.: *Experientia (Basel)* **29,** 1319 (1973).
185. Katzenellenbogen, I.: *Dapim Reffuim* **21,** 299 (1962).
186. Kawai, T., Marsh, D. G., Nagy, S. M. and Norman, P. S.: *Meeting Amer. Acad. Allergol. Chicago 1971.*
187a. Keegan, H. L.: In *Venomous and Poisonous Animals and Noxious Plants of the Pacific Region.* Ed. by Keegan, H. L. and MacFarlane, W. V. Pergamon, Oxford 1963, p. 196.
187b. ibid., p. 165.
188. Kemper, H.: *Proc. 10th int. Congr. Entom.* **3,** 719 (1958).
189. Kern, A. B.: *Arch. Derm.* **65,** 334 (1952).
190. Kern, R. A.: *J. Allergy* **9,** 604 (1938).
191. Kilpio, O. and Pirilä, V.: *Acta derm.-venereol.* **32,** Suppl. 29, 1 (1952).
192. Knicker, W. T., Morgan, P. N., Flanigan, W. J., Reagan, P. W. and Dillaha, C. J.: *Proc. Soc. exp. Biol. (N. Y.)* **131,** 1432 (1969).
193. Kocsis, A. and Selényi, A.: *Derm. Wschr.* **129,** 129 (1954).
194. Konstantinov, D. and Stanoeva, L.: *Dermatologica* **147,** 321 (1973).
195. Krampnitz, H. E.: *Ztsch. Allgemein Med.* **48,** 1221 (1972).
196. Kurban, A. K.: *Brit. J. Derm.* **82,** 76 (1970).
197. Kutzer, E. and Grünberg, W.: *Tierärztl. Wschr.* **82,** 311 (1969).
198. Laarman, J. J.: *Doccum. Med. geogr. trop.* **4,** 268 (1952).
199a. Langlois, C., Shulman, S. and Arbesman, C. R.: *J. Allergy* **34,** 235 (1963).
199b. ibid., **34,** 385 (1963).
199c. ibid., **36,** 12 (1965).
199d. ibid., **36,** 109 (1965).
200. Larrivee, D. H., Benjamini, E. and Feingold, B. F.: *Exp. Parasit.* **15,** 491 (1964).
201. Lee, D. J.: *Med. J. Aust.* **i,** 170 (1968).

202. Lengy, J. and Gold, D.: *Int. Arch. Allergy* **29**, 404 (1966).
203a. Lerner, A. M., Klein, J. O., Cherry, J. D. and Findland, M.: *New Engl. J. Med.* **269**, 678 (1963).
203b. ibid., **269**, 736 (1963).
203c. Lockey, R. F.: *J. Allergy* **54**, 132 (1974).
204. Logan, J. C. P. and Walkey, M.: *Brit. J. Derm.* **76**, 218 (1964).
205. Lucas, T. L.: *J. Amer. med. Ass.* **119**, 877 (1942).
206. Lunsford, C. J.: *Arch. Derm.* **60**, 1184 (1949).
207. Lyon, J. B.: *Practitioner* **200**, 670 (1968).
208. MacConnel, J. G., Blum, M. S. and Fales, H. M.: *Science* **168**, 840 (1970).
209. Mackler, B. F., Russel, A. S. and Kreil, G.: *Clin. Allergy* **2**, 317 (1972).
210. Macpherson, R. K.: *Med. J. Austr.* **2**, 493 (1941).
211. Maguire, H. C. and Kligman, A. M.: *Arch. Derm.* **82**, 62 (1960).
212. Maibach, H. I., Skinner, W. A., Strauss, W. G. and Khan, A. A.: *J. Amer. med. Ass.* **196**, 263 (1966).
213. Makara, G. and Mihályi, F.: *Insects and Diseases* (in Hungarian) MOKT. Budapest 1943, p. 394.
214. Mann, G. T. and Bates G. R.: *Sth. med. J.* **53**, 1399 (1960).
215. Marghescu, S. and Ziethen, H.: *Derm. Wschr.* **154**, 793 (1968).
216. Markland, F. S., Damus, P. S., Davidson, T. M. and Shabley, J. D.: *Lancet* i, 1398 (1970).
217. Marks, R. and Harcourt-Webster, J. N.: *Arch. Derm.* **100**, 683 (1969).
218. Marshall, J.: *Dermatologica* **135**, 60 (1957).
219. Martini, E., Peus, F. and Reichmuth, W.: *Lehrbuch der Medizinischen Entomologie.* 4th ed. Fischer, Jena 1952, p. 60.
220. Mathias, A. P. and Schachter, M.: *Brit. J. Pharmacol. Chemother.* **13**, 326 (1958).
221. Matsumura, T.: *Gunma J. Med. Sci.* **12**, 186 (1963).
222. Maunsell, K.: *Practitioner* **205**, 779 (1970).
223. Maunsell, K., Wraith, D. G. and Cunnington, A. M.: *Lancet* i, 1267 (1968).
224. Mayer, L. D.: *J. Kentucky med. Ass.* **65**, 668 (1967).
225. Mazzotti, L. and Bravo-Becherelle, M. A.: In *Venomous and Poisonous Animals and Noxious Plants of the Pacific Region.* Ed. by Keegan, H. L. and Macfarlane, W. V. Pergamon, Oxford 1963, p. 119.
226. McAllen, M. K., Assem, E. S. K. and Maunsell, K.: *Brit. med. J.* ii, 501 (1970).
227. McCormick, W. F.: *Amer. J. clin. Path.* **39**, 480 (1963).
228. McGovern, J. P., Barkin, G. D., McElhenney, T. R. and Wende, R.: *J. Amer. med. Ass.* **175**, 1155 (1961).
229a. McKiel, J. A. and West, A. S.: *Pediat. Clins. N. Amer.* **8**, 795 (1961).
229b. id., *Canad. J. Zool.* **39**, 597 (1961).
230. McLean, J. A., Terr, A. I. and Cushing, R. T.: *Univ. Mich. Med. Cent. J.* **34**, 40 (1968).
231a. Mellanby, K.: *Scabies.* Oxford University Press, London 1944.
231b. id., *Parasitology* **35**, 157 (1944).
231c. id., *Nature* **158**, 554 (1946).
232. Mendoza, J.: *Ann. Allergy* **28**, 159 (1970).
233. Mészáros, I.: *Z. ges. inn. Med.* **26**, 193 (1971).
234. Metcalf, R. L.: *Natn. malar. Soc. J.* **4**, 271 (1945).
235a. Micks, D. W.: *Texas Rep. Biol. Med.* **10**, 399 (1952).
235b. id., In *Venomous and Poisonous Animals and Noxious Plants of the Pacific Region.* Ed. by Keegan, H. L. and Macfarlane, W. V. Pergamon, Oxford 1963, p. 153.
236. Milner, H. F., Tees, E. C. Dybas, B. and Dean, P. M.: *Acta allerg.* **20**, 379 (1965).
237a. Miyamoto, T., Ishizaki, T. and Sato, Sh.: *J. Allergy* **42**, 14 (1968).
237b. id., *Ann. Allergy* **28**, 405 (1970).
238. Miyamoto, T., Johansson, S. G. O., Ito, K. and Horiuchi, Y.: *J. Allergy clin. Immunol.* **53**, 9 (1974).
239. Miyamoto, T., Oshima, Sh., Mizuno, K., Saza, M. and Ishizaki, T.: *J. Allergy* **44**, 228 (1969).
239a. Molina, C., Aiache, J.-M., Tourreau, A. and Jeanneret, A.: *Rev. franç. Allergol. Immunol. clin.* **15**, 89 (1975).

240. Moretti, C. and Bertamino, R.: *Rass. Derm. Sif.* **21**, 374 (1968).
241. Morgan, R. J., Moss, H. B. and Honska, W. L.: *Arch. Derm.* **90**, 180 (1964).
242a. Mueller, H. L.: *Pediat. Clin. North Amer.* **6**, 917 (1959).
242b. id., *J. Allergy* **30**, 123 (1959).
242c. id., *New Engl. J. Med.* **261**, 374 (1959).
242d. id., In *Immunological Diseases.* Ed. by Samter, M. 2nd ed. Vol. II. Little-Brown, Boston 1971, p. 893.
243. Mueller, H. L. and Hill, L. W.: *New Engl. J. Med.* **249**, 726 (1953).
243a. Mueller, H. L., Schmid, W. H. and Rubinsztain, R.: *Pediatrics* **55**, 530 (1975).
244. Mullaney, P. J.: *Clin. Toxic.* **3**, 613 (1970).
245. Mulvey, P. M.: *Med. J. Austr.* **2**, 1240 (1972).
246. Munjal, D. and Elliott, W. B.: *Toxicon (Oxford)* **9**, 229 (1971).
247. Nash, T. A.: *Trop. Anim. Health* **2**, (1971).
248. Neumann, W. and Habermann: In *Venoms.* Ed. by Buckley, E. E. and Porges, N. Vol. 44, Sympos. American Association for the Advancement of Science, Washington 1956.
249. Nichols, N. and Green, T. W.: *Calif. Med.* **98**, 267 (1963).
250. Norins, A. L.: *Amer. J. Dis. Child.* **117**, 239 (1969).
251. Nosko, L.: *Hautarzt* **4**, 317 (1953).
252. Oberste-Lehn, H. and Baggesen, I.: *Derm. Wschr.* **154**, 437 (1968).
253. O'Connor, R., Stier, R. A., Rosenbrook, W. and Erickson, R. W.: *Ann. Allergy* **22**, 385 (1964).
254. O'Donovan, W. J.: *Brit. J. Derm.* **32**, 297 (1920).
255. Ordman, D.: *Int. Arch. Allergy* **28**, 366 (1965).
255a. Orkin, M.: *Arch. Derm. (Chic.)* **111**, 1431 (1975).
256a. Parrish, H. M.: *Arch. intern. Med.* **104**, 198 (1959).
256b. id., *Amer. J. med. Sci.* **245**, 129 (1963).
257. Pastinszky, I.: *Bőrgyógy. Vener. Szle.* **47**, 108 (1971).
258. Patton, W. S. and Evans, A. M.: *Insects, Ticks, Mites and Venomous Animals.* Grubb, Croydon 1929, p. 786.
259. Pelikan, Z.: *Acta allerg. (Kbh.)* **27**, 167 (1972).
260. Pepys, J.: *Acta allerg. (Kbh.)* **25**, 324 (1970).
261. Pepys, J., Chan, M. and Hargreave, F. E.: *Lancet,* **i,** 1270 (1968).
262a. Perlman, F.: *J. Allergy* **52**, 93 (1961).
262b. id., *Calif. Med.* **96**, 1 (1962).
262c. id., In *Dermatologic Allergy.* Ed. by Criep, L. H. Saunders, Philadelphia 1967, p. 222.
263. Philipp, G. and Jankó, M.: *Zbl. Gynäk.* **92**, 465 (1970).
264. Phillips, I. E.: *Arch. Derm.* **67**, 628 (1953).
265. Pick, F.: *Bull. Soc. Path. exot.* **45**, 60 (1952).
266. Popescu, J. G.: *Allergie u. Asthma* **16**, 242 (1970).
267. Poulson, P. A.: *Acta derm.-venereol.* **32**, Suppl. 29, 296 (1952).
268. Prakken, J. R. and Van Vloten, Th. J.: *Dermatologica* **99**, 124 (1949).
269. Price, H. E.: *Texas Med.* **64**, 38 (1968).
270. Prosser-Thomas, E. W.: *Brit. J. Derm.* **54**, 313 (1942).
271. Rahm, V.: *Rev. suisse Zool.* **64**, 236 (1957).
272. Rajka, E.: In *Allergie und allergische Erkrankungen.* Vol. II. Ed. by Rajka, E. Akadémiai Kiadó, Budapest 1959, p. 664.
273. Reddy, C. R.: *J. Trop. Med. Hyg.* **75**, 98 (1972).
274a. Reisman, R. E.: *J. Allergy* **46**, 254 (1970).
274b. id., *J. Allergy clin. Immunol.* **52**, 257 (1973).
274c. Reisman, R. E., Wypych, J. and Arbesman, C. E.: *J. Allergy clin. Immunol.* **56**, 443 (1975).
275. Reisman, R. E., Wypych, J., Yeagle, I. and Arbesman, C. E.: *J. Allergy clin. Immunol.* **53**, 110 (1974).
276. Rockwell, E. M. and Johnson, P.: *J. invest. Derm.* **19**, 137 (1952).
277. Romagnani, S., Biliotti, G., Passaleva A. and Ricci, M.: *Clin. Allergy* **3**, 51 (1973).
278a. Rook, A. J.: *Pediat. Clins N. Amer.* **8**, 817 (1961).
278b. id., In *Textbook of Dermatology.* 2nd ed. Vol. I. Ed. by Rook, A., Wilkinson, D. S. and Ebling, F. J. G. Blackwell, Oxford 1972, p. 845.

340

279. Rook, A. J. and Frain-Bell, W.: *Arch. Dis. Childh.* **28**, 304 (1953).
280. Rotschild, M.: *Toxicon* **8**, 293 (1970).
281. Rufli, T.: *Dermatologica (Basel)* **140**, Suppl. 2, 45 (1970).
282. Russel, F. E.: *Curr. Probl. Pediatr.* **3**, 1 (1973).
283. Russel, F. E., Wainschel, J., Madon, M. B. and Ennik, F.: *J. Amer. med. Ass.* **224**, 131 (1973).
284. Russel, F. E., Waldron, W. G. and Madon, M. B.: *Toxicon* **7**, 109 (1969).
285. Saelinger, C. B., and Higginbotham, R. D.: *Int. Arch. Allergy* **46**, 28 (1974).
286. Safdi, S. A. and Farrington, J.: *Amer. J. med. Sci.* **214**, 308 (1947).
286a. Saudescu, I. and Durbanca, S.: *Arch. Roumaines Path. Exp. Microbiol.* **31**, 247 (1972).
287. Schaffer, B., Jacobson, C. and Beerman, H.: *Arch. Derm.* **70**, 437 (1953).
288. Schenken, J. R., Tamisieva, J. and Winter, F. D.: *Amer. J. clin. Path.* **23**, 1216 (1953).
289. Schenone, H. and Prats, F.: *Arch. Derm.* **82**, 139 (1961).
290. Schirren, J. M.: *Hautarzt* **21**, 407 (1970).
291. Schwann, J.: *Hautarzt* **16**, 340 (1965).
292. Schwartz, H. J.: *J. Amer. med. Ass.* **194**, 703 (1965).
293. Schwartz, H. J. and Kahn, B.: *J. Allergy* **45**, 87 (1970).
294. Settipane, G. A.: *Acta allerg. (Kbh.)* **25**, 286 (1970).
295. Settipane, G. A. and Hopson, C. N.: *Acta allerg. (Kbh.)* **26**, 121 (1971).
296. Shaffer, B., Jacobson, C. and Pori, P. P.: *Ann. Allergy* **10**, 411 (1952).
297. Shields, T. L. and Walsh, E. N.: *Arch. Derm.* **74**, 14 (1956).
297a. Shkenderov, S.: *Toxicon (Oxford)* **12**, 529 (1974).
297b. Shrank, A. B. and Alexander, S. L.: *Brit. med. J.* i, 669 (1967).
298. Shulman, S.: *Progr. Allergy* **12**, 246 (1968).
299. Shulman, S., Bigelsen, F., Lang, R. and Arbesman, C. E.: *J. Immunol.* **96**, 29 (1966).
300. Shulman, S., Langlois, C. and Arbesman, C. E.: *J. Allergy* **35**, 446 (1964).
301. Shulov, A.: *Trans. Roy. Soc. trop. Med. Hyg.* **33**, 263 (1939).
302. Smart, J.: In *Insects of Medical Importance.* 4th ed. Ed. by Smart, J. British Museum, London 1965.
303a. Smith, C. W. and Micks, D. W.: *Amer. J. trop. Med. Hyg.* **17**, 651 (1968).
303b. id., *Lab. Invest.* **22**, 90 (1970).
304. Smith, F. D., Miller, N. G., Carnazzo, S. J. and Eaton, E. B.: *Arch. Derm.* **77**, 324 (1958).
304a. Sobotka, A. K., Franklin, R. M., Adkinson, N. F., jr., Valentine, M., Baer, H. and Lichtenstein, L. M.: *J. Allergy clin. Immunol.* **57**, 29 (1976).
305. Sobotka, A., Franklin, R., Valentine, M., Adkinson, F., jr. and Lichtenstein, L.: *J. Allergy clin. Immunol.* **53**, 103 (1974).
306. Sobotka, A., Valentine, M., Benton, A. W., Hunt, K. and Lichtenstein, L. M.: *J. Allergy clin. Immunol.* **51**, 97 (1973).
307. Souquet, R., Martoia, R. and Langlet, J.: *Nouv. Presse méd.* **3**, 205 (1974).
308. Spieksma, F. Th. M.: *Rev. franç. Allergol.* **13**, 133 (1973).
309. Spieksma, F. Th. M., Zuidema, P. and Leupen, M. J.: *Brit. med. J.* i, 82 (1971).
310. Stahnke, H. L.: *Scorpions.* Arizona State University, 1956.
311. Staub, H. P., Kimmel, G. C., Berglund, E. B. and Sholler, L. J.: *Pediatrics* **34**, 880 (1964).
312. Stenius, B. and Cunnington, A. M.: *Scand. J. resp. Dis.* **53**, 338 (1972).
313. Stenius, B. and Wide, L.: *Lancet* ii, 455 (1969).
314. Stenius, B., Wide, L. and Seymour, W. M.: *Clin. Allergy* **2**, 303 (1972).
315. Stenius, B., Wide, L., Seymour, W. M., Holford-Strevens, V. and Pepys, J.: *Clin. Allergy* i, 37 (1971).
316. Stephen, W. P.: *Syst. Zool.* **10**, 1 (1961).
317. Tager, A., Lass, N., Gold, D. and Lengy, J.: *Int. Arch. Allergy* **36**, 408 (1969).
318. Tennenbaum, J. I.: *Ohio State Med. J.* **64**, 794 (1968).
319. Theis, J. A. and Budweiser, P. D.: *Experim. Parasit.* **36**, 77 (1974).
320. Theodor, O.: *Trans. R. Soc. Trop. Med. Hyg.* **29**, 273 (1935).
321. Theodorides, J.: *Acta trop.* **7**, 48 (1950).
322. Thompson, F.: *Lancet* ii, 446 (1933).

323. Thone, A. W.: *Dermatologica* **136**, 57 (1968).
324. Toomey, N.: *Urol. cutan. Rev.* **26**, 473 (1922).
325a. Torsney, Ph. J.: *N. Y. St. J. Med.* **68**, 2765 (1968).
325b. id., *J. Allergy clin. Immunol.* **52**, 303 (1973).
326. Touraine, A., Thomas, J. and Caldéra, R.: *Presse méd.* **55**, 654 (1947).
327. Török, L.: *Bőrgyógy. Vener. Szle.* **48**, 103 (1972).
328. Trager, W.: *J. Parasit.* **25**, 57 (1939).
329. Traver, J. R.: *Proc. ent. Soc. Wash.* **53**, 1 (1951).
330. Trinca, J. C.: *Med. J. Austr.* ii, 659 (1964).
331. Valentine, M. D., Sobotka, A. and Lichtenstein, L. M.: *J. Allergy clin. Immunol.* **53**, 105 (1974).
332. Van Bronswijk, J. E. M. H., Jansen, L. H. and Ophof, A. J.: *Dermatologica* **145**, 338 (1952).
332a. Van Bronswijk, J. E. M. H. and Jorde, W.: *Acta allergol.* **30**, 209 (1975).
333a. Voorhorst, R.: *Acta allerg.* **25**, 237 (1970).
333b. id., *Allergie Immunologie* **18**, 9 (1972).
333c. id., *Med. Klin.* **67**, 646 (1972).
334. Voorhorst, R. and Osváth, P.: *Orv. Hetil.* **111**, 1456 (1970).
335. Voorhorst, R., Spieksma, F. Th. M. and Varekamp, H.: *House-Dust Atopy and the House-Dust-Mite*. Stafleu, Leiden, 1969.
336. Voorhorst, R., Spieksma, F. Th. M., Varekamp, H., Leupon, M. J. and Lyklema, A. W.: *J. Allergy* **39**, 325 (1967).
337. Vorse, H., Seccareccio, P., Woodruff, K. and Bennett, G.: *J. Pediat.* **80**, 1035 (1972).
338. Wagner, G.: *Z. Haut-Geschl. Kr.* **10**, 487 (1951).
339. Wakkerman, L. T. B. and Van Rijn, J. F. A.: *Hautarzt* **16**, 37 (1965).
340. Walsh, J. H.: *Ann. Rev. Pharmacol.* **4**, 293 (1964).
341. Ward, W. H.: *Austr. J. Derm.* **12**, 44 (1971).
342. Watt, J. C.: *New Zealand Entom.* **5**, 87 (1971).
343. Weidner, H.: *Zeitschr. Angew. Entom.* **23**, 432 (1936).
343a. Weiss, V.: *Z. ärztl. Fortbild.* **68**, 138 (1974).
344. Wharton, G. W. and Fuller, H. S.: *Mem. ent. Soc. Wash.* **4**, (1952).
345a. W.H.O. Vector Biol. and Control: *Phlebotomine Sandflies* WHO/VBC 71.255 (1971).
345b. id., *Blackflies in the Americas* WHO/VBC 71.283 (1971).
345c. id., *Cockroaches Biology and Control* WHO/VBC 72.354 (1972).
345d. id., *Seminar on the Ecology, Biology and Control of Ticks and Mites. Geneva 1967.* WHO/VBC/68.57.
345e. WHO Expert Commitee: *Insecticide Resistance and Vector Control* WHO Techn. Rep. Ser 443 Geneva (1970).
345f. id., *Application and Dispersal of Pesticides* WHO Techn. Rep. Ser 465 (1971).
345g. id., *The Control of Lice and Louse-borne Diseases. Washington 1972.* Pan. Am. Health Org. Se. Publ. No. 263 (1973).
346. Williamson, D. M.: *Brit. J. Derm.* **76**, 388 (1964).
347. Winer, L. H. and Strakosch, E. A.: *J. invest. Derm.* **4**, 249 (1941).
348a. Winkler, A.: In *Dermatologie und Venerologie.* Vol. II/2. Ed. by Gottron, H. A. and Schönfeld, W. Thieme, Stuttgart 1958. p. 957.
348b. id., *Hautarzt* **21**, 93 (1970).
349. Wirth, L.: *N. Y. St. J. Med.* **53**, 2513 (1953).
349a. Woodiel, N. L., Bennett, S. E., Hornsby, R. P. and Daniel, J. C., jr.: *J. Allergy* **53**, 278 (1974).
350. Wütrich, B.: *Schweiz. med. Wschr.* **100**, 921 (1970).
351. Yarom, R.: *Clin. Toxicol.* **3**, 561 (1970).
352. Yesudian, P. and Thambiach, A. S.: *Dermatologica* **147**, 214 (1973).
353. Yocum, M. W., Johnstone, D. E. and Condemi, J. J.: *J. Allergy clin. Immunol.* **53**, 265 (1973).
354. Young, J. D., Benjamini, E., Feingold, B. F. and Noller, H.: *Exp. Parasit.* **13**, 155 (1963).
355. Young, J. W.: *Arch. Derm.* **49**, 309 (1944).

356. Zimmerman, T. S., Arroyave, C. M. and Müller-Eberhard, H. J.: *J. clin. Invest.* **50,** 103a (1971).

357a. Ziprkowski, L. and Rolant, F.: *J. Invest Derm.* **46,** 439 (1966).

357b. ibid., **58,** 274 (1972).

358. Zumpt, F.: *Myiasis in Man and Animals in the Old World.* Butterworths, London 1965.

359. Zumpt, F. and Graf, H.: *Sth. Afr. J. clin. Sci.* **i,** 196 (1950).

INDEX

acarid 289
Acarus siro 329
Acarus tritici 311
accidental irritative bites of arthropods 311–312
acetylcholinesterase in excretion-secretion antigen of nematodes 218
Achorion schönleinii 129, 149
acquired immunity *see* immunity
acrodermatitis chronica atrophicans caused by venom of castor bean tick 308
ACTH therapy in
trichinellosis 247
tuberculin allergy 46
Actinomyces bovis 170
Actinomyces wolff-israeli 170
actinomycosis 138, 170
active immunization *see* immunization, active
acute rheumatic fever 5–9
acute toxaemic schistosomiasis 235–236
adrenocorticotrophic hormone *see* ACTH
Aëdes aegypti 302
Aëdes maculipennis 302
Aëdes mosquitoes, saliva of 302
African trypanosomiasis 225–226
agammaglobulinaemia
alymphocytic congenital in vaccinia 11
with normal lymphocyte function during vaccination 11
agglutinating antibody (antibodies)
in African trypanosomiasis 226
in amoebiasis 229
in bee venom immunized mice 318
in filariasis 251
in honey bee sting reaction 322
in larval echinococcosis 241
in malaria 232
in South American trypanosomiasis 227
in toxoplasmosis 234
in trichinellosis 247
in trichomoniasis 220, 221
in tuberculosis 54

in visceral larva migrans 248
in visceral leishmaniasis 224
to *Actinomyces wolff-israeli* 170
to Caddis-fly 330
to *Candida albicans* 152, 153
to Chlamydia 211
to *Cryptococcus neoformans* 169
to fungal killed material 136
to *Histoplasma capsulatum* 167
to hyphomycetes 140
to insect, whole body of 279
to mellitin (honey bee venom) 317
to myocardium, human 8
to *Neisseria gonorrhoeae* 189, 192–193, 194
to *Neisseria gonorrhoeae* endotoxin 185
to prostatic extract 10
to *Sporotrichum schenckii*, yeast phase of 164
to *Treponema pallidum* 80–81
Alternaria moulds in inhalant allergy 158
amoebiasis 228–229
anaemia
iron deficiency, in hookworm disease 243
normochromic, in Reiter's syndrome 9
secondary
in erythema nodosum leprosum 113
in visceral leishmaniasis 224
sickle cell, in estivo-autumnal malaria 231
anaphylactic-type reaction
in experimental animal sensitization 157, 242
in fulminant infections 5
to arthropods 276
to bed bug bite 296, 299
to brucellin 19
to fire ant sting 320
to Hymenoptera sting 277, 316, 320
to insect bite or sting in atopic subjects 280
to insect stings 282–283
to mellitin 317, 318
to mosquito bite 302

Australia antigen in lepromatous leprosy 109, 120
autoantibody (autoantibodies) to
  heart, non-cross-reactive with Streptococci 8
  intercellular substances of epithelial cells 116
  myocardium, human 8
  streptococcal cell membrane, cross-reactive with human cardiac muscle, skeletal muscle and arteriolar smooth muscle 8
  streptococcal cell wall, cross-reactive with human glycoprotein 8
  tissue cardiolipins 78, 83
  Wassermann's antigen 77–78, 83, 84, 87, 99
autoantigen(s)
  heart muscle, human 8
  kidney, human 8
  lymph node extract from Reiter's patients as 10
  mitochondrial 99
  prostatic extract from Reiter's patients as 10
  skeletal muscle, human 8
  streptococcal cardiotoxin damaged cardiac tissue 8
  synovial fluid from Reiter's patients as 10
  tissue cardiolipins as 78
  Wassermann's 77–78, 83
autoimmune pathogenesis in
  acute rheumatic fever 7–9
  demyelination process, virus-induced 16
  viral diseases 10
autopsy findings in Hymenoptera sting ∫ reactions 321

bacteriaemia see haemoculture
bacterial diseases, allergic complications of 5–10
bacterial infectious diseases, allergic reactions in 2–10
bacteriocinogenic pattern of Neisseria gonorrhoeae 199–200
BCG vaccination 60–64
  complications of 63
  harmless 63
  protection provided by, against
    leprosy 63–64
    tuberculosis 60–63
bed bug 298–299
Bedsonia-group agent infection in Reiter's syndrome 9
bejel 97
benign leprosy see tuberculoid leprosy
bentonite granuloma model in schistosomiasis 237

β_1 C globulin in
  acute rheumatic fever 6
  biologically false positive reactors for syphilis 83
β_1 E globulin in acute rheumatic fever 6
bilharziasis see schistosomiasis
biologically false positive serum for syphilis 77, 78, 81, 83–84
biting midges 304
blackflies 305
blackfly fever 305
Blastomyces dermatitidis 153, 167, 168
Blattella germanica 328
blister beetles 325–326
Bloch phenomenon 128
blocking antibodies in sera of patients with
  bee whole-body immunization 318
  dermatophytic infections 129, 140
  house dust desensitization 333
blood-sucking flies 305–306
B lymphocytes in lepromatous leprosy 115
Bombus (bumblebees) 315
borderline (dimorphous) leprosy 112
Bordet phenomenon in ascariasis 242
bronchial asthma 152, 154, 158, 159, 220, 229, 250, 320, 325, 329, 330, 331, 332
Brucella abortus 19
Brucella melitensis 19
Brucella suis 19
brucellin test 19–20
brucellosis 3, 4
Brugia malayi 248, 252
Brugia pahangi 251
brugiasis see lymphatic filariasis
Burnet test see brucellin test
burrowing flees 294

Calabar-swellings see loiasis
Candida albicans
  antigenic components of 150
  cell-mediated immune response to 150, 155–156
Candida albicans infection
  candidin skin test in 151–152
  clinical forms of 156–157
  humoral antibodies in 152–155
  immunological responsiveness in 154
  immunological restoration in 156
  predisposing conditions to 150
  vaccination in 152
candida-endocrinopathy syndrome 150
Candida lethal factor, Louria's 152–153
Candida stellatoidea 151
Candida tropicalis 151
candidids 150–157
carriers of
  Ducrey's bacillus 207
  gonococci 198

IgM
  serum level in *(cont'd)*
    malaria 230
    neonatal syphilis 80
    toxoplasmosis 234
IgM producing cells in trichinellosis 246
immobilizin 78–79, 92–93, 98
immune adherence of treponemes 81
immune complexes in
  acute rheumatic fever 7
  acute toxaemic schistosomiasis 236
  Aschoff's bodies 9
  erythema nodosum leprosum 113
  lepromatous leprosy 115
  microfilaraemia 252
  toxoplasmosis 233
  Trichinella spiralis infection 246
  viral diseases 10
immune response, depression of, in
  cryptococcosis 169
  lymphocytic choriomeningitis virus in-
    fection 14
  measles 13
  rickettsial infection 22
  subacute sclerosing panencephalitis 17
immunity
  acquired in
    amoebiasis 229
    arthropod reaction 277
    cysticercosis 239
    dermatophytoses 130
    flea bite reaction 296, 301
    Hymenoptera sting reaction 316,
      322–323
    louse bite reaction 297
    malaria 230
    mosquito bite reaction 296, 302, 303
    mucocutaneous leishmaniasis 222–
      223
    parasitic diseases 218
    sand-fly allergy 304
    syphilis 93–99
    tick bite reaction 308
    tuberculosis 39, 57–58, 60, 64–65
    visceral leishmaniasis 224
  impaired or modified in
    human scabies 288
    Norwegian scabies 290
  natural in
    amoebiasis 230
    arthropod reaction 277
    chancroid 207
    lymphogranuloma venereum 212
    malaria 230
    parasitic diseases 218
    syphilis 92–93
    South American trypanosomiasis
      227
    tuberculosis 38–39
    visceral leishmaniasis 224

immunization
  active
    against bacterial diseases 27–29
    against viral diseases 23–27
    allergic complications of 22–29
    contraindications to 23
    in experimental visceral larva mi-
      grans 248
    in filariasis 251
    in human echinococcosis 241
    in toxoplasmosis 234, 235
    in trypanosome infection 225, 226
    protective antibody production
      during 22
    with *Actinomyces wolff-israeli* 170
    with anti-parasitic vaccine 218
    with BCG 39, 52–53
    with *Coccidioides immitis* 166
    with *Cryptococcus neoformans* 169
    with diphtheria toxoid 17, 18, 27
    with *Haemophilus ducrey* 206, 207
    with *Histoplasma capsulatum* 167–168
    with honey bee venom 318
    with honey bee whole-body 318
    with Leishmania vaccine 223
    with measles virus 12, 13, 17
    with *Neisseria gonorrhoeae* 190, 198–
      200
    with *Mycobacterium tuberculosis*
      vaccine 38
    with rickettsial vaccine 22
    with streptococcal M protein 7
    with *Treponema pallidum* 95–97
    with Treponemes 93–94
    with trichophytin 136, 137, 141
    with *Trichophyton verrucosum* culture
      137
    with vaccinia virus 11
  passive in
    human echinococcosis 241
    Neisseria gonorrhoeae infection 188,
      198–200
    Vespa orientalis sting reaction 323
immunocyto-adherence technique in
  ascaridiasis 242
  filarial infection 252
immunoprophylaxis *see* immunization,
  passive
inclusion bodies in Reiter's syndrome 9
indirect immunofluorescent studies in
  Aspergillus fumigatus infection 160
  cryptococcosis 169
  giardiasis 192
  gonorrhoea 188–189, 192
  lepromatous leprosy 116
inhalant allergens of arthropods 329–330
inhalant test with
  Dermatophagoides culinae 332
  Dermatophagoides pteronyssinus 331, 332
  house dust 332

neurological complications of viral infections 15–17
Neisseria catarrhalis 181, 185
Neisseria flava 194
Neisseria gonorrhoeae 179, 182, 187, 188, 190, 197
  antibodies to 188–190
  antigenic composition of 180–185, 189, 192–194
  endotoxin 184–185
  intracutaneous test for the demonstration of allergy to 196
  pathogenicity of 187–188
  serological tests for the demonstration of 190–196
  virulence of 185–187, 188
Neisseria meningitidis 195
Neisseria perflava 181
Neisseria sicca 193, 194
Neisseria subflava 181
Nippostrongylus brasiliensis 246
nodular leprosy *see* lepromatous leprosy
non-typhoid salmonelloses 3
North American blastomycosis 168
Norwegian scabies 290–291
nummular eczema as chronic reaction to arthropods 280

Onchocerca volvulus 249, 252
onchocerciasis 249–250, 252
ophthalmo-tuberculin reaction, Calmette's 41
opsonin-like factor in South American trypanosomiasis 227

p-aminobenzoic acid, influence on malaria 230
panarama, disease of rubber workers 325
pancarditis 225
papular urticaria, elicited by insect bite 280–281, 301, 307, 309
Paracoccidioides brasiliensis 168
paracoccidioidosis 168
parainfectious encephalitis 16
paramyxovirus, nucleocapsid 17
parasitaemia in
  filariasis 251
  malaria 230
  South American trypanosomiasis 227
  toxoplasmosis 233
paratyphoid fever vaccine 29
passive cutaneous anaphylaxis test in
  bee venom immunized mice 318
  Hymenoptera allergy 284
  larval echinococcosis 240
  visceral larva migrans 248

passive transfer of reactivity
  with lymphocytes in
    coccidioidomycosis 166
    cryptococcosis 169
    LCMV infection 14
    lepromatous leprosy 114
    mucocutaneous leishmaniasis 223
    North American blastomycosis 168
    schistosomiasis 237
    swimmer's itch 235
    tuberculin allergy 42, 47, 48, 49
    tuberculin fever 42, 47
    visceral leishmaniasis 224
  with cells of peritoneal exudate in tuberculin allergy 42, 47, 48
  with patient's serum in
    ascariasis 242
    bed bug hypersensitivity 284, 299
    Candida allergy 152
    Dermacentor variabilis immunization 308
    Dermatophagoides pteronyssinus allergy 331
    honey bee hypersensitivity 285
    Hymenoptera sting reaction 321–322
    LCMV infection 14
    mosquito hypersensitivity 284
    mould allergy 158
    swimmer's itch 235
    trichophytin allergy 133, 140
    wasp hypersensitivity 285
patch tuberculin test, Vollmer's 41
Pediculus humanus capitis 296
Pediculus humanus corporis 296
penicillin, prophylactic use in acute rheumatic fever 5, 7
Penicillium moulds in inhalant allergy 138, 158
pericardium 5, 6
perineural cells with *Mycobacterium leprae* 108
Periplaneta americana 328
persistent insect bite reactions 280, 282
pertussis vaccination 28–29
  demyelinating encephalitis due to 29
  direct toxicity of antigen in 28–29
  encephalopathy due to 29
Phialophora compacta 164
Phialophora pedrosoi 164
Phialophora verrucosa 164
Phlebotomus species 303
phycomycosis 160
pinta 72, 73, 97
plasma cell infiltration in lesions of
  acute rheumatic fever 6
  African trypanosomiasis 225
  cysticercosis 239
  insect bite reaction 282
  insect sting reaction 280
  lepromatous leprosy 109

systemic reaction *(cont'd)*
  to parathyphoid vaccination 29
  to rabies virus vaccine 25
  to spider venom 312
  to tetanus toxoid immunization 28
  to Triatoma saliva bite 300
  to trichophytin injection 131, 132, 133, 145
  to tuberculin injection 38, 41–42
  to typhoid vaccination 29

Taenia saginata 239
Taenia solium 238
Takahashi test in tuberculosis 54
tanned red cell agglutination (Boyden's) test in
  candidiasis 153
  histoplasmosis 167
  tuberculosis 55
target cell destruction in tuberculosis 51–52
tetanus immunization 28
Thaumetopoea wilkinsoni 324
thymectomy, effect on skin reaction 46
tick paralysis 308
ticks 306–309
T lymphocytes in
  carrier-specific helper, in helminthiases 219
  intestinal immuno-expulsion 218
  lepromatous leprosy 115
Toxocara canis 247
Toxocara cati 247
toxocariasis *see* visceral larva migrans
Toxoplasma gondii 232, 233
toxoplasmosis 232–235
  intrauterine 233, 234
  postnatal 232, 234
trachoma inclusion conjunctivitis agent 210
Trambusti's reaction 41
transfer factor, Lawrence's
  administration of, in
    chronic mucocutaneous candidiasis 156
    coccidioidomycosis 166
    lepromatous leprosy 115
  characteristics of 48
transfusion of immunologically competent lymphocytes in chronic mucocutaneous candidiasis 156
Treponema carateum 72, 78
Treponema cuniculi 73, 78, 94, 97
Treponema microdentium 78
Treponema, Nichols strain 94, 96
Treponema pallidum 72, 73, 77, 78, 88–92, 99
  cultivable strains 73
  immunochemistry of 75–76

pathogenic strains of 73–74, 77
  ultrastructure of 74–75
Treponema pallidum haemagglutination test 86–87, 88
Treponema pallidum immobilization test 78–79, 84–85, 87, 88, 92, 93, 98
Treponema pertenue 72, 73, 78, 94, 95, 97, 98
Treponema reiteri 73, 75, 76, 78, 79, 81, 84, 86
Triatoma protracta 299
Triatoma sanguisuga 299, 300
triatomid bugs 299–300
Trichinella spiralis 245, 246
trichinellosis 245–247
Trichomonas foetus 221
Trichomonas hominis 221
Trichomonas tenax 221
Trichomonas vaginalis 220, 221
trichomoniasis 220–221
trichophytia profunda 131, 133, 136, 137, 138, 143, 145
trichophytia superficialis 137
trichophytids 142–149
  classification of 143–144
  clinical forms of 144–149
trichophytin
  antigenic components of 130–131
  cross-reactions of 137–139
  specificity of 130, 135–136
trichophytin allergy 131–139
  cellular defense mechanism in 141
  humoral antibodies in 139–141
Trichophyton infection, lethal, systemic 129
Trichophyton mentagrophytes 129, 130, 133, 134, 136, 137, 139, 141, 147
Trichophyton quinckeanum 128, 134, 149
Trichophyton rubrum 129, 130, 132, 133, 136, 137, 140, 141, 147
Trichophyton verrucosum 130, 137
Trichophyton violaceum 129, 130
Trockentrichophytin 130
tropical pulmonary eosinophilia 250–251
trypanocidal serum factor in African trypanosomiasis
Trypanosoma cruzi 226, 227
Trypanosoma gambiense 225
Trypanosoma rhodesiense 225
trypanosomiasis 225–227
tuberculoid leprosy 110–111, 116, 120
  clinical picture 110–111
  histology 111
  Mitsuda reaction in 115
  reactivity of lymphocytes in 116
  serological reactions in 120
tuberculin fever 42
tuberculin reaction 38, 39–53
  desensitization of 43
  epidemiological significance of 52–53

24*